T0074232

Clinical Cancer Medicine

Treatment Tactics

Also by Jacob J. Lokich:

Primer of Cancer Management

Clinical Cancer Medicine
Treatment Tactics

Edited by Jacob J. Lokich, M.D.
New England Deaconess Hospital
Sidney Farber Cancer Institute
Harvard Medical School
Boston, Massachusetts

 G. K. Hall Medical Publishers
Boston, Massachusetts

G.K. Hall Medical Publishers
70 Lincoln Street
Boston, Massachusetts 02111

80 81 82 / 4 3 2 1

Lokich, Jacob J.
Clinical Cancer Medicine: Treatment Tactics

The authors and publisher have worked to ensure that all information in this book concerning drug dosages, schedules, and routes of administration is accurate at the time of publication. As medical research and practice advance, however, therapeutic standards may change. For this reason, and because human and mechanical errors will sometimes occur, we recommend that our readers consult the *PDR* or a manufacturer's product information sheet prior to prescribing or administering any drug discussed in this volume.

Clinical cancer medicine.

Bibliography: p.
Includes index.
1. Cancer.   2. Cancer—Complications and sequelae.   I. Lokich, Jacob J.   [DNLM: 1. Neoplasms—Therapy.   QZ266   C641]
RC261.C646   616.9'94   79-16587
ISBN-13: 978-94-011-7237-0   e-ISBN-13: 978-94-011-7235-6
DOI: 10.1007/978-94-011-7235-6

To my daughter Emily from whom I took the time

Contributors

Norwood R. Anderson, M.D.
Clinical Instructor in Medicine, Harvard
Medical School
Associate Staff, New England Deaconess
Hospital

Murray M. Bern, M.D.
Assistant Professor of Medicine, Harvard
Medical School
Section Chief of Hematology, Department
of Medicine, New England Deaconess
Hospital

Albert Bothe, Jr., M.D.
Instructor of Surgery, Harvard Medical
School
Assistant Director, Nutrition Support
Service, New England Deaconess
Hospital

Bruce R. Bistrian, M.D., Ph.D.
Assistant Professor of Medicine, Harvard
Medical School
Co-Director, Nutrition Support Service,
New England Deaconess Hospital

R. Bud Dickson, M.D.
Assistant Clinical Professor of Orthopedic
Surgery, University of Arkansas for
Medical Sciences

Michael A. Drew, M.D.
Clinical Instructor of Orthopedic Surgery
Harvard Medical School
Associate in Orthopedic Surgery,
Peter Bent Brigham Hospital
Chief of Orthopedics, Harvard
Community Health Plan

Christopher C. Gates, M.D.
Instructor of Psychiatry, Harvard Medical
School
Associate in Medicine and Consultant in
Surgery, Peter Bent Brigham Hospital

Robert H. Goebel, M.D.
Fellow, Department of Radiation Therapy,
Harvard Medical School
Resident in Radiation Therapy, Joint
Center for Radiation Therapy

Paul Hans, M.D.
Instructor of Psychiatry, Harvard Medical
School
Director of Consultation/Liaison
Psychiatry, Massachusetts Mental
Health Center

Antoinette F. Hood, M.D.
Departments of Dermatology and
Pathology, Washington Hospital
Center, Washington, D.C.
Assistant Clinical Professor of
Dermatology, George Washington
University, Washington, D.C.

Jacob J. Lokich, M.D.
Assistant Professor of Medicine, Harvard
Medical School
Section Chief of Medical Oncology,
Department of Medicine, New England
Deaconess Hospital

Joyce A. McCaffrey, M.D.
Clinical Instructor in Medicine, Harvard
Medical School
Active Staff, New England Deaconess
Hospital
Staff Physician, Section of Medical
Oncology, Lahey Clinic Foundation

James E. Pennington, M.D.
Assistant Professor of Medicine, Harvard
Medical School and Peter Bent Brigham
Hospital
Infectious Diseases Division, Peter Bent
Brigham Hospital

Randolph B. Reinhold, M.D.
Assistant Clinical Professor of Surgery,
    Harvard Medical School
Medical Director, Ambulatory Services,
    New England Deaconess Hospital

Ralph R. Weichselbaum, M.D.
Assistant Professor of Radiation Therapy,
    Harvard Medical School and Joint
    Center for Radiation Therapy
Chief of Radiation Therapy, Peter Bent
    Brigham Hospital

Bruce U. Wintroub, M.D.
Assistant Professor of Dermatology,
    Harvard Medical School
Associate Physician, Robert Breck
    Brigham Hospital
Junior Assistant in Medicine, Peter Bent
    Brigham Hospital
Consultant in Dermatology, Sidney Farber
    Cancer Institute

John H. Wolff, M.D.
Clinical Instructor in Medicine, Harvard
    Medical School
Active Staff, New England Deaconess
    Hospital
Staff Physician, Section of Medical
    Oncology, Lahey Clinic Foundation

Acknowledgments

The individuals who have contributed to the conception, execution, and production of this very special project are innumerable.

Dr. Lloyd Aiello from the Joslin Clinic, Ophthalmology Division, and Dr. Melvin Clouse, Dr. Herbert Gramm at New England Deaconess Hospital, as well as Dr. Arthur T. Skarin, and their staffs provided the resources for many illustrations.

Ms. Rose O'Reilly and Ms. Candice Fullwood organized, edited, and recomposed what must have seemed like countless drafts, and for their excellence and their diligence, I am most grateful.

The enormous case material was graciously provided by my colleagues in the subdivisions of medicine and surgery.

A special thanks is directed to the students and house staff who, for the past 10 years, have provided the inspiration for this undertaking and to the nursing staff at the New England Deaconess Hospital who have, in their collective sensitivity, provided the most important ingredient in treating the patient with cancer—caring.

Preface

With the development of medical oncology as a medical subspecialty, an authoritative and comprehensive text about cancer, *Cancer Medicine* by Holland and Frei, has appeared to explain the bridge between this field and the clinical sciences. In addition, the individual therapeutic disciplines in oncology have developed clinical texts in surgery, radiation, pediatric, and medical approaches to the neoplastic diseases. These texts serve as compendia of information organized and structured for presentation by organ.

This book adds to the growing list of oncologic texts but focuses on pratical tactics in the management of cancer and its complications and incorporates this author's individual philosophy and approach to the cancer patient. In this context, the primary care physician without special training in oncology may find the book a useful reference. A major purpose of preparing the text is to provide an instructional guide for those physicians in training and in practice who are not oriented toward oncology. The organization and structure of this text are designed to reinforce the principles of cancer management and to augment the educational experience.

Initially, this book was conceived specifically to describe the clinical approach to oncologic emergencies. It is clear, however, that those complications of cancer that are not life threatening are equally unique and complex in their management. Furthermore, such complications bridge many of the subdisciplines in medicine and surgery. Thus, the extension from oncologic emergencies to cancer complications at individual organ sites was a natural evolution and one which required collaboration and interaction among the major disciplines of medicine and surgery.

It is hoped that this book will add to the expanding list of oncology texts and will be both an educational tool and a management guide for the treatment of the cancer patient.

Contents

Part I   Introduction

Chapter 1

General Concepts in Cancer Management
J. Lokich

1.0 Introduction

The complications of cancer are myriad, and for those complications with life-threatening potential, the perspective of the therapeutic clinician has been, by and large, one of nihilism. Such an approach has been based on the assumption that the cancer patient will inevitably die and that the acute complication may obviate a long period of suffering. Consequently, it is common for the patient with cerebral metastases, for example, to be allowed to drift into coma without treatment with corticosteroids or for the patient with pneumonia not to receive antibiotics. For many patients, however, adequate therapy for the acute oncologic emergency may result in a prolonged period of disease-free survival without major treatment-related morbidity. Substantial morbidity of a complication in advanced cancer may cause pain or disability over a protracted period, and treatment for the complication may prevent the morbidity of the disease. For example, early treatment of spinal cord compression can prevent paraplegia with prolonged survival. For the less than life-threatening complications of cancer, excessive morbidity can be a consequence of inadequate treatment.

[The goals for treatment of the acute complications of cancer are both to improve the quality of life and to extend the duration of life.]The patient with hypercalcemic coma, acute brain syndrome, or superior vena cava syndrome may be returned to a completely functional state with minimal morbidity through specific therapy.[Effective management of these cancer complications achieves prolonged survival, although the therapy is almost never curative.]

2.0 Therapeutic decision-making

Cancer complications from primary or metastatic tumors involve therapeutic decisions that must be based on characteristics of both the host and the tumor. The host characteristics that play a major role in determining therapy include age, performance status or functional activity, and the presence or absence of concomitant serious disease. Another morbid disease, such as renal failure, chronic heart failure, or cirrhosis, may influence the therapeutic modality to be employed and is often a critical determinant in the choice of specific treatment.

In addition to the host factors, four tumor factors critically influence treatment decisions (Table 1.1). The pathologic category of the tumor—mesenchymal, epithelial, or lymphoma, for example— and the primary site or origin—for example, lung, breast, or colon—greatly influence the therapy by indicating the tumor's potential responsiveness. A second crucial factor in determining therapy is the

Table 1.1 Host and tumor features that influence therapeutic decision-making

Tumor

1. Primary tumor source and pathologic features

2. Stage or extent of disease (quantitative host-tumor burden)

3. Biologic activity of disease (growth rate)

4. Responsiveness or resistance to therapy (prior therapeutic reaction)

Host

1. Age

2. Performance status (functional activity)

3. Other morbid disease

4. Visceral distribution of metastases and functional reserve of organ system

stage or extent of disease. In patients with extensive, local tumor bulk or multiple sites of metastasis, systemic therapy is the treatment of choice unless local complications dominate the clinical picture.

Third, the biologic activity of the tumor—as reflected in growth rates and measured by doubling times for pulmonary nodules, or as measured by the interval from the primary diagnosis to the development of metastasis—may reflect the aggressiveness of the tumor as well as its potential responsiveness to therapy. The fourth determinant of therapy is the potential responsiveness to individual therapeutic modalities. Tumors notoriously resistant to radiation and drug treatment include renal cell carcinoma, colon cancers, and lung cancers. On the other hand, lymphomas and sarcomas become increasingly responsive to both of these modalities. Responsiveness to treatment also depends on response to prior therapy. For example, patients responding to hormonal therapy or chemotherapy are more likely to respond again than patients who have established resistance to one modality or another. Nonetheless, so-called "second-line" therapy is always less likely to induce a response, even in tumors generally responsive to treatment. For example, in advanced ovarian cancer, "first-line" therapy is successful in 40 to 60 percent of patients, while second-line therapy at the time of relapse may induce tumor regression in less than 10 percent of cases.

Second-line therapy is less likely to be successful because of established tumor resistance, increased tumor burden, and decreased host resistance.

First-line therapy contributes to the limitation of response to subsequent therapy not only because of potential induction of tumor cell resistance, but also because of host effects limiting the amount of secondary therapy to be administered. One such example is the reduction of bone marrow reserve by first-line therapy. The corollary to this principle is that tumors which do not respond to primary or first-line therapy also generally fail to respond to the secondary therapy.

These general therapeutic principles relating to features of the tumor are guides, however, and not definitive principles. A common misconception in cancer management is that tumors that are pathologically anaplastic with a high mitotic index are more sensitive to chemotherapy than are well-differentiated tumors. The fact is that such tumors are more likely to develop resistance to therapy more rapidly than do slowly growing tumors, and the initial response will likely be of short duration. No data in humans currently indicate that rapidly growing tumors are more responsive tumors. The most important consideration is tumor type.

The problem of therapeutic decision-making in cancer management is the general question of when to treat, and specifically when to employ chemotherapy or radiation therapy. Combined modality treatment employs complementary methods such as preoperative radiation for rectal cancer or chemotherapy for responsive tumors. Chemotherapy may also be used preoperatively to permit less surgery for patients with locally inoperable tumors that are chemotherapy responsive. Preoperative chemotherapy for soft tissue sarcomas of the extremities has been introduced to promote limb-sparing tumor surgery as opposed to amputation. These approaches involve therapeutic decision-making for primary (local) or regional tumors.

The question of therapy for patients with advanced metastatic disease is often more difficult. The primary reasons for introducing therapy for patients with advanced disease are indicated in Table

1.2. If an established form of therapy is considered "standard," it must be associated with a reasonable degree of effectiveness as measured by tumor regression and improved survival. For example, the use of 5-fluorouracil for colon cancer and dacarbazine (DTIC) for melanoma have been considered "standard therapy" because they are associated with a 20-percent response rate. These drugs do not, however, have a significant impact on the disease because the tumor regressions are invariably partial, and survival is not affected. Tumors for which chemotherapy is associated with a 40- to 50-percent response rate and a substantial incidence of complete regression include lymphomas and cancers of the testicles, ovary, breast, and prostate. For these tumors, the effectiveness of the treatment is a primary indication for therapy even in the absence of symptoms or measurable disease.

Because an improvement in the quality of life is sometimes achieved, symptoms secondary to metastatic disease always justify therapy, even when such therapy is known to have only a marginal effect on the tumor. The presence of measurable disease that may be reasonably monitored to determine the impact of treatment on the tumor is another important component of therapeutic decision-making. Effectiveness of treatment can often be determined within one or two courses of the drug

Table 1.2 Therapeutic decision-making for patients with advanced metastatic cancer

Indications for therapy

1. Standard therapy with known effectiveness
2. Secondary symptoms
3. Measurable lesions
4. Limited prognosis

or radiation. The lack of effectiveness can dictate early withdrawal of therapy and obviate long-term treatment having only marginal effectiveness.

Measurable lesions permit precise monitoring of therapy and withdrawal of morbidity-producing treatment that does not reduce the tumor.

In this context, stable disease is an inadequate "response" to therapy in that survival for such patients is similar to that for patients with unresponding or progressive disease. In fact, it is only in those patients for whom a complete regression of all clinically detectable tumor is achieved that one can measure an improvement in survival.

The last criterion for determining when to introduce therapy is the most difficult to establish. For patients with advanced cancer the prognosis is always limited because incurability is an established fact. But the duration of life varies and predictions depend on biologic factors concerning the host as well as the tumor. In preterminal patients, tumor-specific therapy and even maximally supportive therapy, hyperalimentation, for example, may not be warranted, while for patients with an extended survival expectation, the introduction of morbidity-associated therapy is similarly not warranted. In the absence of known effective drugs, symptomatic disease, or a measurable lesion that can aid in evaluating therapy, the decision to treat must be determined by a delicate interaction between physician and patient. Both biologic and psychologic issues should be considered.

Two special circumstances in therapeutic decision-making for metastatic disease are worthy of comment. The first is the common situation in which the patient has distant metastases at the time of primary presentation. The question then is the primary lesion, which should be treated only if (1) the metastases are controlled or (2) the primary tumor is the source of major symptoms.

Patient A, a 55-year-old woman, presented with shoulder pain and massive hepatomegaly. Needle biopsy of the liver revealed adenocarcinoma, and barium enema demonstrated a lesion at the transverse colon. Hepatic infusion with 5-fluorouracil resulted in dramatic regression of the hepatic metastases, and subsequent resection of the primary lesion was carried out.

Therapy for the primary tumor in the presence of metastases depends on the symptoms produced by the primary tumor and/or the control of the metastatic lesions.

Local therapy for the primary tumor generally involves surgery (see Patient A); conservative surgical procedures are preferable, as incurability is established by the presence of metastases. Adequate surgical palliation, however, may require more extensive surgery.

Patient B, a 36-year-old woman, had a primary breast cancer with a fungating T^3 lesion (10 cm). Routine bone scan revealed multiple lesions. In spite of the bone metastases, a mastectomy was performed as a "toilet" procedure to minimize discomfort and secondary infection in the tumor.

The second special clinical circumstance in therapeutic decision-making for metastatic disease is the unknown primary tumor.

Treatment for the patient with the unknown primary tumor should be based

on the assumption that the tumor is optimally responsive.

All the clinical information should be considered when determing the proper therapy. It is preferable to consider the clinical data and then to integrate the concept that treatment should be directed toward the most treatable (responsive) tumor.

Patient C, a 65-year-old man, had multiple sclerotic bone lesions and a normal acid phosphatase and prostatic examination. Needle biopsy of the prostate was normal, but the patient was treated with estrogens with complete pain relief. At postmortem five years later, he was found to have a small primary tumor in the prostate.

The most treatable metastatic tumors for males are prostate and testicular cancers (response rate 80 percent) and for females are breast and ovarian cancers (response rate 50 percent).

Because few primary tumors are responsive to systemic therapy, and because by and large therapy in responsive tumors is effective regardless of tumor burden, the asymptomatic patient with an undiagnosed primary lesion may not require early systemic therapy.

In addition to therapeutic decision-making for patients with advanced or metastatic disease, the problem of staging or evaluating the extent of disease should be critically considered. Because the presence of metastases establishes the incurability of the disease, additional diagnostic maneuvers such as bone scans, pulmonary tomograms, or intravenous pyelograms are justified only as therapeutic guides. Such procedures are superfluous, not cost-effective, and although not invasive, can produce physical and psychologic discomfort for the patient.

3.0 Concepts of local, systemic, and combined modality therapies.

Cancer therapy may be divided into two categories—local or regional, and systemic. Local or regional disease, such as a stage I carcinoma of the breast or a stage II carcinoma of the rectum, is treated locally, with either radiation therapy or surgery. In circumstances where local therapy is associated with a high incidence of recurrence, a combination of modalities may be effective. For example, preoperative radiation therapy in rectal cancers has added substantially to local control, and prophylatic postoperative radiation therapy to the chest wall following mastectomy decreases the local recurrence rate.

Systemic therapy is treatment distributed not only to the local area but also to other areas throughout the body, excluding the pharmacologic sanctuaries (e.g., central nervous system). Chemotherapy, including cytotoxic drug therapy, hormone therapy, and immunotherapy, is systemic therapy. Its use is based on the tendency for any individual tumor to metastasize outside the local or regional area. For example, osteogenic sarcoma almost invariably leads to pulmonary metastases, and although the management of the local tumor is often uncomplicated, systemic therapy becomes necessary. This combined modality therapy for osteogenic sarcoma usually includes surgery in conjunction with systemic chemotherapy rather than with radiation therapy.

The combination of local and systemic therapy is commonly referred to as "adjuvant therapy" and has resulted in improved local control and prolonged survival for some types of tumors (Table 1.3). For patients with advanced regional disease and presumed occult micrometastatic disease, multiple or combined modality therapy is an evolving area of clinical investigation in cancer management. For

Table 1.3 Effective combined modality therapies with improved local control and/or prolonged survival

Modalities	Tumor
Surgery + Radiation	Rectal cancer
	Sarcoma
Surgery + Chemotherapy	Breast cancer
	Osteogenic sarcoma
Radiation + Chemotherapy	Breast cancer
	Sarcoma
	Pancreatic cancer

breast cancer and sarcoma in particular, adjuvant therapy has demonstrated that combined modality therapy may at least alter the natural course of the cancer.

4.0 Evaluation of response to therapy

The evaluation of the impact of therapy on malignant disease is often difficult because the tumor may reside in such hidden areas as the retroperitoneum, or it may be microscopically distributed and therefore not clinically measurable. Another difficulty in monitoring the impact of therapy on the disease is the subjective evaluation of symptoms. Symptoms associated with cancer may be due to secondary infection or may be related to an ancillary morbid disease. For example, bone pain may be related to arthritis or Paget's disease, and in patients with bone metastases, the nonneoplastic process may be contributing to symptoms. Subjective improvement or deterioration in symptoms does not necessarily confirm the effectiveness or lack of effectiveness of a treatment modality.

As a consequence of these problems, the evaluation of a new therapeutic modality must be as objective as possible.

The comparison between treatment or nontreatment should preferably be performed with a randomized and controlled trial, although in some instances historic controls may be appropriate. Two primary objective criteria determine therapeutic response. Survival, a precise measure of time, is measured from time of primary diagnosis, initiation of therapy, or diagnosis of metastases. One can determine the median survival, or time at which 50 percent of the study sample has died, and compare the median survival to that of an untreated group; alternatively, one can determine the percentage of patients surviving at specific intervals such as two or five years.

Responsiveness to therapy may be determined, in descending order of reliability and objectivity, by survival, tumor regression, and symptom response.

When survival is a criterion, one is evaluating the overall effect of treatment, but the antitumor effect of the therapeutic modality may be undetermined. Objective reduction in tumor size is therefore the criterion primarily employed in chemotherapeutic trials to evaluate the specific effectiveness of a drug or combination of drugs (Table 1.4). The criteria for objective reduction in tumor size are based on measurable parameters and, at least for "partial" and "complete response," as defined in Table 1.4 are almost invariably associated with greater survival. Objective reduction in tumor mass is evidence of response, and in addition, at least one month of sustained regression must be achieved. "Stable disease," "improvement" and "mixed response" are categories primarily used in early-phase drug development studies. A mixed response implies both increasing disease or appearance of new lesions and reduction of disease at another site. Mixed responses are invariably associated with no impact on survival and are therefore inconsequential in the evaluation of a drug or drug combination.

The patterns of measurable metastatic disease are limited; for solid tumor lesions, pulmonary nodules are the most precisely measurable metastases (Table 1.5). Lesions that are determined to be nonmeasurable represent secondary effects of the tumor and therefore do not precisely correlate with tumor mass. Bone lesions, for example, are particularly difficult to evaluate and represent a common metastatic pattern.

5.0 Oncologic emergencies

Oncologic emergencies are those secondary complications of cancer that have either life-threatening potential or major irreversible morbidity if untreated. Within this arbitrary definition, three categories of oncologic emergencies can be established (Table 1.6). The first is clearly life threatening and associated with major morbidity. Neurologic lesions within the nervous system, particularly the central nervous system above the foramen magnum, exemplify this category. Spinal cord compression, if untreated, may cause major morbidity, including paraplegia and conditions requiring prolonged nursing care, but it is not life threatening. The second category of oncologic emer-

Table 1.4 Objective reduction in tumor

Partial response	A 50% reduction in the product of the maximum perpendicular diameters of the most easily measurable lesion without increase in other lesions and with a minimum duration of four weeks.
Complete response	A 100% reduction in all evidence of tumor for minimum of four weeks without appearance of new lesions.
Stable disease	Less than a 25% decrease in measurable disease without other lesions developing.
No response (progressive disease)	More than a 25% increase in the size of the lesion or the development of new lesions.
Improvement	A 25–50% reduction in the product of maximum perpendicular diameters lasting at least four weeks.

Table 1.5 Measurable and nonmeasurable patterns of metastatic disease

Measurable	Nonmeasurable
Discrete pulmonary nodule	Effusions including ascites
Discrete subcutaneous nodule	Neurologic symptoms
Hepatomegaly*	Abnormal liver function tests
Biochemical markers	Pelvic mass
HCG, CEA†	Liver scan lesions
Lymph nodes	Confirmed histologic osseous lesions

*Only if liver is below costal margin in AAL and MCL, in which case criteria of response is a 30 percent reduction in the sum of the measurement from subcostal margin to liver edge at the AAL and MCL
†Only if pretreatment level exceeds 50 ng/ml by Hansen assay

gencies involves mid-line obstruction within the mediastinum with extension to the heart, the venous inflow tracts, or the trachea. Finally, metabolic abnormalities that may be a consequence of primary endocrine dysfunction or secondary paraneoplastic syndromes can result in major morbidity and even in death.

The clinical management of oncologic emergencies often involves immediate therapeutic intervention without specific diagnostic evaluation. For example, a histologic diagnosis or confirmation of cerebral metastases is not generally necessary because of the rarity of other causes of central nervous system lesions. Similarly, the superior vena cava syndrome is almost invariably due to a malignant process, and vigorous diagnostic procedures can be associated with major morbidity and mortality.

All of the oncologic emergencies defined here are treatable so that reversibility of the clinical syndrome may be frequently accomplished with standard, noninvasive, and tolerable therapies. In fact, more than 50 percent of patients with any of the clinical emergencies may have regression. More importantly, the emergency may be effectively treated so that

recurrence is prevented, and prognosis is determined by another site of disease.

6.0 Organ-related cancer complications

The complications of cancer that do not represent emergencies in that they do not have life-threatening potential do have major implications for morbidity. These can be categorized by organ systems (Table 1.7). The categories of complications are related to seven organ systems. Neoplastic lesions affecting the gastrointestinal tract, genitourinary tract, bone, or lung are often diagnostic problems as well as therapeutic dilemmas. Hematologic and dermatologic complications of cancer are commonplace and may cause significant patient morbidity. Nervous system complications comprise a category also included as an oncologic emergency.

Specific pathologic lesions or clinical effects are characteristic for each organ. These include urinary obstruction, pathologic fracture of the bone, lymphangitic infiltration of the lung, and gastrointestinal obstruction. In each visceral organ a benign process may mimic the malignant disease so that definitive diagnostic eval-

Table 1.6 Oncologic emergencies with life-threatening potential

I *Neurologic lesions*

Central nervous system, cerebral hemispheres, cerebellum and brain stem

Spinal cord*

II *Mediastinum or midline structure lesions*

Vena cava obstruction

Laryngotracheal obstruction

Pericardial invasion

III *Endocrinologic or metabolic effects*

Hypercalcemia

Paraneoplastic syndromes, e.g., SIADH

Endocrine organ tumors

*Spinal cord compression is not life threatening but is associated with major morbidity.

uations are necessary. Acquired infections, complications of therapy, incidental degenerative diseases, or unrelated acute or chronic disease are all potential problems that influence the therapeutic approach as well as confuse the diagnostic picture. The patient with cancer is not immune to diabetes mellitus or coronary artery disease and is susceptible to incidental uncommon and rare diseases as well.

7.0 Diagnostic problems in cancer management

The diagnosis of cancer is often simple because pathologic criteria for malignancy are usually clear-cut. Histologic criteria for malignancy are not always unambiguous, and low-grade tumors may represent hyperplastic rather than neoplastic change. Premalignant alterations may further compound the clinical and pathologic considerations.

For many tumors, a diagnosis of malignancy must depend upon organ invasion, since the lesion may be histologically

Table 1.7 Complications of cancer related to organ system involvement

Organ system	Associated complications
Gastrointestinal tract	Infection, obstruction, organ failure
Genitourinary tract	Obstruction, hemorrhage, perforation, serositis, malabsorption
Bone	Pathologic fracture, infection
Lung	Infection, obstruction, serositis
Blood	Anemia, hemorrhage, infection
Skin	Allergy, infection
Nervous system	Seizures, neurologic syndromes, cord compression, altered consciousness

similar to normal or simple hyperplastic tissue. For example, metastatic leiomyomas of the uterus have been observed and have been associated with long-term survival in spite of the presence of multiple implants in the abdomen or lung from histologically benign lesions in the uterus. Presumably such lesions represent low-grade leiomyosarcoma, which although metastatic, does not interfere with organ function. Another example is that of bile duct carcinoma, which is, in the opinion of some pathologists, a progressive form of sclerosing cholangitis. Benign hepatomas, particularly secondary to or associated with estrogen-containing contraceptives, are not metastatic and appear pathologically as hyperplastic hepatic cells, or hepatic adenomas. One confusing entity pathologically is the teratoma, which may be diagnosed as benign teratoma but which, particularly for males, is invariably associated with the capability for malignant invasion and widespread metastasis. In addition to these lesions, low-grade malignancies may be observed in breast cancer, gastric cancer, and tumors of the genitourinary tract. Thus, borderline malignant lesions are a potential diagnostic problem for the pathologist.

Premalignant lesions represent an extraordinarily difficult area in cancer diagnosis. Ulcerative colitis and familial polyposis are premalignant lesions that require careful scrutiny and considered therapeutic judgment. The decision to commence therapy must be made prior to development of the cancer, but only when the potential for cancer is maximum. "Prophylactic" procedures, such as ileostomy, may have a major impact on life style. Prophylactic mastectomy, for example, may be considered for patients with a high risk of developing breast cancer. The procedure is more feasible now than in the past due to the availability of mammary reconstruction and prosthesis.

The major "premalignant lesion" is a history of prior malignancy; patients with one type of cancer have an increased likelihood of developing a second malignancy of unrelated or related types. For bilateral organs, the presence of cancer in one organ predicts the potential development of malignancy in the contralateral organ. This is true for breast cancer, renal cancer, and retinoblastoma. For lung cancer patients, second primary malignancy is common, for all 18 lobes of the lung are at risk with exposure to the carcinogenic stimulus of smoking. Second primary cancers often represent a difficult diagnostic dilemma and may not be clinically distinguishable from a solitary metastasis. Thus, a patient with a history of breast cancer who develops a pulmonary nodule is equally likely to develop a new, primary lung cancer or a solitary pulmonary metastasis. For diagnosis the issues of disease-free interval, stage of the first tumor, adequacy of therapy, and predisposing factors for the development of a new primary cancer are all factors to be considered in establishing whether the lesion is primary or metastatic.

A major diagnostic problem in cancer management is that of the tumor of unknown origin (TUO). Therapeutic management of the TUO is rarely difficult, for by definition the lesion is metastatic and does not arise in the tissue from which a diagnosis is made. The diagnostic implications, however, are substantial in that the search for the primary tumor is often arduous and may not have therapeutic implications; in a major proportion of patients, the primary lesion may not be found at all. In this context, an occult primary neoplastic lesion is presumably microscopic in the presence of macroscopic metastatic deposits. Finally, a common diagnostic problem in cancer management is the inability to obtain a histologic diagnosis. Most commonly this difficulty arises because the morbidity of the diagnostic procedure is exorbitant in relation to the value of the information to be gained.

Patient D, a 48-year-old man, developed shoulder pain and cough. A chest radiograph revealed a superior sulcus tumor with erosion of the vertebral body at T². Sputum cytology was unrevealing and the patient received radiation therapy to the right-upper lobe with rapid relief of pain. Four weeks later a right-upper lobectomy was performed, and an epidermoid carcinoma was identified pathologically.

Antineoplastic therapy (radiation or chemotherapy) may sometimes be employed in the absence of tissue diagnosis.

Other examples of therapy without histologic confirmation include mediastinal mass lesions in children, which almost always represent lymphoma; arteriographically demonstrated brain tumors; and pelvic pain syndromes developing in patients with prior rectal cancers.

8.0 Therapeutic problems in cancer management

Earlier in this chapter, therapeutic decision-making in cancer management was discussed in relation to choices among therapeutic modalities and to timing of therapy. The complexity of the problem increases when the adverse effects of therapy are considered. Such adverse effects as carcinogenicity, acutely and chronically compromised organ function, and tumor resistance to secondary therapy are all crucial issues, particularly in the application of combined modality therapies.

The question of when to treat cancer, previously discussed in the context of advanced asymptomatic disease, can be considered again in the context of sequential versus maximal "up-front" therapy. Sequential therapy is treatment administered as a single modality while holding in reserve other known effective modalities until resistance to the first modality is determined. Then in sequence the next effective modality is employed until it in turn induces resistance. For example, hormone therapy in breast cancer may be introduced at the first evidence of metastasis; after a response and subsequent resistance, hormone ablation may be introduced until, finally, chemotherapy is used when the patient has developed resistance to all hormonal maneuvers. This therapeutic approach allows the patient to have a series of treatments of increasing complexity and risk only in the later stages of disease and permits long-term control with minimal cost. Proponents of the alternative approach, that is, initial use of therapy that employs all effective modalities simultaneously, suggest that sequential therapy is, in effect, palliation and acknowledgment of incurability. The combined use of all effective modalities simultaneously should maximize the impact on the tumor and minimize the ability for growth of resisting clones of tumor cells, thus achieving complete clinical regression and the potential for longer control and possible cure. The resolution of these two divergent therapeutic approaches has not yet been achieved in clinical or experimental trials. It appears clear that sequential therapy is less morbid, but that the potential for long-term control and perhaps for cure is limited and probably nonexistent.

If one presumes that combined modalities are important in treatment, the next question is how the modalities can be effectively combined to maximize therapeutic benefit and minimize adverse effects. Preoperative therapy, particularly preoperative radiation for rectal cancer and head and neck cancers, is applied not only to minimize dispersal of viable tumor cells at the time of surgery but also to promote ease of operation and local control. Preoperative chemotherapy is a new concept applied primarily for local, inoperable lesions or for lesions that would require major disfiguring or mutilating surgery, such as amputation for limb sarcoma. In the context of the modern application of adjuvant therapy, an additional rationale for the use of preoperative chemotherapy is to establish the effectiveness of the adjuvant modality. For example, the patient with breast cancer who is committed to adjuvant therapy for one year or more may be better able to tolerate or endure the adverse effects of therapy when the effectiveness of the drug treatment has been established. The physician administering therapy can also offer more encouragement and sustain the drug treatment if an antitumor effect has been observed by objective measurements.

While considering the when and how of therapy, it is also important to consider the duration of therapy, particularly of adjuvant or combined modality chemotherapy. The issue has not been resolved because adjuvant chemotherapy has not been definitively established as an important and absolute treatment for any tumor. Adjuvant chemotherapy, however, is becoming increasingly popular, and the duration of therapy is still a major question. By and large, for cancers such as acute leukemia or Hodgkin's disease, a finite period of treatment is established (two years and six months, respectively), during which time or at the completion of which the tumor must be in complete clinical remission. In patients with solid tumors and regional disease that has been surgically removed or irradiated, the duration of adjuvant chemotherapy has generally been determined to be the maximum tolerated duration or that period of time during which the maximum rate of tumor reappearance is recognized. For example, most recurrences of breast cancer

develop within the first two years following primary therapy; thus adjuvant therapy never exceeds two years and has been more commonly set at one year. It must be reemphasized, however, that the duration of treatment has at this point not been definitively answered and the issue of maintenance therapy is a major area of controversy. Duration of therapy in patients with metastatic disease may be determined by the degree of response and patient tolerance. No evidence exists that maintenance therapy for any tumor increases the duration of response. Therefore, treatment may be continued simply to the maximal response.

As indicated previously, the therapeutic problems of cancer management relate to the potentially adverse effects of therapy. Whether one is dealing with chemotherapy or radiation therapy, the systemic and local adverse effects may be substantial and must be balanced against the potentially therapeutic effects. Adverse sequelae can be separated into acute and chronic effects. The former relate to the action of the therapeutic modality on the proliferating cells, for example, alopecia and marrow suppression common with chemotherapy. Chronic adverse effects, in contrast, are a consequence of cumulative visceral organ effects and host response. For patients receiving radiation therapy, a decrease in vascular supply related to arteritis can lead to secondary fibrosis within the organ. A major potential long-term effect of chemotherapy and radiation therapy is carcinogenesis. Although it is clear that an increased likelihood of second malignancy is greater with the addition of chemotherapy. Carcinogenesis has not been established for therapeutic doses of radiation administered judiciously. The application of chemotherapy in conjunction with radiation, however, may increase the likelihood of secondary tumors. The long-term effects of chemotherapy have yet to be established, as chemotherapy has largely been employed for patients who have had advanced disease and succumbed early and not for those with early disease and a prolonged prognosis.

9.0 Summary

Cancer treatment involves diagnostic and therapeutic decision-making that bridges many subspecialties of medicine. The development of new diagnostic techniques and improved therapeutic modalities have altered our concepts of the management of malignancy in that the palliation of secondary symptoms is often achievable, and palliation may be translated into an improved quality of life as well as prolonged survival.

Combined modality therapies for patients with primary or regional disease, for whom the prognosis is limited or the statistical likelihood of recurrence high, is a major advance in cancer management. The thrust of such therapy is the promotion of cure or, at the very least, an alteration of the natural course of the tumor. In patients with advanced cancer, the therapeutic goal is palliation rather than cure, and the choice and timing of therapy are complex[It is axiomatic that effective treatment, that is, treatment that induces tumor regression, never simply prolongs life but is invariably associated with an improved quality of life.)

References

Ackerman, L. V., and del Regato, J. A. *Cancer: Diagnosis, treatment and prognosis.* St. Louis: C. V. Mosby, 1970.

Brodsky, I.; Kahn, S. B.; and Moyer, J. H., eds. *Cancer chemotherapy II.* New York: Grune & Stratton, 1972.

Garattini, S., and Franchi, G., eds. *Chemotherapy of cancer: dissemination and metastasis.* New York: Raven Press, 1973.

Greenwald, E. S. *Cancer chemotherapy.* Flushing: Medical Exam. Pub. Co. Inc., 1973.

Higkey, R. C., ed. *Current problems in cancer; rationale and application of immunotherapy for human cancer,* vol. II, no. 11. Chicago: Year Book Medical Publishers, 1978.

Holland, J. F., and Frei, E., III, eds. *Cancer medicine.* Philadelphia: Lea & Febiger, 1973.

Horton, J., and Hill, G. J., II, eds. *Clinical oncology.* Philadelphia: W. B. Saunders Co., 1977.

Lawrence, W., Jr., and Terz, J. J. *Cancer management.* New York: Grune & Stratton, 1977.

Moss, W. T. *Radiation oncology.* 4th ed. St. Louis: C. V. Mosby, 1973.

Salmon-Jones. *Adjuvant therapy in cancer.* New York: American Elsevier, 1978.

Staquet, M., ed. *Cancer therapy: prognostic factors and criteria of response.* New York: Raven Press, 1975.

Cancer chemotherapy: fundamental concepts and recent advances. Proceedings of the 19th annual clinical conference on cancer at the University of Texas System Cancer Center, M.D. Anderson Hospital and Tumor Institute. Chicago: Year Book Medical Publishers, 1974.

Part II   Oncologic Emergencies

Chapter 2

Superior Vena Cava Syndrome
J. Lokich

1.0 Background

The superior vena cava (SVC) syndrome is a unique clinical entity first described by William Hunter in 1757. The syndrome develops as a consequence of a pathologic process within the mediastinum and is considered an oncologic emergency because of the acute cerebral syndrome that results from venous obstruction and increased intracerebral pressure. If left untreated, venous obstruction in the upper thoracic cavity can progress to stasis of blood flow and eventually to intravascular clotting with major secondary sequelae.

Obstruction of the superior vena cava is almost invariably due to malignant disease. In previous reports, a summary of 274 cases of superior vena cava syndrome indicated that 40 percent were secondary to luetic aneurysms of the aorta or to tuberculous mediastinitis. These infectious etiologies of SVC syndrome, however, have been virtually eliminated, and the predominant cause is carcinoma (Table 2.1). In cancer, the two most common causes of SVC syndrome are bronchogenic carcinoma, which accounts for three-fourths of all cases, and lymphoma, including Hodgkin's disease and non-Hodgkin's lymphoma. All tumors, primary and metastatic, are capable of producing the SVC syndrome, although it is reported to be relatively infrequent with extrathoracic tumors. In fact, breast cancer has been associated with only five reported cases in spite of the relative proximity of the breast to the mediastinum and the prevalence of metastases to the internal mammary nodes.

The SVC syndrome is almost invariably due to a malignant disease and is most commonly due to bronchogenic carcinoma.

Benign causes of SVC syndrome, excluding infection, include the obscure diagnosis of "fibrosing mediastinitis" and the relatively infrequent benign goiter, which may impinge upon the superior vena cava. Recently, the increased use of cathe-

Table 2.1 Nonmalignant etiologies of the SVC syndrome

Infectious	Luetic aortitis
	Tuberculous mediastinitis
Idiopathic	Sclerosing (fibrosing) mediastinitis
Vascular	Catheter-, pacemaker-, tubing-induced phlebitis
Traumatic	Mediastinal hematoma
Degenerative	Goiter

ters placed within the superior vena cava either for monitoring cardiac or pulmonary function or for the administration of hyperalimentation solutions has resulted in an occasional thrombosis secondary to the foreign object.

The anatomic orientation of the superior mediastinum and the relationship of the lymph nodes to the venous drainage pattern of the chest, extremities, and neck determine the clinical features of the syndrome (Fig. 2.1). The lymph nodes in the mediastinum encase the superior vena cava as it is formed from the confluence of the right subclavian vein, the azygous vein, and the left innominate vein. The thin vena cava wall and the low intravascular pressure within the venous system allow for the vein to be compressed relatively easily in contrast to arterial structures with the same anatomic distribution. It is evident that the syndrome develops more commonly with bronchogenic carcinoma because of the direct lymphatic drainage of the lung, and more specifically with lesions in the right lung because of the proximity of the right lung to the confluence of veins. In bronchogenic carcinoma, the SVC syndrome is more common with right-sided bronchogenic lesions by a ratio of four to one.

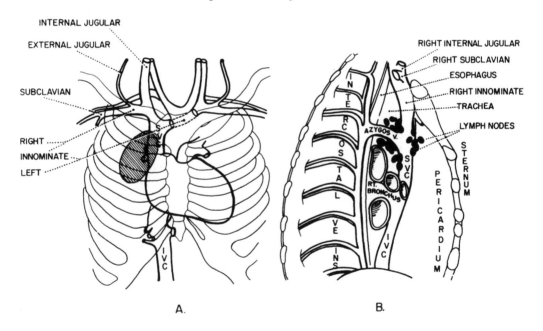

A.   B.

Fig. 2.1 Anterior (A) and lateral or sagittal (B) schematic drawings of thoracic cage and vascular structures within the mediastinum. The most common site of a mass lesion in the mediastinal area is indicated by the shaded oval structure impinging upon the superior vena cava.

Impingement of local node tissue on the vena cava leads to decreased flow rate and subsequent stasis. Caval thrombosis develops eventually and is established in approximately one-third of patients with SVC syndrome at postmortem examination. In addition, the tumor frequently invades contiguous cardiac structures and may form part of the wall of the vascular structures within the mediastinum.

2.0 Clinical presentation of the SVC syndrome

The SVC syndrome is represented by symptoms and physical signs that may be observed individually or collectively (Table 2.2). The obstruction to venous drainage results in secondarily increased venous pressure and dilatation of collateral veins at the upper part of the thorax and neck. Secondarily, edema and plethora of the face, neck, and upper part of the torso develop. Depending upon the site of obstruction above or below the azygous vein, the edema may be confluent or asymmetrical; commonly, edema of one breast develops. The edema of the upper torso may also result in suffusion and edema of the conjunctiva with visual disturbances and proptosis. Finally, symptoms of central nervous dysfunction,

including headache, visual disturbances, and progressive disorientation, and coma may develop. Because of the localization of the tumor in the mediastinum, concomitant obstruction to the trachea and esophageal function can be observed.

Patient A, a 59-year-old woman, had a primary history of dysphagia over four months, progressing to an inability to handle salivary secretions. She denied weight loss but did have an associated cough and on examination had edema of the neck with distended neck veins to the angle of the jaw. Chest x-ray demonstrated an enormous mass of the mediastinum with compression of the trachea and esophagus (Fig. 2.2).

The SVC syndrome may develop with other mediastinal syndromes (dysphagia, dysphonia, dyspnea).

The chest x-ray may demonstrate a large mass in the mediastinum, most often in contiguity with the lung; but particularly with metastatic lesions to the mediastinum, the mediastinal lesion may be quite small and detectable only by tomography.

Patient B, a 45-year-old woman with colon cancer documented five years pre-

Table 2.2 Frequency of signs and symptoms of the SVC syndrome

Physical signs	
Venous distension (neck and thorax)	75%
Facial edema	50%
Thoracic or extremity edema*	40%
Conjunctival edema	25%
Symptoms	
Cough	20–40%
Dyspnea	30%
Headache	70–80%
Visual disturbance	20–40%

*Unilateral or bilateral.

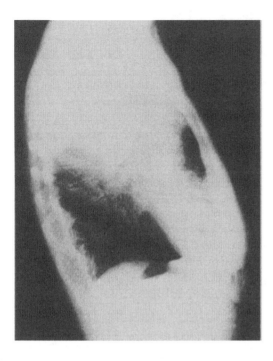

Fig. 2.2 Lateral radiograph of the chest (Patient A) demonstrating large mediastinal mass and tapered air column representing the trachea with obliteration of the esophageal space.

viously, presented with headache and dilated neck veins. Her chest x-ray demonstrated a slight fullness of the left hilum. Carcinoembryonic antigen was 50 ng/ml. Tomograms demonstrated obstruction at the left hilum, and the patient underwent thoracotomy with rapid reversal of the syndrome.

Occasionally the SVC syndrome may be so severe as to suggest Cushing's syndrome. The plethora of the upper torso and the edema, in particular, can create a physiognomy characteristic of Cushing's syndrome.

3.0 Diagnostic evaluation in the SVC syndrome

The SVC syndrome is rapidly controllable

by appropriate therapy. It also represents a clinical diagnosis that need not be confirmed by complex radiographic procedures that are associated with significant complications. Such procedures are designed to establish the site of obstruction, which is in fact already defined by the clinical picture. For example, venography outlines the venous channels in the thoracic inlet and mediastinum, and obstruction can be accentuated.

Patient C, a 49-year-old man, presented with cough, headache, and typical clinical features of the SVC syndrome. Venography via the left arm veins demonstrated the site of obstruction (Fig. 2.3). After the procedure, the patient had an acute exacerbation of headache and cough, and he developed secondary thrombosis of the basilic veins of the arm.

Static blood flow in the dilated venous channels results in delayed flow of the radio-opaque dye and a secondary sclerosing effect on the vein wall. Therapeutic nitrogen mustard can, in a similar man-

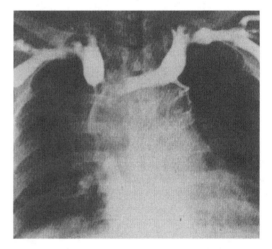

Fig. 2.3 Radiograph demonstrating retarded flow of contrast material into the right ventricle at the site of the conjunction of the left innominate and right subclavian veins.

ner, cause a local sclerosis in the veins. In addition to exhibiting local phlebitis secondary to trauma and the introduction of an irritant, the venous channel may bleed excessively when the needle is withdrawn.

The SVC syndrome is a clinical diagnosis and does not necessitate radiographic procedures for confirmation or for establishing the obstruction site.

In addition to venography, radionuclear flow studies can demonstrate the site of obstruction as well as the rate of flow by a quantitative measure. Again, such studies are unnecessary, and simple manometric measurements based on clinical appreciation of the venous pressure in relation to the heart level are available without compromising the patient.

Venous access in the upper extremities must be avoided, including venipuncture and contrast radiographic studies.

Although the diagnosis of the SVC syndrome is determined on clinical grounds, the histologic diagnosis is not always easily established because of the lack of accessible tumor to biopsy. In fact, the SVC syndrome is almost always due to a malignant disease and should not absolutely require histologic diagnosis for confirmation before initiation of treatment. The tumor is commonly confined to the upper mediastinum, and obtaining a histologic diagnosis may be hazardous.

Patient D, a 35-year-old woman, presented with a typical SVC syndrome. In an attempt to establish a histologic diagnosis, an exploration of the supraclavicular area was undertaken to obtain lymph nodes. The tissue was edematous, and

profuse bleeding ensued upon incision. The bleeding remained uncontrolled for a protracted period during which the patient lost eight units of blood. No lymph nodes were available for analysis.

In addition to the adverse effects and potential complications associated with local biopsy procedures, standard and routine manipulations by esophagoscopy or bronchoscopy can also be associated with catastrophic events.

Patient E, a 62-year-old man, presented with dysphagia and stridor as well as distended neck veins and edema of the upper chest. A chest x-ray demonstrated a typical mass lesion in the parahilar area; an attempt at further evaluation by combined bronchoscopy and esophagoscopy was undertaken. During the procedures no tumor was visible. Within one hour after completion of the procedures, however, the patient developed increasing respiratory distress and died suddenly.

Diagnostic manipulations can accentuate edema in the bronchial tree and as a consequence lead to respiratory compromise. Air flow through the bronchus is related to the fourth power of the radius; therefore, relatively small changes in the caliber of the respiratory tract result in large changes in air flow.

Surgical manipulations in the neck, thorax, and bronchial and esophageal passages are contraindicated.

Because the primary therapy for a local complication is radiation, one can consider therapy without a histologic diagnosis, particularly when the clinical picture is classic.

Patient F, a 14-year-old boy, presented with stridor, headache, and dilated neck veins and was found to have an enormous mass of the mediastinum that impinged upon both right and left lung fields. The patient was immediately given corticosteroids, and radiation therapy was initiated. Rapid resolution of the mass was achieved, and a histologic diagnosis was obtained three months later at biopsy of an axillary node.

Radiation therapy to control acute symptoms may sufficiently alleviate local edema and venous obstruction after a relatively low dose to allow biopsy and further treatment. Alternatively, biopsy of common extrathoracic sources of metastases such as the bone marrow or the liver may be helpful.

Patient G, a 52-year-old male smoker, presented with cough and suffusion of the head. Chest x-ray demonstrated a large mediastinal mass, and radiation therapy was initiated promptly. Subsequent mediastinoscopy was considered, but liver scan demonstrated a mass lesion, and needle aspiration revealed undifferentiated small cell carcinoma (Fig. 2.4).

In children and young adults the SVC syndrome is invariably due to lymphoma, and vigorous attempts at a diagnosis are avoided. In adults the type of tumor-causing SVC syndrome has a broader range, but the therapeutic philosophy should be the same.

Primary treatment for the SVC syndrome is radiation therapy even without a histologic diagnosis.

Occasionally the clinical picture can be obscured or confused by an atypical clinical presentation or by the absence of abnormal findings on chest x-ray.

Patient H, an 83-year-old woman, was diagnosed by node biopsy two years prior to presentation as having Hodgkin's disease. She was treated with radiation therapy to the mantle followed by a booster dose of radiation to the axilla. At the time of secondary presentation, the patient had swelling of the right arm with dilated veins but without palpable nodes in the axilla or neck. Venogram demonstrated

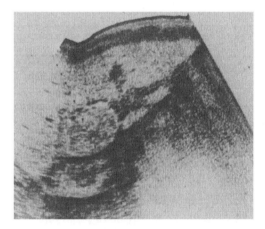 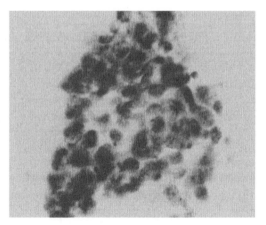

Fig. 2.4 Under ultrasonic guidance (A) a large defect in the deep inferior margin of the liver is identified. Employing ultrasound as a guide for depth, needle aspiration of the mass lesion yielded Class V cytology characteristic for oat cell carcinoma (B).

obstruction at the level of the brachial and subclavian venous access channel. Review of prior radiation portals revealed that she had received 7000 rad to one overlap area precisely at the site of obstruction.

The primary dictum in the diagnosis of the SVC syndrome is that the syndrome is always presumed to be due to malignant disease and does not absolutely require a histologic diagnosis for confirmation, nor is it necessary to establish the site of obstruction by radiographic procedures.

4.0 Therapeutic management of the SVC syndrome

The primary therapy for SVC syndrome is radiation because of the local or regional distribution of the lesion and the responsiveness of mediastinal tumors to radiation therapy. The radiotherapeutic techniques of fractionation, field size, and maximum dose are conditioned, at least in part, by the extent of disease as well as by the type of tumor. Bronchogenic carcinoma and lymphoma are the two primary tumors most often associated with the SVC syndrome.

Patient I, a 36-year-old woman and chronic smoker, presented with cough, headache, and distended neck veins. A chest radiograph demonstrated a large left-upper lobe mass lesion in continuity with the mediastinum. Histologic confirmation of an epidermoid carcinoma resulted in radiation therapy to the mediastinum and left upper lobe to a dose of 6000 rad.

The field of radiation should be restricted but not the dose if bronchogenic carcinoma is the most likely diagnosis.

Patient J, a 28-year-old man, presented with a large mediastinal mass and the typical signs and symptoms of the SVC syndrome. A left axillary node revealed non-Hodgkin's lymphoma, and the patient received mantle radiation including all node-bearing areas in the chest to 4000 rad.

Radiation should include the mantle field if lymphoma is the most likely diagnosis.

The dose fractionation is often variable, and in some instances high-dose intermittent therapy of 400 to 1000 rad may be employed. Normally, however, the standard 150 to 300 rad daily dose is administered. The total cumulative dose is related to tumor type, and for primary tumors of the lung therapeutic doses are used to minimize the likelihood of recurrence. The therapeutic dose is somewhat lower for lymphoproliferative diseases.

The radiation field size and dose are conditioned by the diagnosis of the tumor type. A second consideration is the extent and radioresponsiveness of the tumor. For patients with radioresistant tumors and extensive intrathoracic as well as extrathoracic disease, local radiation at restricted doses and field size is employed as the initial therapeutic modality

Patient K, a 65-year-old woman with metastatic spindle cell sarcoma to the mediastinum, presented with unilateral breast edema, cough, and headache. The patient was treated with a small field of radiation to the mediastinum alone and had partial relief of obstruction. She survived an additional 12 months with intermittent exacerbation of the syndrome.

Chemotherapy has been advocated as an ancillary modality in conjunction with radiation therapy for the management of the SVC syndrome in both lymphoma and bronchogenic carcinoma. Tumor reduction through the use of nitrogen mustard alone or in conjunction with radiation therapy may decrease the likelihood of local edema, according to proponents of the combined modality approach, but neither experimental nor clinical data indicate that the combined modality approach is superior to radiation therapy alone. On the other hand, in exquisitely responsive tumors, chemotherapy as a primary therapeutic modality may be effective and might preclude the need for radiation.

Patient L, a 19-year-old man, presented with a mediastinal mass and clinical components of the SVC syndrome. Histologic examination of the tissue revealed a typical histiocytic lymphoma. In addition to headache, the patient demonstrated retinal changes compatible with the SVC syndrome and was treated with a combination of cyclophosphamide, Adriamycin, vincristine (Oncovin), and prednisone, with rapid resolution of the symptoms (Fig. 2.5).

Patient M, a 62-year-old woman, had primary breast cancer treated with local radiation therapy. She presented one year later with a large lung mass, a lesion in the mediastinum, headache, cough, and dilated jugular veins. Because of the previous radiation therapy to the mediastinum, chemotherapy was employed using a five-drug regimen with rapid resolution of radiographic signs and physical symptoms (Fig. 2.6).

Patient N, a 54-year-old chronic smoker, presented with enlarging cervical lymph nodes and persistent cough. Dilated neck veins without edema were observed, and the patient received four radiation treatments to the general area of the upper mediastinum and neck. Subsequent biopsy on the fifth day of radiation revealed small cell carcinoma, and the patient was treated with a multiple-drug regimen. The clinical syndrome and radiographic evidence of tumor resolved rapidly (Fig. 2.7).

Thus, chemotherapy plays a primary role in the SVC syndrome, which is resistant

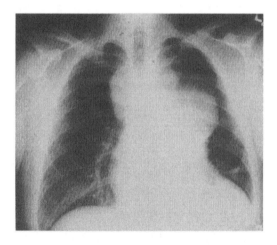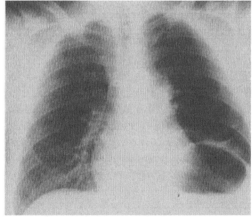

Fig. 2.5 Chest radiographs demonstrating massive mediastinal adenopathy with hilar extension on the left into the left lung field (A). Following one course of chemotherapy, rapid and complete regression of all evidence of mediastinal mass lesions was observed (B).

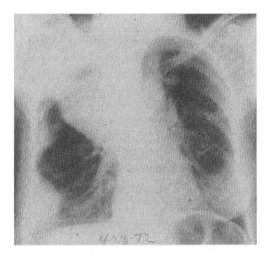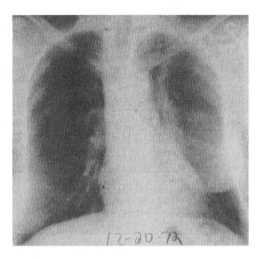

Fig. 2.6 Chest radiograph demonstrating massive mediastinal lesion extending into the right lung field in addition to pleural implants along the peripheral lung margin (A). Within two months major

regression of all evidence of pulmonary tumor had regressed, and the differential breast size reflected radiation to the left breast (B).

to radiation therapy. Chemotherapy is also useful for patients who have received maximum radiation therapy or who have drug-responsive tumors, such as the anaplastic tumors, sarcomas, lymphomas, and breast cancer.

Ancillary modalities of therapy (diuretics, anticoagulants, and corticosteroids) are of no proven effectiveness. Chemotherapy is a primary modality for responsive tumors such as lymphomas.

Surgery for the SVC syndrome should be reserved for localized resistant tumors in the absence of the full clinical picture. Surgical mortality and the incidence of hemorrhage are high. The approach generally employs bypass grafts of the obstruction, radical surgical excision, and venectomy. Surgery can be considered the treatment of choice for the singular but rare circumstance in which sclerosing fibrosis of the mediastinum with second-

ary vascular thrombosis is the primary cause of the syndrome. In this instance bypass graft is a preferable approach.

Surgical intervention is indicated as a secondary procedure only following resistance to other local and systemic modalities.

Ancillary medical measures have been advocated in the management of SVC syndrome, including anticoagulation, fibrinolytic agents, diuretic therapy, and corticosteroids. None of these agents has been singularly successful without definitive local treatment with radiation therapy. Nonetheless, corticosteroids are used routinely to obviate the theoretical induction of radiation edema and an augmentation of the clinical syndrome during early therapy. The presence of edema of the upper torso, including periorbital edema, has often prompted the use of diuretic therapy with some decrease in edema, but

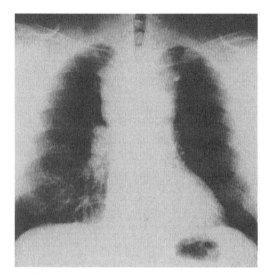 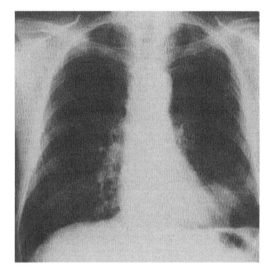

Fig. 2.7 Chest radiograph (Patient N) demonstrated enlarged mediastinal mass with compression of the air column and separate hilar lesion (A). Within three weeks of chemotherapy and radiation total dissolution of the central tumor was evident (B).

it is a temporary measure at most. The use of anticoagulants and fibrinolytic agents is based on the common presence of thrombosis of the venous system that may be observed at postmortem examination. In one series, fibrinolytic agents appeared to increase the effectiveness of local radiation therapy.

5.0 Summary

The SVC syndrome represents an acute oncologic emergency and is rarely chronic and relatively asymptomatic. Major pitfalls in the management of the SVC syndrome are an overexuberant and zealous approach to establishing the obstruction site by diagnostic venography and other contrast procedures, and the surgical pursuit of a histologic diagnosis. The SVC syndrome is invariably due to malignant disease, and routine radiographic procedures generally demonstrate the obstruction. Nonetheless, even in the absence of an obvious site of obstruction, mediastinal radiation can be employed, if one presumes the etiology to be either bronchogenic carcinoma or lymphoma, the two most common etiologies. Early clinical recognition should prompt immediate therapeutic intervention for this oncologic emergency, and additional chemotherapy, surgery, and ancillary medical measures should be applied only when resistance to radiation therapy is established.

Depending upon the primary tumor source, the extent of tumor (metastases), and the responsiveness of the tumor to radiation and/or chemotherapy, the SVC syndrome is not necessarily irreversible. In fact, 10 to 20 percent of patients with the syndrome may survive longer than two years, justifying aggressive therapeutic approaches.

References

Effeney, D. J.; Windson, H. M.; and Shana-
han, M. X. Superior vena cava obstruction: Resection and bypass for
malignant lesions. *Aust. N.Z. J. Surg.*
42:231–237, 1973.

Failor, H. J.; Edwards, J. E.; and Hodgson,
C. H. Etiologic factors in obstruction
of the superior vena cava: a pathologic
study. *Staff Meetings Mayo Clin.*
33:671–678, 1958.

Geller, W. The mandate for chemotherapeutic decompression in superior
vena caval obstruction. *Radiology*
81:385–387, 1963.

Green J.; Rubin, P.; and Holzwasser, G.
The experimental production of superior vena caval obstruction. *Radiology* 81:406–414, 1963.

Howard, N. Phlebography in superior
venal caval obstruction. *Radiology*
81:380–384, 1963.

Perez, C. A.; Presant, C. A.; and Van Am-
burg, A. L., III. Management of superior vena cava syndrome. *Seminars in
Oncology* 5:123–134, 1978.

Roswit, B.; Kaplan, G.; and Jacobson, H. G.
The superior vena cava obstruction
syndrome in bronchogenic carcinoma. *Radiology* 61:722–737, 1953.

Rubin, P.; Green, J.; and Holzwasser, G.
et al. Superior vena caval syndrome.
Radiology 81:388–401, 1963.

Schechter, M. M. The superior vena cava
syndrome. *Am. J. Med. Sci.* 227:46–
56, 1954.

Urschel, H. C., and Paulson, D. L. Superior
vena caval canal obstruction. *Dis.
Chest* 49:155–164, 1966.

Chapter 3

Cardiac Complications of Malignancy

J. Lokich

1.0 Background

Clinical cardiac complications of malignancy are relatively uncommon, although at autopsy heart metastases develop in 10 percent of patients with malignant neoplasms. With some tumor types, cardiac metastases may be present in over 60 percent of patients at postmortem examination. The most common tumors involving the heart are bronchogenic carcinoma by direct contiguous involvement and breast cancer by hematogenous dissemination (Table 3.1). Only 10 percent of patients with neoplasms to the heart develop clinical cardiac dysfunction. Almost 85 percent of the patients with neoplastic cardiac involvement have involvement of the pericardium with or without invasion into the myocardium; therefore, the predominant clinical manifestation of cardiac metastases is the development of a malignant pericardial effusion.

Within the spectrum of cardiac complications and manifestations of malignant disease, rhythm disorders and conduction abnormalities predominate and may develop with or without congestive heart failure but are almost always associated with pericardial tumor implants (Table 3.2). The most critical cardiac complication of malignant disease is malignant

Table 3.1 Relative frequency and incidence of tumors metastatic to the heart

	Relative frequency	Incidence
Bronchogenic carcinoma	20–35%	10%
Breast cancer	15–35%	10%
Lymphoma and leukemia	10–15%	>60%
Malignant melanoma	10–15%	>60%
Other tumors	<5%	—

Table 3.2 Cardiac complications and manifestations in malignant disease

Malignant pericardial effusion

Dysrhythmia with or without congestive heart failure

Marantic endocarditis

Coronary artery disease*

Cardiomyopathy*

    Secondary mural thrombus and embolism

    Congestive heart failure

*Secondary to therapy

pericardial effusion with cardiac tamponade. Another cardiac manifestation of malignancy is marantic endocarditis, which is rarely diagnosed premortem. More recently the relationship of coronary artery disease and cardiomyopathies to cancer therapy have been recognized. The clinical manifestations of cardiac metastases vary from inconsequential arrhythmias, such as sinus tachycardia, to congestive heart failure. Chest pain can develop (1) as a consequence of pericardial involvement, with pericarditis secondary to either tumor implantation or inflammatory response to radiation, or (2) secondary to accelerated coronary arteriosclerosis. Right-heart failure is the usual clinical manifestation of cardiac tamponade secondary to decreased venous return and low-output state. Left-heart failure is the usual clinical manifestation of cardiomyopathy with associated increased pulmonary pressure and congestion.

2.0 Diagnosis of cardiac metastases

The most prevalent clinical manifestation of cardiac metastases is the development of arrhythmias. The type of arrhythmia may vary from ectopic atrial or ventricular beats to persistent and resistant tachycardia of sinus, atrial, nodal, or ventricular origin. Although these arrhythmias are often treated with such standard cardiotropic drugs as procainamide or quinidine, they are notoriously resistant to therapy, and the clinical resistance may be a clue to the etiology of the arrhythmia. The arrhythmia may occur either as a consequence of contiguous pericardial tumor or secondary to hematogenous metastases to the cardiac musculature or conduction system. Endomyocardial metastases are extremely rare.

The majority of the arrhythmic patterns are inconsequential and rarely result in significant morbidity or mortality.

The development of an acute cardiac arrhythmia in patients with neoplastic disease often signals metastases to the heart.

Malignant pericardial effusion is the most important cardiac complication of metastasis. Because of the insidious clinical evolution of effusion, recognition of the life-threatening potential of cardiac tamponade is crucial. The two mechanisms that may result in the production of pericardial effusion are (1) tumor implantation on the serosal surface with secondary exudation of fluid directly from the tumor, or (2) obstruction to the lymphatic flow emanating from the cardiac musculature as a consequence of mediastinal or hilar neoplastic infiltration with transudation of fluid within the pericardial sac. Experimental studies have demonstrated that lymph flow in the heart proceeds from the endocardium to the epicardial surface and, therefore, pericardial effusion represents an accumulation of fluid exuding from the visceral pericardium. Obstruction of the mediastinal lymphatic system draining the heart alone is inadequate to produce pericardial effusion in the experimental model and requires the additional maneuver of ligation of the coronary sinus and the anterior coronary veins. The clinical implication of these data is that mediastinal obstruction with tumor does not produce pericardial effusion in the absence of concomitant neoplastic infiltration of the epicardium and obstruction of the local lymphatic drainage. Furthermore, transthoracic biopsy of the parietal pericardium will generally be inadequate for obtaining tissue, as the neoplastic process must involve the visceral pericardium to generate the secondary clinical effusion.

The diagnostic evaluation of cardiac function in patients with suspected pericardial effusion is supplemented by a number of noninvasive imaging procedures and does not necessarily require cardiac catheterization for confirmation (Table 3.3). The physical examination is the first clue to the presence of pericardial effusion: the classical signs of jugular venous distention and distant heart sounds, and pulsus paradoxicus with or without a pericardial friction rub of two or three components, should prompt additional diagnostic procedures. Actually, it is extremely unusual for the physical examination to reveal the classical signs

in the absence of acute tamponade, and even under those circumstances the physical signs of malignant effusion may be atypical.

The typical clinical signs of pericardial effusion in the absence of acute tamponade are detected by physical examination in a relatively small proportion of patients.

The first clue to the presence of malignant pericardial effusion is often the standard radiograph (Fig. 3.1), which demonstrates a bottle-shaped heart. The heart may be enlarged with or without mediastinal hilar disease, although in patients with bronchogenic carcinoma the primary lesion is commonly identified. In patients with chronic lung disease in whom primary bronchogenic carcinoma is likely to develop, a normal heart size may reflect cardiomegaly because the heart size in patients with chronic lung disease is often relatively diminished. The decrease in cardiac size is related to the expanded chest cavity. An enlarged cardiac border

Table 3.3 Diagnostic evaluation of cardiac function and structure in suspected pericardial effusion

Physical examination

Routine chest radiography and fluoroscopy

Radionuclide scans (including heart; blood pool; combined liver, lung, and heart; and intrapericardial)

Cardiac catheterization

Echocardiography and electrocardiography

Pericardiocentesis

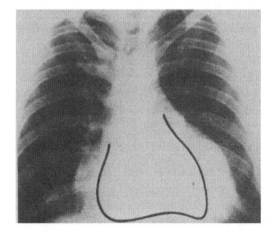

Fig. 3.1 Standard radiograph demonstrating globular bottle-shaped heart. Black line indicates normal heart configuration.

can be confirmed by fluoroscopy, which can demonstrate a poor apical pulsation reflecting encasement of the heart with fluid. Radionuclide scanning of the blood pool is useful in demonstrating pericardial effusion as well, particularly in delineating an expanded space between the heart and the lungs or liver (Fig. 3.2). Other applications of radionuclide scans include direct cardiac scanning, particularly useful in evaluating myocardial injury, and scanning the pericardial space by injection of the radionuclide at the time of pericardiocentesis (Fig. 3.3). The latter technique, however, does not provide important diagnostic or therapeutic information. The electrocardiogram demonstrates diminished voltage; the echocardiogram precisely delineates the posterior heart border as distinguished from the fluid-filled sac and pericardium. The echocardiogram, which is performed at the bedside, is rarely normal in the presence of significant effusion and may be used to quantitate the amount of fluid

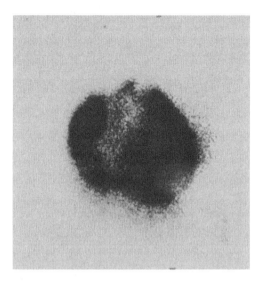

Fig. 3.3 Instillation of technesium (^{99m}Tc) at the time of pericardial fluid aspiration demonstrates an outline of the pericardial space with distribution throughout the pericardial cavity.

present. With manipulation of the patient, ultrasound evaluation may establish the presence of loculation of the fluid. Cardiac catheterization and the use of angiographic dye is rarely necessary except for distinguishing constrictive pericarditis and cardiomyopathy from pericardial effusion.

The concomitant presence of pleural effusion may obscure diagnosis of pericardial effusion by the noninvasive techniques described because of the radiographic obscurity of the cardiac border. In addition, noninvasive diagnostic methods merely delineate the expansion of a cardiac border and do not distinguish pericardial fluid from thickening of the pericardial sac secondary to tumor infiltration or fibrosis.

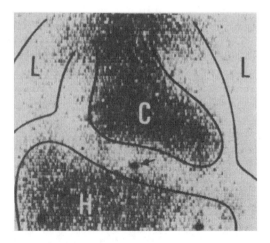

Fig. 3.2 Blood pool scan with simultaneous scan of liver demonstrates a large area between the cardiac blood pool (C) and the liver (H) indicated by the arrow. The space between the cardiac pool and the lungs (L) also reflects pericardial effusion.

Cardiac enlargement in patients with malignancy dictates sonographic evaluation for the presence of pericardial fluid.

Therefore, when pericardial effusion is the suspected diagnosis, a pericardiocentesis is mandatory. Removal of the fluid allows for cytologic analysis, and the simultaneous injection of air after the fluid has been extracted may delineate the tumor implant along the pericardial border (Fig. 3.4)

Table 3.4 Differential diagnosis of the clinical syndrome of pericardial effusion

Intrapericardial hematoma

Myxedema

Constrictive pericarditis

Cardiomyopathy

Pericardiocentesis is an essential diagnostic as well as therapeutic procedure in malignant pericardial effusion.

Patient A, a 64-year-old woman with metastatic malignant melanoma, developed anterior chest pain and on physical examination was found to have a three-component pericardial friction rub without evidence of a paradoxical pulse or cardiomegaly. Within 24 hours the patient developed acute hypotension and a pericardial effusion was identified. Cytologic examination of the fluid demonstrated malignant tumor cells (Fig. 3.5).

The differential diagnosis of pericardial effusion in patients with pericardial disease is relatively concise (Table 3.4). Intrapericardial hematoma may develop as a consequence of cardiac rupture in patients with myocardial infarction. Myxedema with development of a gelatinous fluid in the pericardial sac and a clinical picture of cardiomyopathy has been reported, particularly in patients who have been treated with radiation to the thyroid for Hodgkin's disease. Constrictive pericarditis may develop from radiation to the thoracic structures or in association with prior tuberculosis. It is most important to distinguish the cardiomyopathies from pericardial effusion, since these conditions are increasingly frequent due to the common use of anthracycline antibiotics as cytotoxic chemotherapeutic agents.

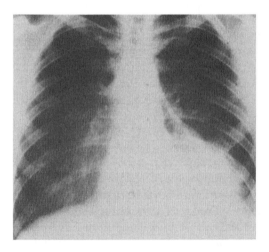

Fig. 3.4 Chest radiograph following removal of pericardial fluid and instillation of 50 cc of air. Note the thickened border of the pericardium reflecting tumor infiltration.

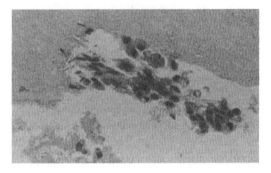

Fig. 3.5 Cytologic preparation of cells obtained from aspiration of pericardial space in a patient with disseminated malignant melanoma and clinical signs of cardiac tamponade.

Additional methods of evaluation for cardiomyopathy include endomyocardial biopsy and cardiac scanning. Biopsy of the endomyocardium may be accomplished with transvenous introduction of a specially designed catheter, which directly samples the endomyocardium of the right ventricle. Specific and characteristic pathologic changes are observed in patients receiving a cardiotoxic dose of Adriamycin. In addition, cardiac scanning has been employed to detect cardiomyopathy, but the scan is rarely positive in the absence of congestive heart failure.

Patient B, a 32-year-old woman with metastatic breast cancer to the pleural and pericardial surfaces, developed acute congestive heart failure after having received a maximum cumulative dose of Adriamycin of 880 mg/M² (normal maximum accumulated dose 450 mg/M²). Endomyocardial biopsy (Fig. 3.6) confirmed the presence of severe cardiomyopathy, and cardiac scanning was characteristic for an active myocardial process (Fig. 3.7).

Echocardiography has been employed in patients with Adriamycin-associated

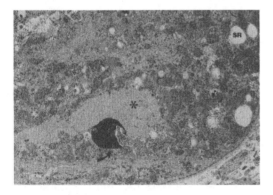

Fig. 3.6 Electron micrograph of an endomyocardial biopsy demonstrating dilatation of the sarcoplasmic reticulum (SR) and lysis of the myofibrils (*). A myeloid body (arrow) is representative of degenerating cellular organelles.

cardiomyopathy to determine the systolic ejection time and the ratio of the presystolic ejection period to the left ventricular ejection time. The usefulness of these procedures is limited because of the inherent variability in the test procedures and the lack of specificity and sensitivity for predicting cardiac toxicity.

3.0 Therapeutic management of malignant pericardial effusion

The therapeutic approach to malignant pericardial effusion (MPE) is contingent on early diagnosis and the need for therapeutic intervention to allay symptoms. The development of acute symptoms of cardiac failure and a low-output state necessitate prompt intervention. In the absence of these critical manifestations of pericardial effusion, however, chest pain or exertional dyspnea may be managed conservatively. In occasional patients the diagnostic pericardiocentesis may provide sufficient therapy without recrudescence or reaccumulation of the fluid.

Patient C, a 55-year-old woman with metastatic breast cancer, presented with acute onset of pericardial effusion and a typical clinical syndrome. She underwent pericardiocentesis at the bedside; cytologic analysis revealed typical Class V malignant cells. The patient subsequently developed metastatic lesions to the bones and was treated with hormonal management. She never developed a recurrence of the pericardial effusion up to the time of her death, 18 months after the initial demonstration of metastases in the pericardium.

Malignant pericardial effusion may be effectively treated for an extended period by a solitary pericardiocentesis.

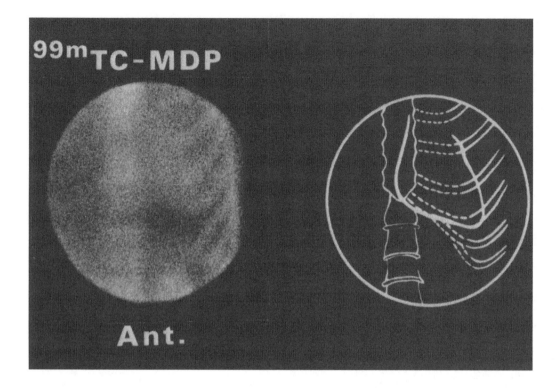

Fig. 3.7 Scintophoto of the anterior thorax demonstrating diffuse myocardial uptake of technesium ^{99m}Tc-methylene diphos- phonate and showing diagrammatic outline.

In addition, pericardial effusion associated with few or no symptoms may persist chronically for months without compromising the patient.

Patient D, a 49-year-old man with metastatic adenocarcinoma of the lung, had progressive dyspnea. Routine evaluation demonstrated a small pericardial effusion. Needle aspiration of the fluid revealed tumor cells, but no specific therapy was employed for the 50-cc effusion. The patient survived an additional six months without cardiac-associated symptomatology (Fig. 3.8).

Patient E, a 64-year-old man with gastric cancer, developed a pleural effusion approximately one year following surgery. Cytologic evaluation of the cells showed them to be consistent with gastric tumor. Because of the concomitant identification of an enlarged cardiac border, the patient had a pericardiocentesis, which demonstrated tumor cells similar to those in the pleural effusion. No specific therapy was administered and the patient survived an additional eight months without cardiac debility.

The basic therapy for malignant pericardial effusion is local regional and the objective is palliation (Table 3.5). Radiation therapy may be employed for patients with radioresponsive tumors, such as breast cancer.

Patient F, a 19-year-old woman, had a clear cell carcinoma of the vagina secondary to fetal diethylstilbestrol exposure

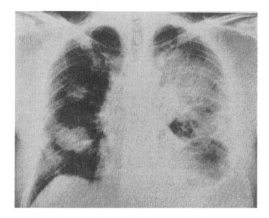

Fig. 3.8 *Chest radiograph (Patient D) demonstrating multiple pulmonary lesions in the pulmonary parenchyma and extending into the left-upper lobe. Following chemotherapy he had regression of the tumor lesions, and the pericardial effusion never recurred.*

and developed a large pelvic mass that responded to radiation therapy. Approximately 12 months later she presented with a malignant pericardial effusion confirmed by pericardiocentesis. The effusion was intermittent, and local radiation therapy provided adequate palliation

Table 3.5 Therapy for malignant pericardial effusion

Pericardiocentesis

Drainage procedure
  Pericardium to pleural space
  Pericardium to peritoneal space

Pericardiectomy (partial)

Talc poudrage

Radiation therapy

Chemotherapy
  Intracavitary
  Systemic

for three months before the patient succumbed to disseminated disease.

In patients with radioresistant tumors or patients who have received radiation therapy previously and for whom the risk of additional radiation to the mediastinum would be significant, a surgical procedure is the treatment of choice.

The therapy for pericardial effusion is pericardiostomy if the tumor is radioresistant or prior radiotherapy precludes further irradiation.

A thoracotomy can be performed to create a "window" in the parietal pericardium to drain fluid into either the pleural space or the abdominal space through a catheter. Because of the tendency for small windows to close over through fibrosis or contiguous tumor growth, a partial pericardectomy involving removal of the pericardium overlying the left ventricle may be necessary. Rarely, surgical introduction of talc to the epicardiac surface may be successful in inducing a vigorous inflammatory response and sealing the potential pericardial space.

Patient G, a 49-year-old woman with acute myelogenous leukemia, was treated with a chemotherapeutic regimen. On the 10th day following initiation of treatment she developed fever, and chest x-ray demonstrated pericardial effusion. Pericardiocentesis revealed a bloody pleural effusion and the systemic circulation platelet count was less than 10,000 cells/mm³. The pericardial fluid reaccumulated within hours, and a thoracotomy provided drainage of fluid into the abdominal cavity without further compromise of cardiac function.

Patient H, a 29-year-old man with Hodgkin's disease, received mantle radiation for Stage IIA disease (mediastinum and cervical nodes). Eighteen months later he developed symptomatic cardiac disease characterized by dypsnea and an enlarged cardiac shadow. At thoracotomy, extensive fibrosis of the pericardium was present without evidence of disease, and a partial left ventricular pericardiectomy was performed.

Chemotherapy in malignant pericardial effusion has a relatively minor role as a therapeutic modality with the exception that in chemotherapy-responsive tumors, such as lymphoma and the hematologic malignancies, chemotherapy may have fewer locally adverse effects and may therefore be superior to radiation.

Patient I, a 45-year-old woman, developed cervical and mediastinal lymphadenopa-thy. Chest x-ray revealed a large pericardial effusion in addition to enlarged mediastinal and hilar lymph nodes, and a left pleural effusion. A node biopsy revealed non-Hodgkin's lymphoma and the patient underwent combination chemotherapy with rapid regression of the pulmonary symptoms (Fig. 3.9). The chest tumor never recurred throughout the course of her disease over the next two years.

In addition to lymphoma, other chemotherapy-responsive tumors include breast and ovarian cancers, testicular and oat cell cancers, and leukemia. In patients previously treated with radiation or those who are not surgical candidates, intracavitary chemotherapy may be employed, although the experience shows that this is more limited than intracavitary therapy

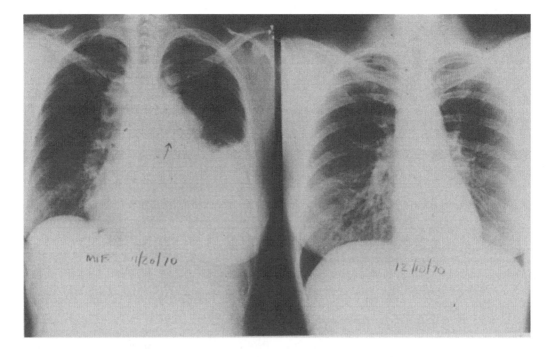

Fig. 3.9 Chest radiographs (Patient I) demonstrating regression of pleural and pericardial effusion as well as mediastinal and hilar adenopathy following combination chemotherapy for non-Hodgkin's lymphoma.

for pleural or peritoneal effusions. Only 5-fluorouracil, gold (^{198}Au), and nitrogen mustard have been employed as local therapy for malignant pericardial effusions.

Patient J, a 49-year-old man with bronchogenic carcinoma, developed an acute pericardial effusion in association with diffuse pulmonary metastases from epidermoid cancer. He underwent a pericardiocentesis, at which time bloody fluid was extracted, and 20 mg of nitrogen mustard was instilled. Within 24 hours an acute cardiac tamponade developed requiring a second pericardiocentesis. Thereafter no recrudescence of fluid occurred.

Frequently with intracavitary therapy, secondary or reactive effusions may develop, and precise cardiac monitoring is essential. In addition, the local irritant effect may result in acute atrial and ventricular arrhythmias. Therefore, intracavitary chemotherapy is not recommended. The primary role of chemotherapy is in the treatment of extracardiac sites of disease.

4.0 Therapy-induced cardiac injury

Cardiac injury as a consequence of either radiation therapy or chemotherapy is a well-recognized complication of antitumor treatment. Radiation therapy in particular routinely affects local tissues by the induction of an obliterative vasculitis with secondary fibrosis and an early acute inflammatory reaction. Radiation-induced pericarditis and myocarditis can be seen routinely in most patients but is rarely of clinical importance. The radiation tolerance level for the heart is 3500 to 4000R beyond which a pericarditis can develop, and therapeutic radiation generally does not exceed these dosages. The increasing

use of combined modality therapy, employing radiation-sensitizing drugs in association with radiation, may potentiate or promote adverse radiation effects on normal tissues.

In addition to radiation-induced pericarditis, premature arteriosclerosis of the coronary arteries and sudden death can occur in young patients with Hodgkin's disease. In these patients the presumption has been that the radiation induces an accelerated atherogenesis, the mechanism for which has not been clearly established.

Chemotherapeutic agents associated with cardiomyopathy include particularly the anthracycline antibiotics, Adriamycin and daunomycin. Cyclophosphamide and 5-fluorouracil have also been associated with carditis, but relatively infrequently, and cyclophosphamide has been implicated only at doses employed primarily for bone marrow transplantation. For the anthracycline antibiotics, cardiomyopathy appears to be dose related and rarely develops at doses less than 550 mg/M^2. Occasionally in patients receiving radiation, cyclophosphamide, or DTIC, the dose at which cardiomyopathy develops may be lower, but the minimal dose at which cardiomyopathy has been observed is 300 mg/M^2. Approximately 30 percent of patients receiving doses beyond 550 mg% develop acute congestive heart failure secondary to cardiomyopathy; approximately 10 percent of these cases are fatal. The therapeutic approach to drug-induced cardiomyopathy is discontinuation of the anthracycline and introduction of digitalis glycosides. In some instances Adriamycin administered at a slower dose rate may permit an increase in the maximum cumulative dose to over 1 gm/M^2. The most important therapeutic principle in drug-induced cardiac injuries, however, is precise monitoring and elimination of the drug at a predetermined drug dose.

5.0 Summary

Cardiac complications of malignancy are uncommon, but with the development of sophisticated chemotherapeutic agents and the combined use of chemotherapy and radiation, the development of therapeutic complications is increasing. The predominant cardiac complication of malignancy is the malignant pericardial effusion, and therapeutic management must establish diagnosis early in order to prevent acute cardiac tamponade. The basic rule of therapeutic management is to employ surgical methods for drainage in radioresistant tumors, and to employ radiation in patients with responsive tumors if the symptoms are not acute or life-threatening. Chemotherapy has a relatively minor role in the overall management of MPE but may be important in patients developing resistant local complications and in patients with chemotherapy-responsive tumors.

References

Biran, S.; Brufman, G.; Klein, E.; and Hochman, A. The management of pericardial effusion in cancer patients. Chest 71:2, 1977.

Charkes, N. D., and Sklaroff, D. M. Radioisotope photoscanning as a diagnostic aid in cardiovascular disease. JAMA 186:920–922, 1963.

Cohen, G. U.; Peery, T. M.; and Evans, J. M. Neoplastic invasion of the heart and pericardium. Ann. Intern. Med. 42:1238–1248, 1955.

Cohn, K. E.; Stewart, J. R.; Fajardo, L. F.; and Hancock, E. W. Heart disease following radiation. Medicine 46:281, 1967.

DeLoach, J. F., and Hagues, J. W. Secondary tumors of the heart and pericardium. Arch. Intern. Med. 91:224–249, 1953.

Groesbeck, H. P., and Cudmore, J. T. P. Intracavitary thiotepa for malignant effusions. Am. Surg. 28:90–95, 1962.

Lokich, J. J. The management of malignant pericardial effusions. JAMA 224:1401–1404, 1973.

McReynolds, R. A.,; Gold, G. L.; and Roberts, W. C. Cornary heart disease after mediastinal irradiation for Hodgkin's disease. Am. J. Med. 60:39, 1976.

Morton, D. L.; Kagan, A. R.; Roberts, W. C.; O'Brien, K. P.; Holmes, E. C.; and Atkins, P. C. Pericardiectomy for radiation induced periocarditis with effusion. Ann. Thorac. Surg. 8:195, 1969.

Nakayama, R. et al. A study of metastatic tumors to the heart, pericardium, and great vessels. Jap. Heart. J. 7:227–234, 1966.

Prichard, R. W. Tumors of the heart: Review of the subject and report of 150 cases. Arch. Pathol. 51:98–128, 1951.

Rose, R. C. Intracavitary radioactive colloidal gold: results in 257 cancer patients. J. Nucl. Med. 3:323–331, 1962.

Scott, R. W., and Garbin, C. F. Tumors of the heart and pericardium. Am. Heart. J. 17:431–436, 1939.

Shuford, W. H. et al. A comparison of carbon dioxide and radiopaque angiocardiographic methods in the diagnosis of pericardial effusion. Radiology 86:1064–1069, 1966.

Silverberg, I. Management of effusions. Oncology 24:25–30, 1969.

Smith, F. E.; Lane, M.; and Hudgkins, P. T. Conservative management of malignant pericardial effusion. Cancer 33:47–57, 1974.

Soulen, R. L.; Lapayowker, M. S.; and Gimenez, T. L. Echocardiography in the diagnosis of pericardial effusion. Radiology 86:1047–1051, 1966.

Suhrland, L. C., and Weisberger, A. S. Intracavitary 5-fluorouracil in malignant effusions. Arch. Intern. Med. 116:431–433, 1965.

Theologides, A. Neoplastic cardiac tamponade. *Seminars in Oncology* vol. 5, no. 2:181–192, 1978.

Weisberger, A. S.; Levine, B.; and Storaalsi, J. P. Use of nitrogen mustard in treatment of serous effusion of neoplastic origin. *JAMA* 159:1704–1707, 1955.

Chapter 4

Central Nervous System Syndromes

J. Lokich

1.0 Background

Metastasis to the central nervous system (CNS) is a common complication of cancer. The incidence of brain metastases appears to be increasing as the longevity of patients with primary and metastatic cancer is prolonged with improved systemic therapies. The increasing frequency of secondary brain lesions in rare and common cancers may be because the brain is a pharmacologic sanctuary from chemotherapeutic agents; therefore, although systemic tumors may be controlled with drug therapy, lesions within the central nervous system are exempt from the drugs' effects. Because of the physiologic inability of most drugs to enter the central nervous system, prophylactic radiation has achieved conspicuous success in the management of some tumors with a tendency to CNS infiltration, such as oat cell carcinoma of the lung.

Metastases to the brain can develop from any primary source. Although uncommon, primary tumors of the ovary, prostate, bladder, and colon can cause brain metastases even in the absence of metastasis to the lungs.

Patient A, a 48-year-old woman, had an endometrioid carcinoma of the ovary removed in 1970. In 1971 she developed metastases to the cervical lymph nodes. The patient was treated with an alkylating drug, and one year later presented with focal weakness of the left side and blurred vision. A lesion in the right posterior hemisphere was demonstrated with standard brain scan; angiogram revealed a solitary mass. At the time of presentation with the CNS lesion, there was no evidence of pelvic recurrence or pulmonary metastasis. Radiation therapy resulted in rapid resolution of the lesion (Fig. 4.1).

Metastatic lesions in the central nervous

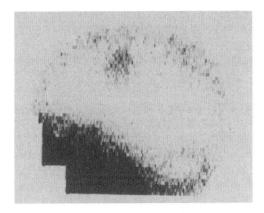 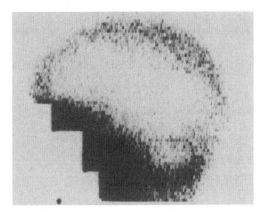

Fig. 4.1 Technesium brain scan demonstrating a solitary lesion in the right hemisphere (A). Following whole-brain radia- *tion therapy the lesion resolved completely (B).*

system do not require the concomitant presence of pulmonary lesions.

CNS metastases are seen in up to 10 percent of cancer patients at postmortem. In collected series, primary tumors of the lung and breast are most commonly associated with cerebral metastases (Table 4.1). Less common tumors, such as melanoma and renal cell cancer, have a relatively high incidence of CNS metastases, and neither are the rare tumors exempt from cerebral invasion.

Tumors metastatic to the central nervous system can be classified on the basis of anatomic distribution (Table 4.2). Intracranial metastases are the most common and result in major clinical symptoms relatively early (see also Chapter 5). Cranial nerve lesions derive from a variety of mechanisms directly and indirectly related to the tumor. The hematologic malignancies, including leukemia and lymphoma, invade the central nervous system by leptomeningeal infiltration rather than by forming mass lesions. Leptomeningeal CNS involvement is most common with lymphomas and leukemia, but breast cancer, lung cancer, and melanoma all may implant on the meningeal surfaces without causing intracerebral mass lesions.

The prognosis for patients with CNS lesions is related in part to the site of the neurologic metastases. For example, survival of patients with leptomeningeal lesions can be measured in weeks, while patients with solitary lesions of the subdural type may survive much longer with appropriate therapeutic management. The primary tumor source and the extra-CNS extent of disease also affect prognosis (Table 4.3). In addition, median survival has been correlated with the anatomic as well as pathologic characteristics of the tumor. The median survival of patients with CNS metastases is comparable to the median survival of patients with the same stage of tumor but without CNS metastases for, at least, some tumors. The longer survival for patients with breast tumors, for example, is related to the greater responsiveness of that tumor to a variety of therapeutic modalities.

Solitary cerebral metastases rarely occur, so that by and large survival data refer to patients with multiple lesions. Isolated or solitary metastases are associated with improved survival, particularly

Table 4.1 Relative frequency of CNS metastases by primary tumor

Primary tumor	Relative incidence of CNS metastases	Frequency of CNS metastases
Lung	25%	
Epidermoid	10%	10%
Adenocarcinoma	3%	10%
Undifferentiated	10%	40%
Breast	20%	15%
Melanoma	5–10%	15%
Kidney	5–10%	10%
Gastrointestinal tract	5–10%	<5%
Stomach		
Colon		
Accessory organs (liver, pancreas)		
Head and neck	<5%	<5%
Genitourinary tract	<5%	<5%
Prostate		
Bladder		
Ovary		
Testicle		
Sarcoma	<5%	5–10%
Hematologic tumors	20%	25–50%
Leukemia		
Lymphoma		
Total	100%	

if the time interval from primary tumor discovery and treatment (disease-free interval) is long and if the extra-CNS metastases are minimal.

More than 75 percent of patients with CNS metastases have multiple rather than single lesions.

2.0 Diagnostic Procedures

The diagnostic approach to CNS syndromes associated with malignancy has become increasingly sophisticated with the development of improved nuclear scanning techniques and computed axial tomography (CAT). Such techniques aid in the detection of CNS lesions and may be important in distinguishing tumors from vascular accidents or congenital from acquired vascular malformations, and further aid in quantifying the size and number of lesions within the cerebral parenchyma. Because patients often present with disorientation and confusion, the initial clinical and laboratory evaluation should exclude metabolic encephalopathy related to electrolyte imbalance and he-

Table 4.2 Anatomic classification of CNS metastatic lesions

A. Intracranial metastases
   1. Intracerebral
   2. Subdural
B. Spinal metastases
   1. Epidural
   2. Intramedullary
C. Cranial nerve lesions
   1. Retinal lesions
   2. Intramedullary lesions of brain stem
   3. Extradural compression (direct)
   4. Nerve compression secondary to increased intracranial pressure
D. Leptomeningeal metastases

patic or renal failure prior to evaluation with expensive and potentially morbid invasive procedures. Conditions that mimic CNS metastasis are diverse, and preliminary screening for such diseases is essential (Table 4.4).

Six diagnostic procedures may be employed to evaluate CNS lesions, but echoencephalography and electroencephalography have only minor diagnostic benefit (Table 4.5). The threshold for detection of brain lesions with these methods is relatively high, and encephalographic interpretations are not specific; nor are they qualitative or quantitative. Arteriography by way of the carotid artery is now largely replaced by the CAT scan, which has been complemented by the recent availability of emission computed tomograms (ECAT) in addition to transmission computed tomograms (TCAT). The brain scan employing technetium radionuclides is a standard screening procedure with the highest detection rate for its simplicity and economic costs. The superiority of CAT scanning over standard scanning relates to the area of the posterior fossa that is often obscured in standard brain scanning. The CAT scan is useful as a more specific quantitative tool than standard brain scanning, and sequential examinations may provide diagnostic information as well as a means of monitoring the effectiveness of treatment.

Patient B, a 69-year-old woman with disseminated endometrial cancer to the liver and lung, presented with a one-day history of falling down, an acute onset of right-side hemiplegia, and right-facial paralysis. Diagnostic evaluation included a brain scan, which demonstrated focal lesions of the right frontal and left parietal areas. The TCAT scan was normal, but ECAT scans on day one and day eight

Table 4.3 Comparative survival with advanced stage disease related to primary tumor type with and without CNS metastases

| Tumor type | Median survival (months) | |
	With CNS metastases	Without CNS metastases
Lung	4–6	6–12
Breast	8–14	8–36
Melanoma	4	4–6
Leukemia	<12	12–24

Table 4.4 Non-CNS causes of cerebral syndromes for patients with malignancy

Systemic sepsis	Hypercalcemia
Diabetes mellitus with acidosis or nonketotic hyperosmolarity	Hyponatremia (e.g., syndrome of inappropriate antidiuretic hormone)
Pulmonary insufficiency with respiratory acidosis or anoxia	Drugs Narcotics
Hepatic precoma with alkalosis	Chemotherapeutic agents (e.g., mithramycin)
Renal failure with metabolic acidosis	Antibiotics (e.g., amphotericin)
Electrolyte imbalance Hypokalemia	Psychotropic drugs

demonstrated an expansion effect suggesting a vascular lesion. The ECAT thus made the distinction between a vascular stroke with localized hemorrhage and tumor (Fig. 4.2).

Computed tomographic techniques may be complementary to standard scans and radiographs in defining an intracerebral process.

Patient C, a 55-year-old woman with known chronic arteriosclerosis, had been treated intermittently for metastatic breast cancer over the previous year. She presented with a short history of progressive disorientation and withdrawal. Standard brain scan demonstrated two lesions thought to be metastatic deposits. CAT scan by the transmission technique, however, demonstrated that both lesions were centrally necrotic and represented old vascular infarcts.

Computed scanning techniques complement standard radionuclide scanning but should not be employed alone.

Table 4.5 Diagnostic procedures in the evaluation of CNS syndromes

Procedure	Application	Complication
Echoencephalography	Nonspecific	None
Electroencephalography	Nonspecific	None
Carotid arteriography	Quantitative	Increased edema
"Standard" Tc^{99m} scan	Qualitative	None
Computed axial tomography	Qualitative and quantitative	None
Emission (ECAT) Transmission (TCAT)		
Lumbar puncture	Meningeal carcinomatosis	Cerebellar herniation

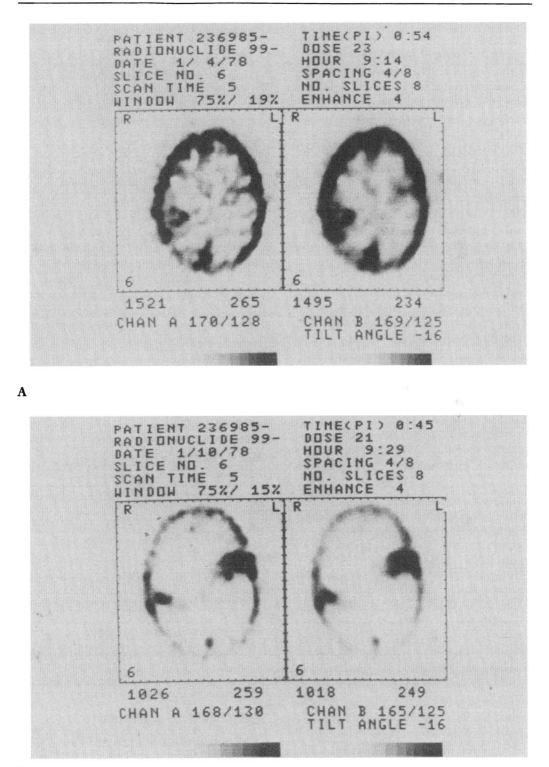

A

B

Fig. 4.2 Sequential ECAT scans at seven-day intervals demonstrating an expansion of the radionuclide uptake in both the right and left hemisphere (A and B).

Lumbar puncture is an important procedure in the evaluation of potential CNS lesions and should be performed to rule out secondary infection for the majority of patients with CNS lesions or syndromes. It is also important to identify leptomeningeal neoplastic disease, which is treated differently from mass lesions within the cerebral parenchyma. Lumbar puncture may be performed with complete safety in the absence of increased intracranial pressure. In the presence of papilledema, lumbar puncture should be undertaken only after administration of corticosteroids to decrease intracerebral edema. Furthermore, a small-gauge needle (not larger than 26-gauge) should be used, and only a small amount of fluid should be withdrawn. With such guidelines the development of "coning" or cerebellar herniation following lumbar puncture should be essentially nil. Cerebral spinal fluid obtained from lumbar puncture should be replaced with Elliot's B solution and in anticipation of the possibility of leptomeningeal tumor, the local instillation of methotrexate at a standard dosage of 12 mg should be available.

In the presence of a known or suspected CNS lesion, lumbar puncture must be preceded by brain scan evaluation and prophylactic corticosteroids.

The diagnostic procedures employed in the evaluation of CNS lesions are intended not only to detect but also to evaluate and quantitate the CNS lesions. For these reasons the use of computed tomography is important; the procedure allows for the delineation of the number and size of the lesions as well as the extent of secondary cerebral edema. In addition, information about the secondary enlargement of the ventricular system may be obtained.

3.0 General principles of therapy

The therapy for CNS metastases can involve neurosurgery, radiotherapy, chemotherapy, or all three modalities. The rationale for employing one or another is based on a number of host as well as tumor factors (Table 4.6). The therapeutic determinants can be separated into local and systemic features of the tumor. The local features include the size, number of lesions (solitary vs. multiple), site of lesions (dominant vs. nondominant hemisphere), and the depth of the lesion. Such factors aid in determining whether a local neurosurgical approach would be indicated. For lesions that are solitary, small, superficial, and in the nondominant hemisphere, surgery is associated with minimal morbidity and contributes substantially to longevity.

Systemic, extra-CNS clinical features reflect the aggressiveness of the tumor and, by and large, determine whether or

Table 4.6 Clinical and tumor-specific features that determine therapy for CNS metastases

---

Local features of the tumor

Size

Number of lesions

Site of lesion

Depth of lesion

Systemic features of the tumor

Biologic activity as measured by growth rate

Disease-free interval

Quantitative extent of tumor

Responsiveness to therapy

---

not surgery should be employed. Biologic tumor activity can be determined by the growth rate, which is ascertained either by the doubling times of pulmonary nodules or by the disease-free interval (the time from the diagnosis of the primary tumor to the development of cerebral metastases). Survival of patients with tumors for which the disease-free interval is less than 12 months generally does not increase with surgery, even in the presence of solitary lesions. The quantitative extent of tumor and distribution within more than one organ, such as lungs, bone or liver, similarly provides an estimate of the aggressiveness of the tumor. Finally, the singular systemic feature of crucial importance in determining local therapy is the responsiveness of that tumor to nonsurgical treatments, including chemotherapy and radiation therapy. For example, tumors that are exquisitely responsive to radiation therapy may be treated in the central nervous system with radiation even when the lesion is solitary, superficial, and surgically accessible.

Neurosurgery. Neurosurgical approaches to CNS metastases include palliative decompression for increased intracranial pressure resistant to osmotherapy, definitive tumor extirpation for solitary lesions, and cerebral spinal fluid shunt for obstructive lesions, especially of the posterior fossa. Neurosurgical excision of CNS lesions is reserved almost exclusively for solitary lesions in accessible sites (i.e., superficial, slowly growing tumors in the nondominant hemisphere that cause minimal systemic burden to the host).

Patient D, a 30-year-old woman, developed acute focal seizures; brain scan demonstrated a left parietal lobe lesion. At the time of presentation, the patient had a mass that had been present for two years in her right leg and had multiple pulmonary lesions evident on chest x-ray. Tumor biopsy revealed an alveolar soft tissue sarcoma; arteriography demonstrated the CNS lesion to be solitary and peripheral but impinging on the dominant hemisphere. In spite of disseminated tumor and the presence of the lesion in the dominant hemisphere, the patient underwent neurosurgical extirpation of the lesion because of the long growth period of the tumor and the insensitivity of the tumor to radiation and other forms of treatment. The patient survived over the next two years without recurrence of CNS symptomatology and in spite of extensive pulmonary metastases (Fig. 4.3).

Neurosurgery is thus reserved for metastatic tumors that are generally resistant to other forms of treatment. Included in this category are renal cell tumors, the sarcomas, and malignant melanoma. CNS lesions are rarely discovered prior to the clinical detection of a primary lesion, and

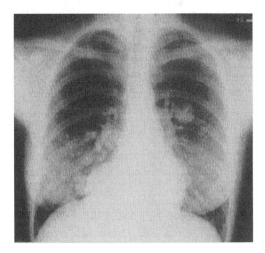

Fig. 4.3 Chest radiograph demonstrating multiple pulmonary metastases (Patient D) who survived brain metastases and progressive pulmonary metastases over two years.

rarer still is a mass lesion in the central nervous system that may be unrelated to the primary systemic cancer. In either case neurosurgery is an appropriate diagnostic and therapeutic procedure.

Patient E, a 55-year-old woman, had primary breast cancer (Stage I) three years previous to admission. She presented with a four-week history of progressive vertigo and tingling of the right hand. A brain scan demonstrated two lesions, one in the left parietal lobe and a second deep in the right parietal lobe. No other evidence of metastasis was established. The patient underwent neurosurgery in spite of multiple lesions, as the diagnosis was unclear. At operation a single meningioma was discovered. The second lesion was not palpable and was presumed to be an artifact.

Neurosurgery for CNS lesions is indicated in superficial and solitary lesions resistant to other forms of treatment (renal cancer, melanoma, sarcoma).

Radiation Therapy. Radiation is the most important treatment for intracerebral metastases because solitary lesions conducive to neurosurgery are uncommon, and chemotherapy is generally ineffective. Radiation therapy induces symptomatic relief for more than 50 percent of patients and is most effective for those tumors that are radioresponsive (i.e., ovarian and breast cancers).

Patient F, a 45-year-old woman, presented with progressive headache and disorientation. She had had a carcinoma of the breast removed two years previously. Physical examination revealed papilledema, and the patient was initiated on corticosteroids with rapid relief of her headache. A brain scan demonstrated a solitary parietal lobe lesion and the patient received radiation therapy to a dose of 3000 rad, whole brain, and a cone down to a boost of 1000 rad (Fig. 4.4). The patient remained alive and well for 12 months, during which time there was no exacerbation or recurrence of the brain lesion.

In spite of the solitary lesion, the therapeutic approach for this patient involved radiation therapy because of the exquisite sensitivity of the tumor to radiation.

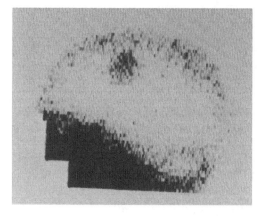 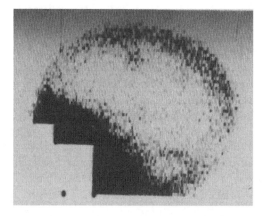

Fig. 4.4 Technesium brain scan demonstrating solitary parietal lobe metastasis (Patient F) (A) which receded in follow-up scan following radiation therapy (B).

Radiation therapy is the treatment of choice for patients with multiple or deep lesions and in those with radioresponsive tumors.

Principles of radiation therapy for CNS lesions are outlined in Table 4.7. Uniformly, patients are pretreated with corticosteroids to obviate the development of cerebral edema in response to radiation. In some reported series the combined application of radiation and corticosteroids has yielded increased survival over radiation therapy alone. Dose-fraction schemes are quite variable and are conditioned primarily by the habit of the radiation therapist. Single-dose radiation therapy has been employed to increase tumor cell kill, but the superiority of single-dose over dose-fraction schemes over short or protracted periods has not been established. Because of the frequency of multiple lesions in spite of clinical detection of only single sites, whole-brain radiation is commonly used for treatment with a cone down to the site of symptomatic metastases.

Chemotherapy. The use of chemotherapy for metastatic cancer in the central nervous system has not been encouraging, possibly because of the inability of most drugs to cross the blood-brain barrier. A number of agents have, however, been recently developed that have lipid solubility and therefore the potential for passage across the blood-brain barrier. These drugs have demonstrated activity predominantly in primary rather than metastatic brain tumors (Table 4.8). The podophyllotoxins are experimental drugs, but the nitrosoureas, particulary the intravenous preparation BCNU (carmustine) and the oral capsule CCNU (lomustine) are commercially available. Both nitrosoureas have been employed with limited success in metastatic tumors. The limited success is related to the relatively restricted spectrum of tumors against which these drugs have specific activity.

Table 4.7 Principles of radiation therapy of CNS lesions

1. Pretreatment with corticosteroids

2. Dose-fraction schemes
   Low dose (<150rad/d) over
     protracted period
   Moderate dose (200–400rad/d) over
     5 to 10 days
   High dose (600–1000rad) in a single
     dose

3. Field at risk (whole brain) with cone
   down to lesion

4. Maximum whole brain dose of 4500rad

Table 4.8 Chemotherapeutic agents for the treatment of CNS metastases

Systemic administration

Active drugs with known access to the
  central nervous system
  Nitrosoureas
  Podophyllotoxins

Variably active drugs, unknown transport
  to the central nervous system
  Mithramycin
  Vincristine

Inactive drugs, no known transport to
  the central nervous system
  Methotrexate
  5-Fluorouracil
  Cyclophosphamide
  Unevaluated drugs

Intrathecal administration
  Methotrexate
  Cytosine arabinoside
  Thiotepa
  Mitomycin C
  Cyclophosphamide

Some drugs, including mithramycin and vincristine, have been known to cause secondary effects in the central nervous system and have therefore been used to treat CNS metastases. Because of the limited activity of these agents, their effect on CNS metastases has been only minimal. At least three drugs are definitely inactive in spite of their systemic activity, because of the lack of transport across the blood-brain barrier (methotrexate, 5-fluorouracil, and cyclophosphamide).

Intrathecal administration of drugs is generally reserved for leptomeningeal carcinomatosis, and may be administered by frequent lumbar puncture or by an Ommaya reservoir into the intraventricular system to bathe the cerebral lesion. The drugs most commonly introduced by the intrathecal route are methotrexate, cytosine arabinoside, and thiotepa. Although these drugs are effective against CNS lymphomas and leukemias, their activity in CNS solid tumors has been marginal.

4.0 The use of corticosteroids and osmotherapy

Corticosteroids are a major asset in interrupting the acute clinical effects of CNS metastases. Corticosteroid therapy will produce relief of neurologic symptoms in 60 to 75 percent of patients with CNS metastases. Response to corticosteroid therapy is often a good prognostic indicator, and although not definitively established, it is also a possible gauge of the therapeutic benefit to be expected from radiation. The mechanism of the corticosteroid effect has been attributed to a reduction in cerebral edema related to secondary alterations in blood flow. In general, the immediate value of corticosteroids is most evident in patients with severe or overwhelming neurologic symptoms.

Clinical response to corticosteroids is possibly predictive of the patient's response to radiation therapy.

The use of corticosteroids should be precisely regulated to preclude the profound secondary effects that can occur with prolonged steroid use. In addition, prophylactic use of steroids in conjunction with radiation therapy should be carefully monitored to taper corticosteroids early and thereby preclude the development of adverse secondary effects. In patients with life-threatening CNS effects, the standard approach has been to introduce dexamethasone in dosages up to 16 mg per day, in divided doses. This is done despite the fact that dexamethasone has a long half-life. Some evidence indicates that increasing the dose beyond this level may be effective when a patient becomes resistant at 16 mg, and occasionally as much as 64 mg has been employed to control CNS symptoms. In general, corticosteroids are used as a protective mechanism and should be withdrawn or at least tapered as soon as the local therapy has been introduced. A schematic approach to the tapering of steroids following the initial introduction is illustrated in Fig. 4.5. The plan involves a dose decrease of 50 percent at seven-day intervals following introduction of steroids so that by week seven only maintenance corticosteroids are employed. Antacids should be used in conjunction with steroid therapy, particularly because of the potential complication of Cushing's ulcers of the stomach and steroid ulcers.

Osmotherapy is the use of dehydrating agents to interrupt cerebral edema. These drugs produce dramatic results in patients developing acute cerebral herniation. Mannitol is administered intravenously while the urinary output is monitored precisely, because the osmotic diuretic effect may result in peripheral as well as

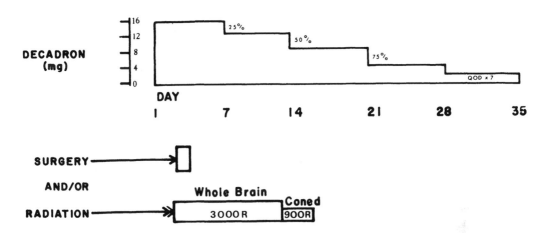

Fig. 4.5 Dexamethasone (Decadron) is administered at a dosage of 16 mg distributed throughout the day, one day prior to surgery or initiation of radiation therapy. Subsequently, at seven-day intervals a 25 percent decrement dose is achieved so that by day 35 corticosteriod may be withdrawn completely with impunity.

cerebral dehydration. More recently, glycerol has been used because it can be administered orally and it produces a modified diuresis with less likelihood of electrolyte imbalance. Many complications have been associated wtih glycerol therapy, including neurologic rebound, nausea and vomiting, and hyperosmolality with coma, but precise monitoring will prevent these complications. Modulation and combination of osmotherapeutic drugs can minimize the adverse effects of one or another of the agents; for example, the dose of corticosteroids can be reduced to levels unassociated with side effects.

5.0 General clinical features of CNS lesions

The clinical syndromes associated with CNS metastases may be separated into three basic categories (Table 4.9). Each symptom may occur alone or in combination with another. Confusion or disorientation is observed as a solitary manifestation or a primary complaint of the patient or family in 30 percent of cases; it is demonstrated, however, by detailed examination of cognitive function in an additional 40 percent of patients. The headache syndrome predominates in 25 percent of patients and is often characteristic in that the headache appears upon awakening in the morning and recedes within a short time only to return on each subsequent morning. The headache is often localized to the apex of the scalp and is persistent rather than throbbing in character. It may be resistant or occasionally sensitive to analgesic therapy. An additional 25 percent of patients with CNS metastases will have nonspecific headache of minor importance. Almost 50 percent of all patients with CNS metastases develop a focal neurologic syndrome. These patients experience either seizure activity or focal neurologic signs and symptoms such as motor loss, sensory loss, or ataxia. On examination, an additional 30 percent will have focal motor weakness, so that neurologic signs actually occur in as many as 75 percent of the patients examined.

Table 4.9 Clinical features of CNS metastases

	Solitary	Combined
Confusion syndrome	30%	70%
Headache syndrome	25%	50%
Focal neurologic signs	45%	75%
Seizure activity	15%	
Hemiparesis; sensory loss		
or ataxia	30%	
Total	100%	

Three neurologic syndromes are characteristic of CNS metastases: confusion, headache, and focal neurologic signs.

One important aspect of the clinical examination of patients with potential CNS metastases is the demonstration of papilledema. Papilledema may in fact be observed in only 25 percent of patients and may be subtle even in those patients. The papilledema may be only unilateral, and the absence of venous pulsations, which has traditionally been the first sign of increased intracranial pressure, is not consistently observed. Furthermore, confusing eyeground changes such as hypertensive or diabetic retinopathy may impede the identification of papilledema.

The clinically distinct syndromes associated with cerebral metastases are largely related to the pattern and anatomic site of tumor implantation. Six categories of CNS lesions can be identified on the basis of anatomic distribution (Table 4.10). Each of the six presents with a distinctive clinical syndrome, and each requires specific therapeutic management.

6.0 Lesions of the cerebral hemispheres

The cerebral hemispheres are the most common sites of metastasis to the central nervous system. A mass in the cerebral hemisphere may be clinically manifested as a nonspecific state of confusion or disorientation without a localizing neurologic component. Commonly associated with a state of confusion are headache and blurred vision secondary to increased intracranial pressure and papilledema.

Patient G, a 64-year-old man, presented with a solitary oat cell carcinoma in the left lung, which was resected. Because of the presence of mediastinal nodes, the patient received postoperative radiation therapy. Five months later he developed nodules in the skin incision. During physical examination, he was extremely agitated and had difficulty with time orientation. The family indicated that he was extremely irritable at home and was intermittently somnolent. A superficial screening for potential metabolic causes of encephalopathy revealed a serum sodium of 127 mEq/liter with a disparity in the serum and urine osmolalities suggesting the syndrome of inappropriate antidiuretic hormone. In spite of this abnormality, which could account for a confused state, the patient had a brain scan, which demonstrated multiple cerebral metastases in the frontal and parietal lobes. Steroid therapy and subsequent radiation caused a resolution of the confused state

Table 4.10 Potential distribution of
lesions within the central nervous system

Cerebral hemisphere
    Frontal
    Parietal
    Temporal-occipital

Cranial nerves

Posterior fossa (cerebellum)

Brain stem

Retina

Leptomeninges

but his agitation and increased anxiety
persisted.

The patient demonstrated a relatively
small tumor burden, having had only cutaneous nodules within the incision.
Therefore, pursuing a diagnosis and therapy for a CNS lesion was warranted. The
clinical confusion created by the syndrome of inappropriate antidiuretic hormone, concomitant with a brain lesion, is
common in patients with oat cell
carcinoma.

    A second syndrome associated with
cerebral lesions is motor seizures or paresis, which is associated with lesions
along the motor strip in the frontal parietal
area. Seizures are almost never associated
with simple increased intracranial pressure, so that the development of Jacksonian seizures and Todd's postictal paralysis
are helpful in localizing lesions.

**Seizures secondary to CNS metastases
may or may not be associated with increased intracranial pressure.**

---

*Patient H, a 45-year-old woman, had a
primary resection for a Stage II carcinoma
of the lung. Eight months following sur-*

*gery, she developed a seizure that was
associated with an aura of dysethesia in
the left hand; subsequently Jacksonian
seizure activity that proceeded from the
left hand to the arm and shoulder, and
finally generalized seizure activity. A
brain scan demonstrated a solitary lesion
in the right hemisphere overlying the
motor cortex. There was no evidence of
systemic metastases but, because of the
short disease-free interval, the patient was
treated with a whole-brain radiation therapy, and corticosteroids were administered in the pattern previously described.
Five months after the initial episode the
patient remained well.*

In the presence of seizure activity the
adjuvant use of dyphenyl hydantoin or
other anticonvulsant therapy is essential
with radiation therapy, but anticonvul-
sants should not be continued beyond the
time when tumor control is clearly established unless seizure activity persists.

*Patient I, a 64-year-old woman with meta-
static breast cancer to the bones, lungs
and liver, developed acute episodes of
"loss of reality contact" and dysphasia
for specific words. A brain scan demonstrated at least four lesions and the patient
was placed on steroids and dyphenyl
hydantoin after which radiation therapy
was directed to the central nervous system. Steroid withdrawal was accomplished by the completion of radiation, at
which time the patient developed a diffuse drug rash. Seizure activity was suppressed by the alternative, phenobarbital.*

    Sensory, temporal, and occipital lobe
seizures are unusual manifestations of
metastatic disease to the central nervous
system. More commonly, lesions in the
temporal or occipital lobes are found
incidentally on routine brain scanning in
patients with clinical indications of CNS
tumors at other sites.

7.0 Lesions of the cranial nerves

Solitary cranial nerve palsies are uncommon manifestiations of CNS metastases. Of the several cranial nerve abnormalities, oculomotor palsies occur most often. Increased intracranial pressure may result in a VIth nerve palsy of no localizing value related to the length of the VIth nerve in its transit from the brain stem through the cranial vault to the ocular muscles, making it more susceptible to compression. Thus, a VIth nerve palsy cannot pinpoint the site of metastasis; the lesion may occur anywhere in the central nervous system. Third nerve palsy is also a common manifestation of CNS metastases; the mechanism is generally related to direct tumor compression of the brain stem or along the path to the oculomotor muscles. The VIth and IIIrd cranial nerves are also those most commonly involved as a consequence of metabolic disease (e.g., diabetes) or other nonneoplastic diseases of the central nervous system.

Patient J, a 45-year-old woman with known breast cancer and multiple bone metastases, developed diplopia and decreasing visual acuity gradually over seven days. She also had insulin-dependent diabetes, which became increasingly difficult to control with progression of the tumor. Neurologic examination was completely normal except for the right IIIrd cranial nerve palsy. Brain scan and EEG were essentially normal. The palsy disappeared slowly over the ensuing four months.

Another type of cranial nerve involvement in patients with malignancy is direct tumor invasion of the nerves from tumors of the oral cavity. The tumor may spread to the base of the skull or invade the retromolar triangle with secondary growth along the cranial nerve pathway. Nasopharyngeal tumors commonly invade locally into the cranial vault and may

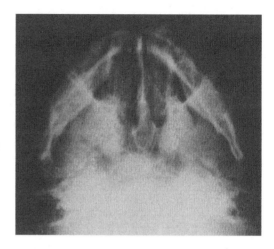

Fig. 4.6 Radiograph of the base of the skull demonstrating expansion of the foramen ovale.

cause secondary meningitis in addition to cranial nerve involvement.

Patient K, a 62-year-old man, had a recurrent nasopharyngeal carcinoma treated with local radiation over four years. He presented in coma with fever and was found to have a peripheral VIIth nerve palsy bilaterally with extensive retropharyngeal tumor extension. Tomography demonstrated bone erosion at the skull base (Fig. 4.6). Lumbar puncture revealed a purulent cerebrospinal fluid that grew pneumococcal pneumonia in culture.

Involvement of the VIIIth through XIIth cranial nerves is distinctly unusual and is generally related to a process in the brain stem. Occasionally, extensive radiation therapy of the oral cavity may result in peripheral neuronal degeneration and nerve paralysis.

8.0 Lesions of the retina

The retina is the Ist cranial nerve and is distinct from the other 11 because it is available for direct visual inspection; thus, visualization of tumor implants in a neural structure is possible. In spite of the complex vascular network that pervades the retinal structures, however, it is distinctly uncommon for retinal lesions to develop in patients with malignancy. The most common tumor to metastasize to the retina is breast cancer. Of the hematologic malignancies, leukemia is by far the most common to affect the retina. Primary tumors of the ophthalmic structures are retinoblastoma and melanoma of the choroid plexus. Neither of these primary tumors will be considered in this discussion.

Two distinctive lesions and pathophysiologic mechanisms are involved in leukemic infiltration of the retina. The most common clinical manifestation is a decrease in visual acuity related to hemorrhage, which develops following vascular leukostasis within the arterial supply to the retina.

Patient L, a 40-year-old man with diabetes mellitus, had been treated for three years with oral hypoglycemic agents. He noted decreasing visual acuity over two months and was evaluated for laser beam therapy. Ophthalmic examination revealed multiple areas of hemorrhage without evidence of diabetic retinopathy or microaneurysm formation (Fig. 4.7). A routine complete blood count revealed a white blood cell count of 370,000 cells/mm³. Further laboratory examination and cytogenetic analysis confirmed chronic myelogenous leukemia. The patient was treated with radiation therapy to the retina and systemic chemotherapy using busulfan; a gradual decrease in the peripheral white blood count occurred over the next three weeks. His visual acuity improved moderately, from 20/400 to 20/200, but a persistent abnormality in visual acuity was documented at 10 weeks, when the patient was in clinical remission from the leukemia.

Leukostasis is a common phenomenon in patients with leukemia with extremely elevated white blood counts. In this patient with chronic myelogenous leukemia, the treatment of the central nervous system by whole-brain radiation or cranial-spinal radiation, in addition to radiation directed at the retina, is not indicated. In contrast to the treatment for acute leukemic ophthalmic infiltration, the inability to correct visual acuity completely with radiation is related to the slow pro-

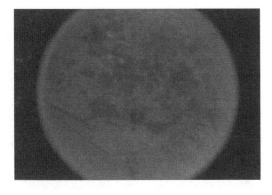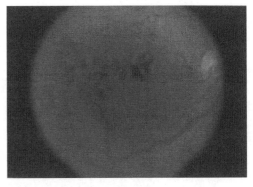

Fig. 4.7 Fundoscopic view (Patient L) demonstrating multiple hemorrhages without evidence of microaneurysm (A), which receded with leukemia-specific therapy (B).

cess of resorption of the secondary hemorrhage, which contributes in a major way to decreased acuity.

Retinal lesions associated with leukemia may be treated with local radiation and systemic chemotherapy.

Acute leukemia, and particularly acute lymphocytic leukemia in children, is commonly associated with CNS invasion. For this reason, prophylactic therapy is routinely employed for patients entering complete remission. Patients with lymphocytic leukemia who develop acute ophthalmic lesions often have disease recurrence in the bone marrow and central nervous system. For these patients, both systemic and local therapies are indicated.

Patient M, a 24-year-old man, presented with a white blood count of 284,000 cells/mm³, which were predominantly lymphoblasts, and fever. Remission was promptly induced with a standard chemotherapeutic regimen, but relapse with multiple cutaneous lesions occurred at four weeks. In addition, a hypopyon and decreased visual acuity developed. Multiple leukemic infiltrates were noted on the retina (Fig. 4.8). The patient was treated with *local radiation to the whole brain and retina as well as systemic chemotherapy.*

Retinal lesions from hematogenous metastases of solid tumors are uncommon. The lesions are observed most commonly in the peripheral margins of the retina and appear as simple raised areas with central umbilication and pallor surrounded by erythema (Fig. 4.9). Because breast tumors are radioresponsive, this is the treatment of choice.

Other, less common lesions in the retina may develop as a consequence of secondary or associated systemic diseases, such as hypertension or diabetes, or in association with secondary infection. In addition, coagulation abnormalities may result in arterial or central vein thrombosis. Abnormalities of the retinal vasculature are also observed in patients with malignant disease of the lymphoproliferative system and dysproteinemias. Retinal lesions due to these diseases may be treated by plasmaphoresis or leukophoresis.

9.0 Lesions of the posterior fossa and brain stem

The posterior fossa includes the cerebellum and the brain stem from the medulla

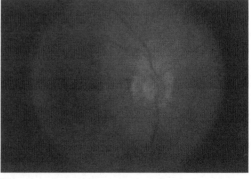

A

Fig. 4.8 Fundoscopic image (Patient M) demonstrating multiple leukemic infiltrates with associated hemorrhage and **B**

appearance of papilledema (A); improved within five days of chemotherapy (B).

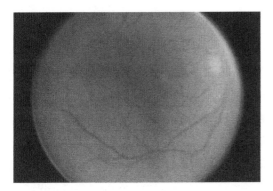

Fig. 4.9 Fundoscopic view of bulging retina lateral inferior margin secondary to metastatic tumor implant from breast carcinoma.

to the thalamus. Malignant lesions in these areas are distinctly uncommon, and diagnosis of disease in this area is particularly difficult. It is, for example, difficult to evaluate brain scans of an area in which vascular structures, including the draining venous sinuses, abound. In addition, computed tomographic evaluation must use special techniques to focus on the posterior fossa.

The clinical manifestations of posterior fossa and brain stem lesions are often subtle. Increased intracranial pressure from obstruction of the foramina prevents egress of fluid from the ventricular system and leads to headache and ocular motor palsies. Symptoms of specific cerebellar dysfunction may develop as well. The therapies are similar to those directed at cerebral lesions.

Patient N, a 26-year-old woman, two weeks postpartum, was discovered to have a choriocarcinoma with extensive metastasis to the lungs and liver. Systemic chemotherapy was administered. Ten days after initiation of treatment, she complained of headache and nausea and was bedridden. Neurologic examination demonstrated nystagmus on right lateral gaze and bilateral papilledema. CAT scan

revealed a lesion of the left hemisphere of the cerebellum (Fig. 4.10). Intrathecal methotrexate was administered as well as radiation to the whole brain and left cerebellar hemisphere. The patient's symptoms completely resolved, although the lesion persisted on CAT scan four months following therapy.

Ataxia and cerebellar dysfunction are also common manifestations of posterior fossa involvement. The cerebellar degeneration associated with malignancy and the cerebellar abnormalities associated with other diseases such as alcoholism may be clinically confusing.

Patient O, a 59-year-old man, was a chronic smoker and alcohol abuser. He developed a pulmonary lesion which, on biopsy, was found to be small cell carcinoma of the lung. The patient received local radiation therapy and was well for eight months when he began falling to the right. A standard brain scan was normal; neurologic examination revealed subtle cerebellar signs. A CAT scan demon-

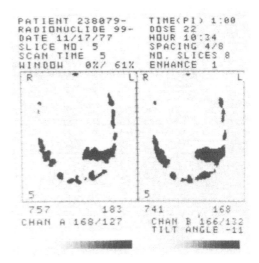

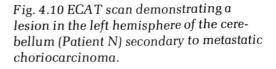

Fig. 4.10 ECAT scan demonstrating a lesion in the left hemisphere of the cerebellum (Patient N) secondary to metastatic choriocarcinoma.

strated a large left hemisphere lesion of the cerebellum with involvement of the vermis (Fig. 4.11). Radiation therapy resulted in partial clearing of the symptoms.

Posterior fossa lesions are associated with headache and clinical signs of cerebellar dysfunction.

Intramedullary tumor involvement is unusual in the brain stem, but occurs particularly with carcinoma of the breast. These rare lesions are important because radiation therapy to the base of the brain is extremely effective. Manifestations of brain stem lesions are most commonly reflected in cranial nerve abnormalities, such as parasthesias along the facial nerve,

in the jaw, or periorally. Brain stem invasion along the thalamus into the pituitary may result in hormonal syndromes as well.

10.0 Lesions of the leptomeninges

Carcinomatous meningitis, or metastasis to the meninges, is an uncommon complication of the central nervous system. Although most common in leukemia and lymphoma, carcinomatous meningitis does occur, although rarely, in patients with lung cancer, breast cancer, and malignant melanoma. The prognosis is dismal, with median survival measured in weeks from time of diagnosis of meningeal involvement.

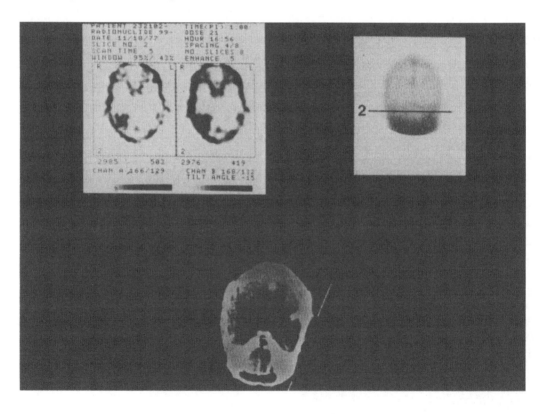

Fig. 4.11 Three scan studies (Patient O) demonstrating a left cerebellar lobe lesion by ECAT for which the standard brain scan (B) and TCAT scan (C) were normal.

Patients with leptomeningeal lesions generally present with seizures and coma, in contrast to patients with mass lesions, who often manifest disorientation and focal neurologic signs. Because of nerve entrapment in carcinomatous meningitis, cranial nerve abnormalities are also common. Leptomeningeal disease from solid tumors develops by contiguous bone involvement in the vertebral column and does not respond effectively to therapy. In contrast, leptomeningeal lesions from leukemia implant hematogenously and are exquisitely sensitve to therapy. Leukemic meningeal disease is often occult or subclinical and may be discovered only by routine lumbar puncture in the course of evaluation for treatment. The laboratory evaluation of the cerebrospinal fluid often reveals, in addition to the leukemic cells, a decreased glucose content. This depletion of cerebrospinal fluid glucose is related to the high metabolic rate of the implanted tumor cells. The cells themselves are often difficult to distinguish from lymphocytes, but in cytocentrifuge and millipore filter preparations the histologic features of the cells can be observed.

Meningeal carcinoma is often manifested by seizures and obtundation, and may mimic infectious meningitis.

Patient P, a 42-year-old woman with breast cancer diagnosed two months prior to admission, was admitted with progressive coma. She had no focal neurologic signs, but on lumbar puncture was found to have increased protein and decreased glucose in the cerebrospinal fluid. Cytocentrifugal analysis revealed tumor cells without an inflammatory component (Fig. 4.12). The patient was treated with intrathecal methotrexate followed by radiation to the cranial-spinal axis. She died two and one-half weeks following initiation of treatment.

In spite of vigorous attempts at therapy, including intrathecal drugs, the prognosis for leptomeningeal invasion by tumor is dismal. The recent development and general application of the Ommaya reservoir for continuous perfusion of the central nervous system may be superior to intrathecal administration because with increased intracranial pressure it is unlikely that a lumbar puncture would allow a drug access to the cerebral hemisphere.

11.0 Remote effects of cancer

In addition to the neurologic syndromes associated with metastasis and impingement on central and peripheral neurologic structures, remote neurologic effects occur as a consequence of systemic cancer that is not metastatic to the brain or spinal cord. These effects (Table 4.11) are extremely rare, but they raise difficult diagnostic issues. Because the syndromes are uncommonly reversible, even when the tumor can be controlled, the mechanism of the neurologic effects is not clear. It is possible that remote neurologic effects are due to nutrituional losses as

Table 4.11 Neurologic effects in patients with non-CNS metastasis

---

Central nervous system
    Multifocal leukoencephalopathy
    Subacute cerebellar degeneration
      (polioencephalopathy)

Spinal cord syndromes
    Amyotrophic lateral sclerosis

Neuropathy

Myopathy

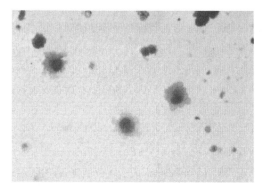 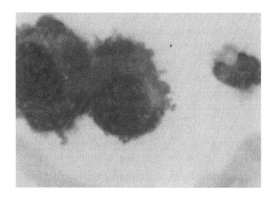

Fig. 4.12 Cytocentrifuge specimen from cerebral spinal fluid (Patient P) demonstrating large reticulum-like cells with features of anaplastic malignancy (A–low power, B–high power).

a consequence of cancer cachexia, but the literature is controversial and at the very least inconsistent.

The tumors most commonly associated with remote neurologic effects are lung and breast cancers. Although any tumor may occur with distant neurologic manifestations, only oat cell carcinoma of the lung has been reported to be associated with the myasthenic syndrome.

Central nervous system lesions include multifocal leukoencephalopathy (MFL) and a polioencephalopathy or ganglion dropout disease involving predominantly the cerebellum or the brain stem. Multifocal leukoencephalopathy has been associated with the papova virus and is clinically manifested as a rapidly progressing dementia with focal neurologic signs but without seizures. Subacute cerebellar degeneration has been associated with Hodgkin's disease and the lymphomas as well as lung and ovarian cancers. This syndrome also evolves very rapidly with predominantly cerebellar signs. Amyotrophic lateral sclerosis (ALS) has been associated with cancer and may be an independent disease rather than a remote effect of the tumor. Neuropathies associated with cancer vary from purely sensory to the combined sensory-motor neuropathies and are distinct from the myasthenia typical of oat cell carcinoma. Myasthenia is discussed in Chapter 19.

12.0 Summary

Metastatic lesions to the central nervous system are common and are occurring even more frequently as a result of extended survivals of patients with cancer. Diagnosis of these lesions is becoming increasingly sophisticated with the development of computed tomography for evaluation of the central nervous system. Therapies have also proved increasingly successful and can effectively reverse CNS symptoms caused by tumors, such as ovarian and breast cancers and the leukemias and lymphomas, that are known to be radioresponsive or sensitive to chemotherapy. Malignant melanoma, lung cancer, and sarcoma continue to be resistant tumors, although radiation is effective in a small proportion of patients with CNS lesions. For the occasional patient with a solitary metastasis, neurosurgery should be considered, particularly in the context of limited or slowly growing disease.

References

Bedikian, A. Y.; Valdivieso, M.; and Withers, H. R. *Glycerol (G), a new alternative to dexamethasone (d) in patients receiving brain irradiation (XRT).* Houston: The University of Texas System Cancer Center, M.D. Anderson Hospital and Tumor Institute, 1977.

Deely, T. J., and Edwards, J. M. R. Radiotherapy in the mangement of cerebral secondaries from bronchial carcinoma. *Lancet* 1209–1212, 8 June 1968.

Deutsch, M. ; Parsons, J.; and Mercado, R. Radiotherapy for intracranial metastases. *Cancer* 24:1607–1611, 1974.

Fewer, D.; Wilson, C. B.; and Boldrey, E. B. et al. The chemotherapy of brain tumors: clinical experience with carmustine (BCNU) and vincristine. *JAMA* 222:549–552, 1972.

Galluzzi, S., and Payne, P. M. Brain metastases from primary bronchial carcinoma: a statistical study of 741 necropsies. *Br. J. Cancer* 10:408–414, 1956.

Gawler, J.; Bull, J. W. D.; Du Boulay, G. H.; and Marshall, J. Computer-assisted tomography (EMI scanner): its place in investigation of suspected intracranial tumours. *Lancet* 419–424, 1974.

Hazra, T.; Mullins, G. M.; and Lott, S. Management of cerebral metastasis from bronchogenic carcinoma. *Johns Hopkins Med. J.* 130:377–383, 1972.

Hildebrand, J. *Lesions of the nervous system in cancer patients.* European organization for research on Treatment of Cancer Monograph Series. New York: Raven Press, 1978.

Horton, J.; Baxter, D. H.; Olson, K. B., and the Eastern Cooperative Oncology Groups. The management of metastases to the brain by irradiation and corticosteroids. *Am. J. Roentgenography* 111:335–336, 1971.

MacGee, E. E. Surgical treatment of cerebral metastases from lung cancer: the effect on quality and duration of survival. *J. Neurosurg.* 24:416–420, 1971.

Marty, R., and Cain, M. L. Effects of corticosteriod (dexamethasone) administration on the brain scan. *Radiology* 107:117–121, 1972.

Newman, S. J., and Hansen, H. H. Frequency, diagnosis and treatment of brain metastases in 247 consecutive patients with bronchogenic carcinoma. *Cancer* 33:492–496, 1974.

Nisce, I. Z.; Hilaris, B. S.; and Chu, F. C. H. A review of experience with irradiation of brain metastasis. *Am. J. Roentgenography* 111:329–333, 1971.

Order, S.; Hellman, S.; and van Essen, C. et al. Improvement in quality of survival following whole brain irradiation for brain metastases. *Radiology* 91:149–153, 1968.

Perese, D. M. Prognosis in metastatic tumors of the brain and the skull: an analysis of 16 operative and 162 autopsied cases. *Cancer* 12:609–613, 1959.

Posner, J. B. Management of central nervous system metastases. *Seminars in Oncology* 4(1):81–91, 1977.

Renaudin, J., and Fewer, D. et al. Dose dependency of decadron in patients with partially excised brain tumors. *J. Neurosurg.* 29:302–305, 1973.

Stier, M. Metastatic tumors of the brain. *Acta. Neurol. Scand.* 41:262–278, 1965.

Wilson, W. L., and de la Garza, J. G. Systemic chemotherapy for CNS metastases of solid tumors. *Arch. Intern. Med.* 115:710–713, 1965.

Yap, H. W. et al. Meningeal carcinomatosis in breast cancer. *Cancer* 42:283–286, 1978.

Chapter 5

Spinal Cord Compression
J. Lokich

1.0 Background

Spinal cord compression is one of the most devastating complications of cancer. Palliation for this complication is of paramount importance, for survival is frequently prolonged, and the paralytic effects of cord compression can be an overwhelming ordeal for both the patient and the family. Nursing care, physical therapy, rehabilitation, and psychosocial attention are all part of the expanded health care needs of patients with residual neurologic damage from spinal cord compression. The two critical determinants of successful palliation are early clinical recognition of the syndrome and maximum combined modality therapy once the syndrome is diagnosed.

The most common tumors with which spinal cord compression develops are lung and breast cancers, because of the high general incidence of these tumors. Prostate cancer, renal cell carcinoma, lymphoma, myeloma, and sarcoma are the next most frequent tumors in sequence. Spinal cord compression occurs as a complication of the individual tumors, commonly, in multile myeloma (15 percent) and prostate cancer (10 percent); for the other common tumors the relative frequency of spinal cord compression is approximately 5 percent. Spinal cord compression occasionally occurs as the first manifestation of a primary tumor that may be occult or not yet clinically apparent.

Patient A, a 69-year-old man, presented with spinal cord compression at T_4. He underwent laminectomy for undifferentiated tumor and received postoperative radiation therapy with complete relief of symptoms. Two years later, on routine checkup for diabetes, he was found to have supraclavicular adenopathy which, on biopsy, was consistent with histiocytic lymphoma.

The incidence of spinal cord compression is increasing, and the clinical consequences are devastating so that it represents a major clinical problem. Anatomically, the two types of spinal cord compression are (1) extradural compression and (2) intramedullary compression from metastases within the spinal cord proper. The mechanism of tumor implantation is generally through hematogenous metastasis, first to the vertebral body, from which point the tumor moves out to compress the dura, compressing the cord directly (Fig. 5.1).

The mechanisms of spinal cord compression are: 1) contiguous extension from vertebral mestastases and 2) retroneural growth from the paraspinal area through intervertebral foramina.

Thus, more than 80 percent of patients with spinal cord compression from the extramedullary or extradural mechanism will have radiographic evidence of vertebral bone lesions, determined either with routine radiography or with nuclear scans. A second pathogenetic mechanism of spinal cord compression is retroneural growth from paraspinal areas through the intervertebral foramina with the development of secondary compression by direct impingement on the cord. In this instance, the tumor grows from the retroperitoneal or retrothoracic space in continuity with the paraspinal musculature, but along the

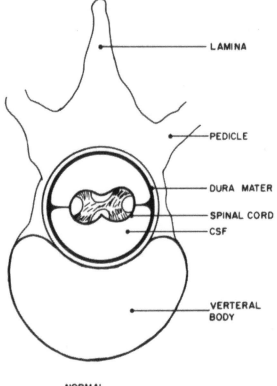

LAMINA

PEDICLE

DURA MATER

SPINAL CORD

CSF

VERTERAL BODY

NORMAL

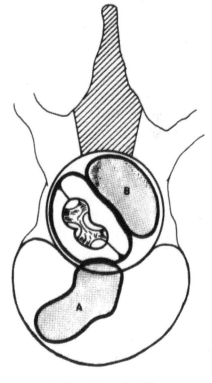

EXTRA DURAL TUMOR

Fig. 5.1 Schematic diagram of the spinal cord and spinal vertebral body (normal). Laminectomy involves removal of the shaded area representing the dorsal process (extra dural tumor). Tumor A results in spinal cord compression from contiguous growth within the bone lesion, and tumor B is hematogenously implanted. Both tumors are extradural in anatomic localization.

nerves emanating from the spinal canal. This is the most common mechanism for intramedullary spinal cord compression. It is sometimes suggested that spinal cord compression and other central nervous system lesions must be associated with pulmonary lesions because the latter represent the bed from which the central nervous system is seeded, but this is refuted by the frequency with which these lesions develop in the absence of pulmonary disease. The presence of a vertebral venous system extending from the pelvis to the cranial vault and carrying blood from the neuraxis to the cranial circulation was described by Batson. With increased systemic circulating pressure, the implantation or reverse flow allows tumor cell penetration in the neuraxis without arterial access.

Central nervous system lesions (cerebral hemispheres and spinal cord) may develop in the absence of pulmonary lesions.

2.0 Clinical patterns of presentation

The clinical presentation of spinal cord compression is quite variable, but early recognition is important. The specific clinical syndrome may be related to (1) the site of obstruction (thoracic, lumbar, or cervical), (2) the acuteness of obstruction, or (3) the mechanism of obstruction either from an extradural or an intramedullary process.

The primary symptom associated with spinal cord compression is pain, which may develop as a preclinical symptom in up to 90 percent of patients.

Pain is the singular initial symptom of spinal cord compression and can vary in intensity and site of origin.

The pain may be insidious and is most

often attributed to a low-back pain syndrome or, in patients with known bone lesions, as simple bone involvement with tumor. The pain commonly becomes radicular, particularly in those instances in which the tumor enters through the intervertebral foramina. Following the development of pain, paresis and paralysis evolve in sequence in the lower extremities. Sensory loss in the extremities develops after motor weakness; the last neurologic insult is autonomic dysfunction with bladder and bowel incontinence. Urinary retention and constipation rarely develop as the first clinical syndrome, but neurologic signs are variably present. In the elderly group of patients with spinal cord compression, the clinical picture may be complicated by mundane neurologic abnormalities, including strokes or diabetic peripheral neuropathy, thus making it more difficult to identify specific neurologic signs.

A summary of clinical neurologic signs and symptoms is detailed in Table 5.1 The clinical picture is primarily related to the site of cord involvement, and may be asymmetric or complicated by multiple sites of compression.

Extradural and intramedullary compression. The most common mecha-

Table 5.1 Neurologic signs and symptoms in spinal cord compression

Symptoms	Frequency
Pain	90%
Muscle weakness	70%
Sensory loss	50%
Autonomic dysfunction*	50%
Signs	
Sensory level	30–40%
Hyperactive reflexes†	70%
Pathologic reflexes	60%

*Bowel, bladder, or genital dysfunction.
†Generally "super" hyperactive.

nism of spinal cord compression is through extradural compression, and fewer than 100 cases of intramedullary spinal cord metastasis have been reported. The most common tumors to be associated with intramedullary tumor metastasis are lung cancer, melanoma, and lymphoma. Clinical characteristics of intramedullary spinal cord compression include radicular pain, muscle atrophy and fasciculations, associated sensory loss, evolution of sensory loss from distal to proximal areas, early autonomic dysfunction, and normal myelography in up to one-half of reported cases. The importance of identifying intramedullary tumor is that decompression laminectomy is generally not indicated in the absence of documented edema of the cord, and local radiation therapy alone may provide major palliation. An important clinical clue to the diagnosis of intramedullary tumor is that most previously reported patients have had associated cerebral metastasis.

Superacute evolution of spinal cord compression implies vascular injury and cord infarction.

Acute and chronic spinal cord compression. Acute spinal cord compression occurs most typically in trauma with secondary hematoma of the cord or vertebral fracture and direct tumor compression. The development of acute spinal cord compression generally indicates a compromise in the arterial supply to the cord with secondary cord infarction. If infarction develops, the prognosis is ominous. Alternatively, in rapidly growing tumors the clinical syndrome may appear over a short interval without vascular infarction.

Patient B, an 18-year-old man with Stage III lymphosarcoma, had been in remission except for persistent retroperitoneal adenopathy. On routine follow-up his examination appeared to be unremarkable, but he returned 12 hours later with acute urinary retention and early motor paresis. He was begun on corticosteroids and local radiation therapy, which brought rapid regression of his symptoms.

Multiple sites of spinal cord tumor implants are common and necessitate radiologic evaluation of the entire cord.

Patient C, a 23-year-old man with mediastinal teratoma, developed quadriplegia from extension of the tumor through the retrothoracic space into the thoracic spinal cord. The patient developed radicular pain and underwent a surgical decompression, at which time the tumor was noted to be on the anterior as well as the posterior cord surface. The pain regressed rapidly, but four days following operation the patient developed a dense paraplegia; at reoperation the tumor was found to encircle the cord completely with compression of the anterior spinal artery. No recovery of extremity function was achieved.

In contrast, the most typical manifestation of spinal cord compression is slow evolution of back pain over two to three weeks before neurologic signs and symptoms may be observed and after which a more rapid clinical progression may occur over days. This slowly evolving syndrome may be referred to as "subacute spinal cord compression." Chronic or stable cord compression is unusual because a growing tumor in the confined space of the spinal canal eventually impinges upon the cord.

Spinal cord compression relative to site of obstruction. Spinal cord compression can develop as a consequence of tumor implantation anywhere along the entire length of the spinal cord, from the cauda equina to the foramen magnum, but in order of frequency implantation occurs at the level of the thoracic, lumbar, and cervical spine. Multiple sites of tumor implantation are commonly observed even when clinical symptoms are related to only a single site. The clinical implications of multiple sites of involvement are that diagnosis and treatment with radiation must often involve the entire spinal cord. Furthermore, surgical decompression must extend beyond the upper and lower limits of the defined lesion by at least one vertebral space, and can promote instability of the vertebral column, particularly when the vertebral body is compromised anteriorly by tumor.

Motor, sensory, and sphincter symptoms may be observed independently without evolving in a chronologic sequence.

Thoracic cord compression is the most common type of involvement, and the clinical picture is typically one of girdle pain beginning in the back and radiating around to the anterior chest or upper abdomen. Localized pain over the vertebral process can frequently be elicited.
In the older literature it was suggested that herpes zoster may precede the development of localized spinal cord compression, particularly in patients with Hodgkin's disease, and may therefore warrant local radiation therapy to the root site of herpes zoster involvement. In patients suspected of having herpes zoster pain but without a typical rash or vesicular eruption, spinal cord compression should be considered. Neurologic examination in thoracic cord lesions should demonstrate abnormalities of the motor and sensory systems with weakness and paresis as well as a decrease in normal reflex and the appearance of pathologic reflexes (Babinski reflex and its variants). The sensory level is typically two or three segments lower than the

actual site of obstruction and may not be symmetrical. In addition, the paresthesias may precede the development of specific neurologic signs.

Autonomic dysfunction occurs most commonly with lesions of the conus medullaris.

Lesions at the level of the lumbar vertebrae are often associated with sphincter abnormalities because the spinal cord ends at L_3, and the conus medullaris carries the neuronal supply to the bladder. In addition, lesions at this level are often associated with root compression and radicular pain syndromes. The differential diagnosis involves a consideration of benign herniated disk because of the frequency with which disk disease develops in the lumbar area.
The autonomic dysfunction commonly associated with lumbar lesions is incontinence secondary to overflow with inadequate sphincter competence. Thus, the absence of bladder detrusor muscle contractability and bowel peristalsis results in constipation and urinary retention followed by overflow incontinence for both stool and urine.

The cord may be compressed anteriorly, posteriorly, or laterally as a consequence of dural impingement, but the neurologic signs and symptoms generally do not permit specific localization. Occasionally patients present predominantly with cerebellar signs as a consequence of compression of the spinal cerebellar tract.

Patient D, a 55-year-old woman with breast cancer metastatic to multiple bones, was controlled on hormonal management and had relatively minor residual pain in the lumbar and thoracic spine. She complained of losing her balance intermittently for approximately three weeks, during which time she often fell and sustained multiple leg bruises. On neurologic examination she demonstrated profound ataxia with weakness of the proximal muscles. There was no sensory deficit, and reflexes were intact. Myelogram demonstrated a lesion at T_{12}. The patient underwent decompression laminectomy and had a partial recovery.

The clinical picture is therefore variable and related to the extent to which one or another neurologic pathway is interrupted.

Cervical cord lesions are the least frequent type of metastases and are invariably associated with local pain and pain extending into the shoulder with radiographically evident bone destruction. The pain may radiate down the spinal column in response to neck flexion (Lhermitte's sign), but more importantly, the appearance of long tract signs or symptoms of the distal extremities or bladder dysfunction heralds progression to quadriplegia.

Spinal cord compression, and primary tumor source. The primary tumor type influences the clinical picture of spinal cord compression because the rapid rate of tumor growth, distribution of metastases, and survival are all influenced by the primary source of the tumor. For example, rapidly growing tumors such as the lymphomas can cause acute compression that is rapidly reversible because of the tumor's responsiveness to treatment.

Patient E, a 24-year-old man with known Hodgkin's disease in the retroperitoneum, had a normal examination without evidence of tumor dissemination approximately three years after initial treatment for Stage III disease. Two days after examination the patient developed pain, followed within hours by unstable gait. He was immediately placed on corticosteroids and received radiation therapy

to the site of obstruction demonstrated by myelogram. Within 2 hours of corticosteroid therapy and within 24 hours of initial irradiation, the pain subsided and the patient's gait returned to normal.

Multiple myeloma is the most common cause of spinal cord compression in an unrecognized primary tumor. Furthermore, decompression laminectomy is contraindicated for this disease.

When spinal cord compression occurs, the primary tumor is generally known (i.e., spinal cord compression appears metachronously). In multiple myeloma, however, cord compression may be the initial presentation of the tumor, and the diagnosis may be obscured by radiographs that are consistent only with osteoporosis.

Patient F, a 57-year-old man, presented with typical symptoms of spinal cord compression secondary to metastatic cancer. There was no evidence of a primary tumor site. An elevated serum calcium, erythrocyte sedimentation rate of 110, and anemia suggested the diagnosis of multiple myeloma. Radiographic studies of the bones were essentially normal except for mild osteoporosis. Because of the suspicion of myeloma, the patient underwent a bone marrow biopsy; the presence of sheets of plasma cells established the diagnosis. Therapy for the spinal cord compression involved local radiation therapy and corticosteroids.

Multiple myeloma affects the bone homogeneously, and a decompression laminectomy may accentuate instability and promote compression of the vertebral body. It is not possible to stabilize the bone surgically, as all of the vertebrae are, for the most part, compromised. In addition, surgery involves an immobilization period that can lead to hypercalcemia.

Spinal cord compression due to prostate or breast cancer is often heralded by increased and resistant bone pain.

The responsiveness of multiple myeloma to chemotherapy and radiation accentuates the need for avoiding surgery. The possibility that a localized plasmacytoma will compress the cord without bone disease can be considered, but the rarity of such a lesion and its exquisite sensitivity to radiation preclude the necessity of surgical decompression in myeloma-associated spinal cord compression.

Breast and prostate cancers represent the female and male counterparts of a tumor that is exquisitely responsive to hormonal therapy and uniformly associated with osteolytic as well as osteoblastic bone lesions. Both tumors therefore have a high incidence of spinal cord compression. The clinical picture is often obscured because the patients may have had bone lesions over a long period with intermittent back pain, and the development of recalcitrant pain in the setting of multiple previous episodes of pain is often attributed merely to tumor resistance. Nonetheless, the cardinal rule must be that persistent localized pain that is resistant to therapy and that develops a pattern of radiation to the legs, arms, or chest may indicate spinal cord compression.

Myelography is indicated in all patients with back pain and malignancy even in the absence of neurologic signs, and especially if bone lesions are not detected.

The clinical picture of spinal cord compression in these "solid tumors" frequently evolves over weeks and sometimes over months, but lack of neurologic recovery after treatment is generally an ominous prognostic sign for survival.

Patient G, a 55-year-old man with metastatic prostate cancer and multiple osteoblastic lesions, had been treated with hormonal manipulation for known bone lesions over the previous two years. His analgesic requirement had increased over the two weeks prior to observation and necessitated his confinement to bed. On neurologic examination he was found to have a profound paraparesis with abnormal pathologic reflexes. He underwent a decompression laminectomy with incomplete recovery, necessitating bladder drainage for the next four months.

Although bone involvement in these tumors is diffuse, and the tumor is responsive to systemic as well as local radiation therapy, the most direct therapy is often surgical decompression.

Two primary tumor types associated with long survival after spinal cord compression are the soft tissue sarcomas and renal cell carcinoma. These tumors are often characterized by local growth and solitary metastasis. Renal cell carcinoma is almost invariably associated with bone lesions; sarcoma is not unless it is derived from the bone in proximity to the cord. These tumors are notoriously resistant to both radiation and systemic therapy and therefore necessitate surgical intervention as a primary approach.

Patient H, a 57-year-old man with a large chondrosarcoma of the ribs, had a chronic complaint of local back pain. Radiation therapy was ineffective in controlling the pain, and the patient gradually developed typical spinal cord compression. Decompression laminectomy was instituted when the patient developed paraplegia, but restitution of function was not possible. He lived an additional two years as a total paraplegic.

Prolonged survival in such patients necessitates early diagnosis because of the devastating effects of paraplegia.

Spinal cord compression and lepto-meningeal carcinoma. Meningeal carcinomatosis must be distinguished from spinal cord compression and has been reviewed with the acute central nervous system syndromes (see Chapter 4). The pathophysiologic distinction of the two complications is sometimes difficult, but leptomeningeal tumor generally involves hematogenous implantation on the under surface of the dura, directly bathing the cord with cells deposited within the cerebrospinal fluid. Tumor implants may evolve along the cord and the under surface of the dura, with secondary entrapment of nerves and the development of a neuropathy sometimes associated with pain. In contrast, the typical spinal cord lesion is implanted on the external surface of the dura, and cells are not generally found in the cerebral spinal fluid.

3.0 Diagnosis of spinal cord compression

The diagnosis of spinal cord compression depends on a clinical awareness of the typical symptoms and of the classic and atypical neurologic signs. Confirmation of the diagnosis is achieved by myelography. As previously indicated, intramedullary tumors may have a normal myelogram in 50 percent of patients. Ancillary procedures, including examination of the cerebrospinal fluid and radiographic evaluation of osseous structures, are incidental to the myelogram but provide additional information that may guide the therapy.

Myelography not only establishes the definitive diagnosis but also delineates the level of cord compression and establishes the amount and distribution of tumor. The morbidity of myelography is minimal even in association with multiple lesions and a dense clinical syndrome secondary to spinal cord compression. Therefore, myelography should be performed on all patients in whom spinal cord compression is suspected, even in the absence of neurologic signs and in the presence of pain or weakness as the only symptom.

Patient I, a 79-year-old man, had had prostate cancer for four years. During that time, the tumor had metastasized to most bones, giving an "ivory" appearance to all osseous structures (Fig. 5.2). He developed progressive weakness of the lower extremities without pain and without neurologic signs of hyperactive reflexes. Myelogram demonstrated a block at T_{10}

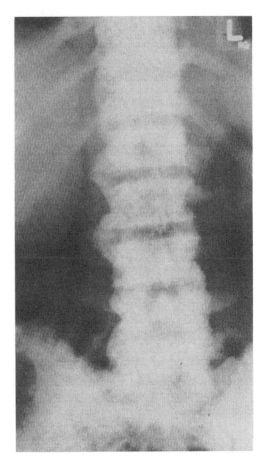

Fig. 5.2 Lumbar spine (Patient I) demonstrating ivory appearance secondary to prostatic cancer metastases.

(Fig. 5.3). Steroids and local radiation therapy resulted in gradual improvement in quadriceps strength.

Clinical spinal cord compression and a normal manometric examination are common and do not imply a vascular lesion.

The myelographic procedure is performed in two steps (Table 5.2). Lumbar puncture permits introduction of the dye below the site of obstruction; a second cisternal puncture allows for introduction of the dye above the obstruction site. The upper and lower levels of obstruction are thus

Table 5.2 Myelographic procedure

1. Enter lumbar space to obtain cerebrosinal fluid for analysis.
2. Introduce radio-opaque dye in lumbar space.
3. Tilt patient to head-down position to establish lower level of obstruction.
4. Introduce radio-opaque dye into cisterna, and tilt patient to head-up position to establish upper level of obstruction.
5. Remove most but not all radio-opaque dye from lumbar puncture site.

established, and in addition, the identification of multiple sites of implantation can be defined. The field of radiation can be defined completely if radiation is the therapy to be used (Fig. 5.4). The characteristics of the cerebrospinal fluid can be analyzed to define the lesion. One of the important applications of myelography is in the sequential monitoring of patients. If residual dye is maintained in the spinal canal, the flow and contour of the spinal canal can be evaluated repeatedly.

The cerebral spinal fluid in patients with extradural or epidural compression almost always demonstrates an increased protein content of more than 100 mg%. The cerebrospinal fluid glucose is generally normal except in those instances in which leptomeningeal carcinoma is observed. Although immediate manometric evaluation of the lumbar puncture generally demonstrates a block, the absence of a defined obstruction by manometric manipulation does not preclude spinal cord compression. The clinical syndrome in the presence of normal manometrics does not necessarily imply a vascular as opposed to a neoplastic lesion.

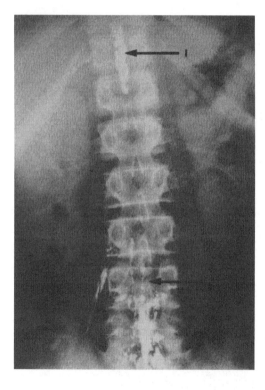

Fig. 5.3 Myelogram demonstrating obstruction of dye at Level 1 (injected into the lumbar space). Extent of tumor obstruction is therefore over five vertebra.

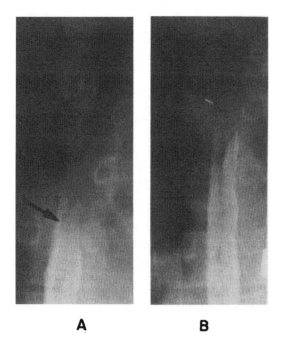

A   **B**

Fig. 5.4 Myelogram demonstrating obstruction indicated by arrow (A). Following radiation therapy (B) the dye extends beyond the original point of obstruction.

Radiographically demonstrated bone lesions and back pain necessitate detailed neurologic examination and/or myelography.

Because spinal cord compression is commonly associated with tumors that have metastasized to the vertebral bodies, radiographic evaluation of the vertebral structure frequently establishes the tumor site. Radiographic confirmation of local bone lesions can complicate and delay diagnosis, because pain is often attributed to the bone lesion rather than to spinal cord compression. A cardinal rule, therefore, in evaluating patients with back pain is that the confirmation of vertebral bone lesions in patients with recent onset

of pain should prompt a detailed neurologic evaluation to rule out concomitant spinal cord compression. An important corollary is that for patients with back pain and no radiographically demonstrable bone lesions, spinal cord compression should be suspected and a myelogram performed, particularly if subtle or equivocal neurologic abnormalities are present.

Spinal cord compression, unlike CNS metastases, is not sheltered within a pharmacologic sanctuary.

Radiologic evaluation of the bones is therefore potentially confusing, although the extent of the tumor can be more precisely defined. Radionuclide bone scans can be helpful in identifying the site of the lesion before standard radiographs are abnormal.

The importance of the neurologic examination must be emphasized. Neurologic deficits or signs appear in classic sequence: sensory, motor, and finally autonomic dysfunction. The examination may be atypical, however, in its chronology and the quantitative deficit. The distal loss of motor strength and reflex abnormality may be asymmetrical, for example, and hyperactive or pathologic reflexes will often fluctuate. The critical neurologic examination involves repetitive, sequential follow-up over a short time to guide therapy and determine the appropriate time for therapeutic intervention.

4.0 Therapies for spinal cord compression

The attitude toward spinal cord compression secondary to metastatic carcinoma is often nihilistic, particularly when considering surgery, but such a generalization is not tenable without a consideration of the total clinical picture. For example, the traditional rule for determining surgical intervention has been based on the density and duration of the neurologic deficit. The quantitative neurologic deficit, however, is only one component in the determination of therapy; other considerations include the primary tumor source, the potential responsiveness of the tumor to radiation or chemotherapy, the extent of the tumor, and the presence of other morbid disease. The chronology and rate of evolution of the neurologic deficit are important variables as well. The principles of treatment for spinal cord compression involve an interdigitation of the primary therapeutic modalities: surgery, radiation, and chemotherapy (Table 5.3).

Surgical decompression is accomplished by laminectomy or removal of the osseous structures that encompass the cord posteriorly. The purpose of laminectomy is to allow for expansion of the edematous cord within a confined space, thus relieving the pressure on the neurologic tissue. In addition, the tumor mass may be

Table 5.3 Treatment principles in spinal cord compression

1. Surgical decompression is the primary modality of therapy for most tumors.

2. Radiation is the treatment of choice for multiple myeloma (without laminectomy).

3. Postoperative radiation therapy is always applied independent of the primary tumor source.

4. Chemotherapy for responsive tumors should be employed for presumed disease outside the nervous system, but intrathecal drug therapy is not indicated.

wholly or partially excised. The tumor mass commonly encircles the cord and may extend up and down additional vertebral spaces, necessitating laminectomy of multiple, contiguous vertebrae. Silver clips are placed at the extreme ends of the laminectomy site to guide postoperative radiation therapy.

Surgical morbidity is related to cerebrospinal fluid leakage and wound dehiscence, but the most important complication is the development of an unstable vertebral column resulting from the removal of the posterior supporting lamina. In the presence of anterior disease in the vertebral body, the result may be complete instability of the vertebral column. Previously reported mortality from spinal cord compression is more often related to tumor complications than to the decompression procedures. Decompression laminectomy itself is associated with low morbidity and mortality.

Radiation therapy is the treatment of choice for spinal cord compression secondary to such radioresponsive tumors as multiple myeloma and lymphoma. In such patients laminectomy may be contraindicated because tumor responsiveness is rapid and often complete. Radiation therapy is invariably indicated after laminectomy even for patients with radioresistant tumors. The presence of residual disease is uniformly assumed in these patients, and the potential presence of multiple, asymptomatic tumor implants should be treated prophylactically. The radiologic techniques are variable but are generally similar to the doses and fractions employed in the treatment of cerebral metastases. In rapidly evolving spinal cord compression, high-dose fractions (400 rad to 1000 rad), are employed in conjunction with corticosteroid therapy, which can minimize the edematous reaction to radiation. Alternatively, for some patients the dose fractionation scheme may be initiated at low doses and gradually built up or administered as a standard fraction at 150 rad to 200 rad per day for a total dose of 3000 rad to 4000 rad.

Corticosteroids are used routinely as a prophylactic measure in patients receiving radiation therapy, although the necessity for these drugs has not been established in a controlled study. Corticosteroids are, however, primary cytolytic agents in both lymphoma and multiple myeloma and therefore play a dual rule in the management of spinal cord compression due to these tumors.

Little if any role has been established for systemic or intrathecal chemotherapy in the management of spinal cord compression. Because this is a regional complication of malignancy, direct therapy must involve surgery, radiation, or a combination of both. Chemotherapy should be used to control systemic disease that seeds the spinal cord, particularly if the tumor is responsive to chemotherapy. Spinal cord compression occurs secondary to contiguous growth from extraneural sites and does not involve a pharmacologic sanctuary as do the other central nervous system complications of malignancy. Therefore, systemic therapy in chemotherapy-responsive tumors can be expected to augment the effects of surgery or radiation in spinal cord compression.

Surgical decompression laminectomy can be used regardless of the duration or density of the neurologic deficit.

Therapy for spinal cord compression can be summarized by basic principles. The primary approach is immediate surgical decompression regardless of the neurologic deficit. Postoperative radiation therapy to the entire obstruction site is indicated in almost all patients. In patients with dense hemiplegia, radiotherapy may achieve at least partial and possibly

complete recovery. Only for patients with a slowly evolving or stable spinal cord compression should radiation be used as a primary modality to the exclusion of surgery.

In the series reviewed by Gilbert, Kim, and Posner (1978), patients undergoing laminectomy with or without radiation therapy consistently achieved a higher level of function than those receiving radiation therapy alone, although the data were not statistically significant. But any added increment achieved by surgical decompression even in a rare patient is worthwhile, considering the devastating alternative and the minimal adverse effects of surgery.

The two primary determinants of prognosis in spinal cord compression are the duration of the neurologic deficit and the density or quantitative severity of the neurologic deficit. Quantitation of the density of neurologic deficit is difficult, but flaccid paralysis is considered an advanced stage beyond that of spastic or hyperactive paralysis. The latter circumstance generally indicates stimulation of a responsive neurologic arc; the flaccid state reflects an incapacitated or infarcted neurologic arc. The duration of a neurologic compromise beyond 24 hours is associated with irretrievability in more than 90 percent of patients. Nonetheless, recovery in isolated cases has been reported, and this singular criterion should not preclude an aggressive surgical and radiotherapeutic approach.

Patient J, a 37-year-old woman who had had Hodgkin's disease for 10 years, presented with progressive back pain over approximately two months. Upon presentation she was found to have hyperactive reflexes, and within two hours developed flaccid paralysis. At 36 hours she came to decompression laminectomy, which produced rapid recovery of neurologic function.

The total clinical situation must therefore be considered in evaluating the therapeutic alternatives.

5.0 Summary

Spinal cord compression, although one of the most devastating complications of cancer, is always reversible if detected before irretrievable neurologic compromise occurs. Therapy is invariably applicable, but the most important modality to be considered is surgery, the choice of which is guided by the total clinical picture and not by considerations of the neurologic deficit alone. The retrievability of occasional patients even in the presence of dense neurologic deficits mandates the application of neurosurgery with only rare exceptions. The major contraindications to surgery are the disease type (i.e., multiple myeloma, Hodgkin's disease, and non-Hodgkin's lymphoma, which are exquisitely responsive to radiation therapy), and the development of cord infarction from compression of the anterior spinal artery, which is rarely possible to diagnose clinically. Intramedullary tumor is a unique but rare form of spinal cord compression, which nonetheless requires decompression to allow edematous expansion of the cord and to prevent cord infarction.

References

Bansal, S.; Brady, L. W.; Olse, A.; Faust, D. S.; Osterholm, J.; and Kazen, I. The treatment of metastatic spinal cord tumors. *JAMA* 292:686–688, 1967.

Botterell, E. H., and FitzGerald, G. W., Spinal cord compression produced by extradural malignant tumors: early recognition, treatment and results. *Can. Med. Assoc. J.* 80:791–796, 1959.

Bruckman, J. E., and Bloomer, W. D. Management of spinal cord compression. *Seminars in Oncology* 5:135–140, 1978.

Edelson, R. N.; Deck, M. D. F.; and Posner, J. B. Intramedullary spinal cord metastases; clinical and radiographic findings in nine cases. *Neurology* 22:1222–1231, 1972.

Friedman, M.; Kim, T. H.; and Panahon, A. M. Spinal cord compression in malignant lymphoma; treatment and results. *Cancer* 37:1485–1491, 1976.

Gilbert, R. W.; Kim, J-H.; and Posner, J. B. Epidural spinal cord compression from metastatic tumor: diagnosis and treatment. *Ann.Neurol.* 3:40–51, 1978.

Haddad, P., Thaell, J. F.; Kiely, J. M.; Harrison, E. G., Jr.; and Miller, R. H. Lymphoma of the spinal extradural space. *Cancer* 38:1862–1866, 1976.

Jameson, R. M. Prolonged survival in paraplegia due to metastatic spinal tumors. *Lancet* 1209–1211, 1974.

Kahn, F. R.; Glicksman, A. S.; Chu, F. C. H.; and Nickson, J. J. Treatment by radiotherapy of spinal cord compression due to extradural metastases. *Radiology* 89:496-500, 1967.

Millburn, L.; Hibbs, G. G.; and Hendrickson, F. R. Treatment of spinal cord compression from metastatic carcinoma: review of the literature and presentation of a new method of treatment. *Cancer* 21:447–452, 1968.

Mullan, J., and Evans, J. P. Neoplastic disease of the spinal extradural space (a review of 50 cases). *Arch. Surg.* 74:900–907, 1957.

Mullins, G. M.; Flynn, J. P. G.; El-Mahdi, A. M.; McQueen, J. D.; and Owens, A. H., Jr. Malignant lymphoma of the spinal epidural space. *Ann. Intern. Med.* 74:416–423, 1971.

Parker, J. C., Jr. Intramedullary spinal cord involvement in Hodgkin's disease with an atypical systemic distribution. *Cancer* 30:545–552, 1972.

Perese, D. M. Treatment of metastatic extradural spinal cord tumors (a review of 30 cases). *Cancer* 11:214–221, 1958.

Rubin, P.; Mayer, E.; and Poulter, C. Extradural spinal cord compression by tumor: part II: high daily dose experience without laminectomy. *Radiology* 93:1248–1260, 1969.

Silverberg, I. J., and Jacobs, E. M. Treatment of spinal cord compression in Hodgkin's disease. *Cancer* 27:308–313, 1971.

White, W. A.; Patterson, R. H., Jr.; and Bergland, R. M. Role of surgery in the treatment of spinal cord compression by metastatic neoplasm. *Cancer* 27:558–561, 1971.

Wild, W. O., and Porter, R. W. Metastatic epidural tumor of the spine (a study of 45 cases). *Arch. Surg.* 87:825–830, 1963.

Chapter 6

Hypercalcemia of Malignancy
J. Wolff

1.0 Introduction and background

Patients with cancer frequently have an increased serum calcium concentration. Hypercalcemia can occur at any point in the course of the disease and may be the first clue to the presence of malignancy. The condition can be clinically silent and detected only by automated multiphasic blood chemistry determinations; conversely, it can be the most debilitating aspect of the disease. The disorders of calcium homeostasis that underlie this condition are similarly varied. Fortunately, a variety of therapeutic modalities is available for patients who require reduction of their serum calcium.

Hypercalcemia developing in association with malignancy may be directly related to the tumor (secretion of parathyroid hormone) or to osseous metastases, or it may be related in a nonspecific way to another morbid process such as primary hyperparathyroidism. The latter disease is associated with an increased incidence of malignancy. Whatever the mechanism, hypercalcemia develops in as many as 10 percent of patients with advanced malignancy.

To facilitate detection of hypercalcemia as early as possible, it is necessary to be familiar not only with the signs and symptoms that may be produced, but also with those tumors commonly associated with this complication. Certain tumors will produce hypercalcemia much more frequently than others; for these patients the physician's "index of suspicion" for hypercalcemia should be higher. In a series of 156 consecutive cases of hypercalcemia secondary to malignancy, 46 percent were cases of lung or breast cancer, with a variety of other tumors responsible for the remaining portion. For patients with bone involvement, most instances of hypercalcemia are due to breast cancer or multiple myeloma. Virtually any tumor, including leukemia and lymphoma, can produce hypercalcemia under these circumstances. In patients free from bone metastases, most cases of hypercalcemia are due to bronchogenic carcinoma and renal cell carcinoma. A number of other tumors characteristically produce this syndrome, although less frequently than the two major histologies (Table 6.1). Isolated cases have been reported for virtually every tumor producing hypercalcemia in the absence of bone metastases.

The most common histopathologic class of tumor associated with hypercalcemia is squamous cell carcinoma at any site, including lung, head and neck, and bladder.

2.0 Clinical presentation

Hypercalcemia can produce altered physiology in a number of organs and can give rise to a variety of signs and symptoms (Table 6.2). Many of these symptoms are commonly found in cancer patients with normal serum calcium, but the appearance of any one should prompt a calcium determination.

In the gastrointestinal tract, hypercalcemia is often associated with constipation, a manifestation of a general tendency toward depression of neuromuscular activity. Hypercalcemia can also be responsible for anorexia, nausea, vomiting, and vague abdominal pain. In evaluating these symptoms, the physician should recall that hypercalcemia is associated with an increased incidence of peptic ulcer. Calcium stimulates gastrin secretion, which in turn causes increased acid production; this is the probable link between the two conditions. (A similar link between hypercalcemia and pancreatitis is less well established.) If nausea, vomiting, or pain does not respond quickly to correction of the serum calcium, an upper-GI series is indicated; conversely, excessive or unexpected gastrointestinal symptoms may be attributed to alterations of calcium homeostasis.

Table 6.1 Tumors associated with hypercalcemia in descending order of frequency

In the absence of bone metastases
    Bronchogenic carcinoma
    Renal cell carcinoma
    Head and neck cancers
    Carcinoma of the female genital tract
        Ovary
        Endometrium
        Cervix
        Vulva
    Bladder carcinoma
    Pancreatic carcinoma
    Breast cancer

In the presence of bone metastases
    Head and neck cancer
    Breast cancer
    Lung cancer
    Multiple myeloma
    Renal cell cancer
    Prostatic cancer

Table 6.2 Clinical signs and symptoms of hypercalcemia

Organ system	Symptoms
Gastrointestinal tract	Anorexia, nausea, vomiting, constipation
Genitourinary tract	Polyuria, polydipsia, no renal stones
Central nervous system	Disordered mental state progressing to coma, no seizures

Patient A, a 35-year-old man with meta-static malignant melanoma, had extensive bone lesions but had not had hypercalcemia. He had a brief response to dacarbazine (DTIC), but then failed both this treatment and other drug therapies. He was started on a new chemotherapeutic regimen and was told that nausea and vomiting were among the potential side effects but that these would last only a few hours. Three days after beginning the new regimen, he continued to have severe nausea with occasional vomiting, and hypercalcemia was suspected. The serum calcium was 13.2 mg%.

In the kidney, hypercalcemia causes an inability to concentrate the urine. Consequently, polyuria, polydipsia, and dehydration occur. Nephrolithiasis will appear only when the hypercalcemia is long standing. Thus, stone formation is seen in hypercalcemia due to such benign disorders as hyperparathyroidism; stones are rare in the patient with hypercalcemia due to cancer.

Signs of extraskeletal calcification such as band keratopathy or nephrocalcinosis are uncommon in patients with hypercalcemia secondary to malignancy, also because hypercalcemia must be long standing to produce these signs.

Central nervous system manifestations of hypercalcemia include apathy, weakness, personality change including psychosis, and headache. Seizures and focal neurologic signs are rare. Patients with elevation of serum calcium may present with stupor or coma.

Patient B, a 44-year-old woman, had a past history of depressive psychosis but had been well for eight years. At that time, apathy, anorexia, and forgetfulness returned. Although insomnia had been a prominent symptom of her earlier disease, she now exhibited constant drowsi-ness. The physical examination revealed an ovarian mass; the serum calcium was 15.0 mg%. At laparotomy, an 8.0-cm ovarian carcinoma was removed; there was no evidence of metastatic disease. Following operation, the calcium fell to normal, and the patient's mental condition cleared.

The symptoms of hypercalcemia are gastrointestinal, urinary, or neurologic, and the extent of the symptoms does not necessarily correlate with the quantitative serum calcium level.

3.0 Pathophysiology of hypercalcemia

A variety of pathophysiologic mechanisms is responsible for hypercalcemia in malignancy. The details of each have not been completely elucidated, and it is likely that other mechanisms, about which we are unaware, are operating. In spite of these deficiencies in our knowledge, an understanding of the pathophysiology of a particular case can help in the selection of optimum therapy.

The majority (>90%) of patients with hypercalcemia have bone metastases.

The most common mechanism of hypercalcemia is local destruction of bone by invading tumor. As bone is destroyed, calcium is released into the blood at a rate that exceeds maximal renal clearance. Clearly, factors other than the simple presence of tumors in bone are operating here. For example, given a patient with bone metastases, the histology is important in determining whether hypercalcemia will occur. Breast cancer is frequently associated with hypercalcemia, but only when the patient has bone disease. In contrast, another tumor commonly metastatic to bone, oat cell carcinoma of the lung, very rarely causes hypercalcemia. Bone involvement is most readily detected by whole-body radionuclide scanning. The bone scan will generally become abnormal before conventional radiographs, but it lacks specificity and will become positive in any area with increased osteoblastic activity. Degenerative, metabolic, and neoplastic bone disease are all associated with a positive bone scan. Healing (nonpathologic) fractures will show increased uptake on bone scan for prolonged periods of time. Therefore, it is necessary to study roentgenograms of bones that are abnormal on scan. These will usually provide the specific diagnosis, but in rare cases, needle biopsy may be required to establish the presence of bone metastases. Biochemically, hypercalcemia associated with metastatic tumor in bone is accompanied by normal or increased serum phosphorus, increased alkaline phosphatase, and normal serum chloride. Parathyroid hormone (PTH) production will be suppressed by the hypercalcemia, although perhaps not totally, as a component of PTH secretion is not sensitive to serum calcium. If measured, the serum PTH level will be found to be low or undetectable, but occasionally it is increased because of a response to therapeutic measures to decrease the serum calcium level.

Parathyroid hormone. In contrast to direct bone destruction by metastatic tumor is hypercalcemia that is mediated by humoral substances. The first substance proposed for this role was PTH. In these cases, PTH is produced by tumor tissue just as other hormones are produced in similar "ectopic hormone" syndromes. Hormone production is autonomous (i.e., not responsive to the usual negative feedback control by serum calcium). Biochemically, this syndrome closely resembles

that of primary hyperparathyroidism, with decreased serum phorphorus and tubular resorption of phosphate. Hyperchloremic acidosis may be seen as well. Pseudohyperparathyroidism has thus been defined as the constellation of increased serum calcium and decreased serum phosphorus in a patient with nonparathyroid malignancy without bone metastases. The role of PTH in these cases, however, is still under debate. In the older literature such cases were often simply noted to lack autopsy evidence of bone metastases and parathyroid neoplasia, and a pathophysiologic role for PTH was assumed. More recently, radioimmunoassays for PTH have become available. At present, a well-studied case would ideally include: (1) simultaneous measurement of serum calcium and PTH, (2) simultaneous measurement of PTH in the arteries supplying and veins draining the tumor bed (A-V gradient), and (3) measurement of PTH concentration in tumor tissue and surrounding normal tissue. Such completely documented cases are rare, and the currently available data are inconsistent.

Ectopic secretion of PTH by a tumor has not been definitively demonstrated to date.

Powell and co-workers reported 11 cases of the putative PTH-mediated syndrome that were studied with radioimmunoassays using a variety of antisera (1973). The investigators stated that these antisera collectively recognized a number of antigenic sites along the entire length of the PTH molecule in addition to detecting pro-PTH and PTH fragments. In the reported cases, no detectable PTH was present in peripheral blood, venous blood from the tumor bed, or tumor extracts. Yet tumor tissue extracts did cause bone resorption in vitro. They concluded that at least one-half of all cases of pseudohyperparathyroidism was mediated by a humoral substance other than PTH. On the other side, Benson and co-workers studied a series of 108 patients with hypercalcemia and malignancy and found that for over 95 percent of them the serum PTH concentration was inappropriately high for the level of serum calcium (1974). Furthermore, patients with bone metastases, who might be presumed to have hypercalcemia from some other mechanism, had PTH levels similar to those without bone metastases. This study would seem to indicate that most patients had hypercalcemia mediated by PTH.

It is not currently possible to reconcile these studies. Differences in radioimmunoassay technique undoubtedly contribute to differences in results. Normal PTH might differ immunologically from that produced by tumor. In addition, the assumption that even a low PTH level is inappropriately high for a given serum calcium will have to be reevaluated; recent data show that a low level of PTH secretion may not be suppressible at any calcium level. A development that may help to clarify this issue is the measurement of urinary excretion of adenosine 3', 5'-monophosphate (cyclic AMP). This compound is relatively easy to measure, and its measurement may supplant (or at least supplement) the radioimmunoassay for PTH, which is technically difficult. Cyclic AMP is produced in the kidney in response to PTH and mediates the renal effects of PTH. Urinary cyclic AMP represents both glomerular filtration of plasma cyclic AMP and tubular secretion of cyclic AMP. Only the latter portion is a reflection of PTH activity. By measuring plasma cyclic AMP and creatinine clearance, the filtered portion of urinary cyclic AMP can be calculated and subtracted from the total, leaving the nephrogenous portion. There are few data on patients with malignancy and hypercalcemia using

this new technique, but Shaw and co-workers studied 16 such patients, and related the cyclic AMP levels to serum calcium and PTH (1977). Two groups of patients were evaluated. One group of 6 patients had urinary cyclic AMP levels similar to those of normal volunteers given calcium infusion or to those of patients with hypercalcemia not mediated by PTH. Most of these patients had bone metastases; 4 patients had bone scans, and all were positive. In this group, the mechanism of hypercalcemia is likely due not to PTH but to bone metastases. The second group (10 patients) had urinary cyclic AMP levels similar to those of patients with primary hyperparathyroidism. Most of these patients had no evidence of bone metastases; 6 had bone scans and all were negative. In this group, the hypercalcemia may well be mediated by PTH.

Prostaglandins. It now appears that PTH is not the only humoral mediator of hypercalcemia in malignancy. Evidence exists that prostaglandins of the E series, especially prostaglandin E_2 (PGE_2), may be responsible for hypercalcemia in some cases. Interest in this role for prostaglandins stemmed from studies by Tashjian and co-workers of a mouse fibrosarcoma that regularly produced hypercalcemia. In this model, PGE_2 is secreted by the tumor; tumor-bearing animals have high blood levels of PGE_2 and hypercalcemia. The PGE_2 causes resorption of bone in vitro and produces hypercalcemia when infused into normal rats. Furthermore, indomethacin, an inhibitor of prostaglandin synthesis, corrects hypercalcemia in mice bearing the fibrosarcoma and lowers the serum level of PGE_2.

A human tumor in which hypercalcemia was apparently mediated by prostaglandins was first reported by Brereton and co-workers in 1974. Their patient had renal cell carcinoma metastatic to liver and lung, but not to bone. Hypercalcemia was refractory to conventional management but responded on two occasions to indomethacin. Assays for prostaglandins in plasma showed no detectable amounts; liver metastases had greatly increased amounts of prostaglandins as compared to normal liver, while lung metastases had less than normal lung tissue.

This initial case report was followed by other isolated reports, and then by two small series. Robertson and co-workers studied prostaglandin E (PCE) in 21 patients with malignancy. Of 11 hypercalcemic patients, 4 had elevated plasma PGE. Of 10 normocalcemic patients, 1 had a minimal elevation of PGE. Seven patients received indomethacin for hypercalcemia, and 6 had a significant decrease in PGE. Two of the 7 treated patients were in the group with elevated pretreatment PGE; these 2 had a decrease in serum calcium with indomethacin.

Seyberth and co-workers measured the excretion of the major urinary metabolite of the prostaglandin E series (PGE-M). In 14 patients with hypercalcemia and solid tumors, 12 had markedly increased PGE-M; none of the 14 patients had detectable serum PTH. Thirteen patients with normal serum calcium had urinary PGE-M that was normal (8 patients) or slightly increased (5 patients); again, PTH was low. Six patients with primary hyperparathyroidism had normal PGE-M. Seyberth's group has analyzed treatment results according to pretreatment PGE-M levels and the presence or absence of bone metastases. Hypercalcemic patients who did not have an elevation of PGE-M prior to therapy did not respond to treatment with a prostaglandin synthesis inhibitor (aspirin or indomethacin). Of 9 hypercalcemic patients with increased PGE-M, all responded to treatment, with a decrease in PGE-M and serum calcium. Five of these did not have bone metastases; serum calcium in these patients fell to normal. Four patients with bone metastases had a decrease in serum calcium, but not to normal levels.

Combining the two series of patients, one finds that 13 of 24 hypercalcemic cancer patients had increased PGE in the plasma or urine. The conclusion that prostaglandins are involved in 50 percent of cancer patients with hypercalcemia must await the study of many more cases. What is more impressive is the effectiveness of treatment in appropriately selected cases. All 11 patients with hypercalcemia and increased PGE had a reduction of serum calcium in response to treatment with aspirin or indomethacin. Response to drugs that inhibit prostaglandin synthesis does not identify the exact role of these compounds in hypercalcemia. It may be that prostaglandins are not the tumor product that causes hypercalcemia, but rather are produced by normal tissues in response to some other stimulus from the tumor. Yet the available data in animals and humans suggest otherwise. The distinction is not pragmatically crucial so long as the therapy is effective.

Osteoclast-activating factor. A third tumor cell product that can cause hypercalcemia has been studied in patients with multiple myeloma and other hematologic malignancies by Mundy and co-workers (1974). Short-term cell cultures were derived from tumor tissue of seven patients with myeloma; supernatant fluid from six cultures showed bone-resorbing activity in vitro. The active factor was determined by a variety of techniques to be most similar to osteoclast-activating factor (OAF) rather than to PGE, PTH, or vitamin D analogs. A product of normal human leukocytes, OAF is released in response to challenge with antigen or mitogen, but plasma and normal leukocytes from myeloma patients did not contain an excess of this factor. Morphologic studies showed that prominent osteoclastic activity occurred along bone surfaces adjacent to myeloma deposits. The degree of this activity paralleled the extent of infiltration by myeloma in the immediate area. Thus, in this tumor it appears that the malignant cells secrete an excess of a factor similar to the OAF of normal leukocytes. This factor does not appear in large amounts in plasma but achieves high concentrations near substantial tumor deposits and thus stimulates osteoclasts in the immediate vicinity of these deposits. The resulting bone destruction produces hypercalcemia. Whether this mechanism applies for other tumors has not been settled; it may be operative in some cases of Burkitt's lymphoma (another B-cell neoplasm) and perhaps in other lymphomas.

Finally, osteolytic vitamin D-like sterols have been mentioned as another humoral mediator of hypercalcemia. Evidence for an excess of such sterols in the plasma of cancer patients has not, however, been corroborated.

Hypercalcemia unrelated to tumor. When a patient with known malignancy develops hypercalcemia, the disturbance in calcium metabolism is almost always secondary to the malignancy. In a small number of cases, however, the hypercalcemia will not be related to cancer; thus, it is always necessary to consider the entire differential diagnosis of hypercalcemia (Table 6.3). This is particularly true for the patient who has had a cancer in the past and who has apparently been cured. For example, in the patient who has had a mastectomy for breast cancer and who develops hypercalcemia two years later, the hypercalcemia may represent the initial manifestation of metastatic bone disease, but this must not be presumed. In the patient known to have cancer at the time hypercalcemia develops (synchronous), the odds that hypercalcemia will be due to any cause other than malignancy are small, yet this possibility must be considered. The cause of hypercalcemia not related to cancer and most difficult to establish is concurrent primary hyperparathyroidism. A few well-documented cases of incidental primary parathyroid

Table 6.3 Differential diagnosis of hypercalcemia

Primary hyperparathyroidism
Malignancy
Vitamin D intoxication
Hypophosphatasia
Addison's disease
Sarcoidosis
Milk-alkali syndrome
Immobilization

disease have been reported, and these may provide some helpful clinical clues. For example, primary parathyroid hyperplasia is almost invariably associated with decreased phosphate and with increased serum chloride and calcium. The most critical observation is the comparison of the clinical courses of the hypercalcemia and the tumor. If the tumor is responsible for hypercalcemia, the onset of the latter condition should come at a time when the tumor burden has increased. Similarly, if a patient has a good response to antitumor therapy of any sort and has a reduction in tumor burden, the hypercalcemia should become more easily controlled or should disappear entirely. Any discrepancy between the clinical severity of hypercalcemia and the tumor burden should suggest the possibility that the two are not causally related and should stimulate appropriate investigation. In the patient suspected of concurrent primary hyperparathyroidism, selective venous catheterization of the neck and measurement of PTH concentrations in venous effluent from both the tumor bed and the parathyroid glands comprise the most definitive diagnostic approach.

Patient C, a 53-year-old woman, was referred because of jaundice. Seven years previously she had had a mastectomy, and four years previously had had a duodenal ulcer. Physical examination revealed nodular cutaneous lesions of the chest wall, jaundice, and hepatomegaly. Serum calcium was 12.6 mg% and phosphorus 2.1 mg%. Liver scan was consistent with metastasis; bone scan was normal. Chemotherapy was begun; complete regression of the skin lesions occurred, and her liver chemistries improved. Serum calcium and phosphorus remained essentially unchanged. A peripheral venous PTH was at the upper limit of normal, inappropriately elevated for the serum calcium. Venous sampling from various sites revealed PTH production from the neck but none from the liver. A parathyroid adenoma was removed, and subsequently the serum calcium and phosphorus became normal.

Parathormone-mediated hypercalcemia (secondary to primary parathyroid disease) is suggested by decreased phosphate and increased chloride levels.

Primary parathyroid disease is commonly associated with the familial endocrinopathies that have neoplastic evolution; these are referred to as the neurocristopathies. Thus multiple tumors of the pancreas, adrenal gland, thyroid, and pituitary are associated with parathyroid tumors. The multiple endocrine neoplasia (MEN) syndromes were previously limited, but other forms of MEN have been described, including associations with lung and thymic tumors.

Patient D, a 40-year-old man, presented with a large mediastinal mass and a serum calcium of 13 mg%. He underwent exploratory thoracotomy and removal of a large carcinoid tumor of the thymus. Four weeks later he had three of four hyperplastic parathyroid glands removed. The mediastinal tumor recurred five years later. The patient's family was then evaluated: one daughter and the mother of the propositus had elevated calcium and variable PTH levels.

Primary hyperparathyroidism in association with malignancy may be related to multiple endocrine abnormalities and may be familial.

Spurious hypercalcemia. One must also consider the possibility of "spurious" hypercalcemia or an increase in the concentration of protein-bound calcium without an increase in the ionized calcium concentration. Since calcium bound to protein is biologically inactive, no ill effects occur from processes that affect only the protein-bound calcium and leave ionized calcium unchanged. This situation is encountered most frequently in patients with intravascular volume loss. Cancer patients often have anorexia, nausea, and vomiting secondary to their disease and its treatment. With decrease of intravascular volume, the concentration of serum proteins rises, producing an increase in the total calcium concentration. Such increases in calcium are generally small and will respond immediately to fluid replacement. Adrenal insufficiency is associated with hypercalcemia: its mechanism is thought to be intravascular fluid depletion. Adrenal insufficiency is commonly encountered in the patient who has had long-term corticosteroid therapy or who takes replacement steroids after adrenalectomy or hypophysectomy, and who either abruptly discontinues steroids or does not increase the steroid dose appropriately in response to stress. An interesting case of "spurious" hypercalcemia in a myeloma patient has been reported in which serum-ionized calcium was normal in spite of severely elevated levels of calcium (thus the lack of symptoms). The increase in total serum calcium was due to an increased protein-bound calcium associated with the abnormal serum globulin produced by the myeloma cells.

Immobilization as a cause of hypercalcemia is not generally symptomatic. Nonetheless, patients with bone metastases may be bedridden because of pain, and the combination of bone disruption by tumor and immobilization can accentuate the calcium problem. The only critical difficulty that develops with immobilization occurs with multiple myeloma. In this disease, patients must be mobilized to prevent potentiation of hypercalcemia, which rarely occurs in the solid (nonmyelomatous) tumors.

Patient E, a 69-year-old man, developed a plasmacytoma of the chest wall and then rapid dissemination of disease associated with hypercalcemia (14.3 mg%). Fluids and corticosteroids reduced the calcium to 11.9 mg% over seven days, but when the patient ambulated after day seven, the calcium promptly fell to 9.5 mg%.

Hypercalcemia associated with multiple myeloma is especially prone to fluctuations related to ambulation.

4.0 Treatment of hypercalcemia

A variety of methods and agents is available for the treatment of hypercalcemia of malignancy. Each has its own mechanisms of action and side effects; thus each has its own indications and contraindications. The most important approach to the patient with hypercalcemia of malignancy is to gain control of the underlying tumor. A reduction of the tumor burden, however achieved, will alleviate the hypercalcemia. If the reduction in tumor burden is sufficient, treatment directed at the serum calcium alone may not need to be continued. In almost every situation, effective control of the malignancy will result in the most complete and durable

control of the serum calcium while producing the fewest side effects.

Patient F, a 46-year-old premenopausal woman, was well for four years after mastectomy when she presented with bone pain, nausea, and anorexia. A bone scan showed multiple areas of increased uptake of the radionuclide. The serum calcium was 14.2 mg%. The hypercalcemia was treated with six liters per day of intravenous normal saline, and the serum calcium decreased to 13.0 mg%. The patient then had therapeutic oophorectomy, and the serum calcium declined to normal over the first seven postoperative days. Fluid therapy was tapered and discontinued, and the calcium remained normal.

Treatment of the tumor is the most important component of hypercalcemia therapy.

It is generally helpful to consider the treatment of hypercalcemia in two stages. The first stage is the treatment of newly discovered or acutely exacerbated hypercalcemia. Therapy is usually performed in the hospital with all the available technical resources that are required to deal with an acute, life-threatening problem. When control of the serum calcium is achieved, and the patient's condition has stabilized, out-patient therapy begins. At this point, the patient requires a stable schedule of medications that will control serum calcium on a week-to-week rather than hour-to-hour basis.

Patients must be evaluated individually with respect to the quantitative elevation of serum calcium, for they have a markedly variable tolerance to a particular level of hypercalcemia. Other factors that may be important are the chronicity of the hypercalcemia and the rate of evolution. A slowly rising calcium may be well tolerated to rather high levels; an acute rise in calcium can produce symptoms at a lower level. The total clinical circumstances must be evaluated to determine how aggressive treatment must be.

Patient G, a 56-year-old woman with breast cancer metastatic to bone, pleura, and lymph nodes, had been treated initially with combined oophorectomy-adrenalectomy. After therapy, she had done well for 18 months but then had progression of her disease. She was given a trial of progesterone therapy but experienced increasing pain. In addition, her alkaline phosphatase rose sharply to 367 IU per liter, and her serum calcium rose to 14.3 mg%. There were no symptoms of hypercalcemia. She was begun on an antiestrogen, tamoxifen, and the pain diminished. The alkaline phosphatase declined to 204 IU per liter and the calcium became normal without recourse to the usual calcium-specific methods.

The quantitative level of hypercalcemia does not necessarily relate directly to the secondary clinical symptoms (i.e., a serum calcium of 18 mg% may be associated with only mild anorexia).

Some general guidelines for therapy may be helpful. An elevation of serum calcium less than 12.5 mg% is often asymptomatic and readily managed with fluids only; hypercalcemia of greater than 15 mg% may be life threatening and generally requires more than one therapeutic agent; possibly all five will be needed (diuretics, fluids, steroids, mithramycin, and phosphates).

Of the various therapeutic options for hypercalcemia, the one most frequently used as the initial treatment is the promotion of calcium excretion. This is accomplished by the infusion of large quantities of intravenous fluids that contain sodium.

Saline infusions cause increased urinary sodium losses, and renal calcium excretion parallels sodium excretion. The other benefit of this regimen is that dehydration is corrected. Patients with significant hypercalcemia generally have anorexia, nausea, and vomiting and are unable to concentrate their urine; thus they are nearly always dehydrated. Restoration of intravascular volume can produce significant clinical improvement. In addition, correction of dehydration will result in some lowering of total serum calcium. The decrease in serum calcium, however, is due to the lowering of the concentration of protein-bound calcium and may not significantly alter the calcium-induced symptoms.

To increase the rate of calcium excretion associated with saline infusion, diuretics are added to the regimen. Thiazides are contraindicated because they can retard urinary excretion of calcium and can aggravate the hypercalcemia; furosemide and ethacrynic acid are the agents of choice because they increase calcium excretion. With a combination of intravenous fluids and diuretics, large volumes of fluid can be passed through a patient. It is common to begin with three liters of intravenous normal saline or the equivalent per day and to work up to six or eight liters, depending upon the patient's cardiac reserve. Initial doses of the diuretics may be 20 to 40 mg of furosemide or 5 to 10 mg of ethacrynic acid intravenously. This may be repeated hourly if necessary or escalated to 100 mg furosemide or 40 mg ethacrynic acid.

The potential toxicity of aggressive fluid therapy is related to iatrogenic fluid overload. Patients with diminished cardiac or renal function will not tolerate such a program and must be treated with a much lower infusion rate. Even patients with unimpaired cardiac and renal function must be closely monitored with frequent vital sign determinations and care-

ful hour-by-hour accounting of input
and output. For most patients receiving
high volumes of infusate, a central venous
pressure line will facilitate monitoring
and enable earlier detection and correction
of hyper- or hypovolemia. In addition,
patients undergoing this kind of therapy
are prone to losses of other electrolytes
such as potassium and magnesium; serum
levels of these must be carefully monitored and appropriate replacement given.
Urinary concentrations of electrolytes
provide an easy indication of the appropriate rate of replacement, but usually the
regimen is constantly changing, and the
utility of these measurements is then
limited.

**Serum potassium is commonly decreased
in patients with malignancy and hypercalcemia so that diuretic therapy must be
associated with simultaneous potassium
replacement.**

---

*Patient H, a 58-year-old woman, had had
a modified radical mastectomy for carcinoma of the breast. She had been well
for four and one-half years after which
liver and bone metastases appeared. Con-
currently, the serum calcium rose to 14.6
mg%. She was admitted to the hospital,
and intravenous fluid therapy was begun
with five percent dextrose in half-normal
saline at a rate of four liters per day. Furosemide was added to the regimen to maintain fluid balance. In spite of the addition
of 40 mEq of KCL to each liter of infusate,
the serum potassium fell to 3.1 mg per
liter. Further potassium supplementation
was given orally. The serum calcium
fell to 11.0 mg%; serum potassium rose to
3.5 mEq per liter.*

Aggressive fluid therapy requires constant vigilance and is potentially hazardous. Furthermore, its effect on serum
calcium, although often dramatic, is tran-

sient, and serum calcium will begin to
rise within a few hours after discontinuing
treatment. Therefore, fluid therapy can
be only an initial step in gaining control
of the serum calcium and must quickly be
replaced by another treatment modality.

An alternative to saline infusion is the
use of sodium sulfate infusion. With this
preparation, a sulfate-calcium complex
that is nonreabsorbable forms in the urine;
the additional effect of the natriuresis
makes sulfate infusion more potent than
saline infusion. A disadvantage of sulfate
infusion is its lack of ready availability
in most pharmacies. Isotonic sodium
sulfate is generally used and is prepared
as 38.9 g of sodium sulfate decahydrate
per liter. Generally, one to three liters are
infused per day; greater volumes can be
used for very severe cases. Because of the
greater potency and the generally smaller
volumes required with sulfate, the problems associated with massive saline infusions are avoided. The side effects of sulfate infusion are generally similar to those
of a saline infusion at a similar rate. There
may be a tendency toward the development of hypernatremia, but this is generally not symptomatic.

The administration of inorganic phosphate provides a rapid and dose-depen-
dent decrease in serum calcium by promoting precipitation and deposition of
calcium into bone. An intrinsic advantage
of phosphate therapy is the availability
of dose forms for intravenous, oral, and
rectal administration. Intravenous phosphate is reserved for initial management of
acute hypercalcemia and has largely been
supplanted by other agents such as mithramycin but oral phosphate is ideal for
chronic out-patient therapy. In calculating
doses, care must be taken to distinguish
between phosphorus and phosphate. The
contents of pharmaceuticals are often
listed as milligrams of phosphate, while
doses of these preparations are generally
given in milligrams of phosphorus. In

addition, pharmaceutical preparations differ in the cations that accompany the phosphate anion; one can choose from products containing only sodium, only potassium, or both.

Phosphate therapy is generally well tolerated. Some patients taking oral phosphate may have diarrhea, particularly during the first few days of treatment, but this is generally self-limited and may be avoided by slowly accelerating the dose. Shock and renal failure due to cortical necrosis have been reported as consequences of intravenous phosphate. Infrequently, the major complication of phosphate therapy is the development of metastatic calcification. The role of phosphate therapy in producing metastatic calcification is difficult to evaluate, as hypercalcemia is also a cause of calcium deposition in soft tissues. There are no means to ensure that metastatic calcification will not be aggravated by phosphate therapy, but to minimize the problem, the serum phosphate concentration is used as a guide to phosphate dose. For a given calcium concentration, a higher serum phosphate level will be associated with an increased risk of the complication. Thus the patient with hyperphosphatemia has a relative contraindication to phosphate therapy. In general, one can start with a dose of 1000 mg inorganic phosphorus daily for intravenous use and 1500 mg daily for oral or rectal administration.

Patient I, a 59-year-old man with laryngeal carcinoma that was metastatic to the lung, had chronic hypercalcemia with a serum calcium concentration of 12 to 13 mg% and a serum phosphorus in the low normal range. He had had no symptoms related to hypercalcemia but with advancing disease he became depressed, and intravenous fluids were required to maintain adequate intake. He was started on oral phosphate and received 1.5 g of elemental phosphorus per day. Over five

days, the serum calcium fell from its previous value to 11.4 mg%. The patient became more alert, began to drink sufficient fluids, and eventually was discharged.

Phosphates may be associated with metastatic calcification and diarrhea but are the most useful agents for out-patient management, particularly with diuretics.

The effectiveness of corticosteroids in hypercalcemia of malignancy is debatable, and the steroid suppression test (to distinguish primary hyperparathyroidism) is in disrepute. Steroids are undoubtedly effective in cases where the underlying tumor is responsive to the drug, in which case the hypocalcemic effect is due to antitumor action. Data also indicate, however, that steroids can inhibit prostaglandin synthesis in animal tumors, thus suggesting a more direct effect on calcium metabolism. Steroids also reduce absorption of calcium in the gut and increase renal excretion of calcium, but these are not dramatic effects. The usual dosage is 60 mg of prednisone (or equivalent) per day in divided doses. The maximal hypocalcemic effect will be seen within four to five days. Because of the toxicity of steroids and their disputed effectiveness, they are reserved for cases in which a direct antitumor effect is anticipated, as for lymphoma, or for secondary or tertiary therapy, where other measures have failed.

Mithramycin, an antibiotic derived from *Streptomyces plicatus*, was developed as a cytotoxic agent that has particular activity against certain testicular carcinomas, but it directly affects the skeleton where it inhibits bone resorption. Because of this site of action, the drug is useful in all cases of hypercalcemia of cancer regardless of the pathophysiologic mechanism. The drug is given in a dosage of

25 mcg/kg intravenously as a "push" or infused over a few hours. The initial fall in serum calcium can be observed in 6 to 12 hours, and the maximum hypocalcemic effect will be seen by 24 to 48 hours after a dose. The effect can last from two days to several weeks. Mithramycin toxicity can be severe.

When the drug was first investigated as an antitumor agent, doses of 25 to 50 mcg/kg were used daily for five days. Toxicities included nausea and vomiting, fever, encephalopathy, and bleeding diathesis. Thrombocytopenia and prolongation of the prothrombin time were common. Azotemia occurred due to damage of renal tubular epithelium, but the toxicity was markedly reduced if the drug was given every other day. Therefore, daily doses of mithramycin must be avoided, but weekly or twice-weekly therapy is generally possible. Hypocalcemia is not often seen with mithramycin therapy but may develop surreptitiously. When used with prudent cautions, mithramycin is safe and dependable and is a mainstay of therapy for hypercalcemia.

Patient J, a 64-year-old man with metastatic hypernephroma, had severe muscle weakness due to hypercalcemia. Initial therapy with intravenous fluids and diuretics failed to lower the serum calcium to normal levels. Oral therapy with phosphate, indomethacin, and steroids also failed to decrease his serum calcium by day seven. Mithramycin was begun with intravenous bolus doses of 25 mcg/kg, and twice-weekly doses were necessary to control the serum calcium without other thrapy. He was maintained on this regimen as an out-patient, and his calcium levels were monitored on a weekly basis.

A major concern in using mithramycin as a hypocalcemic agent is the additive effect with the secondary introduction of cytotoxic antitumor chemotherapy. As mithramycin is a myelosuppressive drug, the marrow effect may be accentuated.

Patient K, a 56-year-old man, had extensive bladder cancer with bone metastases and a serum calcium of 15 mg%. The calcium was resistant to steroids and fluids, and the patient received mithramycin; his calcium fell to 10.5 mg% by day 3. On day 7, the patient received cyclophosphamide and Adriamycin at full therapeutic doses; on day 12 he developed severe leukopenia and thrombocytopenia.

Mithramycin should not be used without dose adjustment to treat hypercalcemia in association with cytotoxic chemotherapy.

Patients with bone metastases have a decreased marrow reserve related to tumor replacement, and the addition of multiple cytotoxic drugs is a major physiologic insult.

The potential role of prostaglandins in the production of hypercalcemia of malignancy has already been discussed; drugs that inhibit prostaglandin synthesis may be potent hypocalcemic agents in such cases. Although measurements of prostaglandins and their metabolites in serum and urine are not generally available, indomethacin and aspirin may deserve an empiric trial for any patient with hypercalcemia, as the side effects are minimal. Beneficial effects of these drugs have been observed in patients with hypercalcemia presumably mediated by the antiprostaglandin effect. Any effect will be seen within three or four days of therapy, so that if no clinical improvement is observed, the drugs can be discontinued.

Prostaglandin-blocking agents (indomethacin and aspirin) should not be used

for patients with hypercalcemia secondary to bone metastases but should be used only when a hormone mediator is suspected.

Aspirin has a less potent effect on prostaglandin synthesis; it is given in dosages of 1.8 to 4.8 g per day. Although its side effects are quite familiar, special mention should be made of its deleterious effect on platelet function; this is particularly hazardous for a patient who already has thrombocytopenia from tumor invasion of bone marrow or from antineoplastic therapy. Indomethacin is given in dosages of 75 to 150 mg per day in three divided doses. The most common side effects are gastritis and gastrointestinal ulceration with bleeding; these can be avoided in some cases by giving the drug with meals or an antacid. A variety of other side effects has been seen, notably blood dyscrasias.

Calcitonin, a hormone derived from the C cells of the thyroid, is secreted in response to hypercalcemia, and causes subsequent lowering of serum calcium and phosphorus. Like mithramycin, the mechanism of action is inhibition of bone resorption. Experience with this agent for patients with hypercalcemia of malignancy has been limited, although the response rate has been high. If the results of two series are combined, 22 of 26 patients showed a hypocalcemic effect with calcitonin therapy, and essentially no side effects occurred. The responses were incomplete, and the duration of action was quite short, so that even with the preparation having the longest duration of action (salmon calcitonin, 200 to 400 MRC units per day), administration at six-hour intervals is required. Therefore, the usefulness of calcitonin is confined to the hospital setting, where other more effective agents are available. This drug has not been approved by the U.S. Food and Drug Administration for the treatment of hypercalcemia.

Serum calcium can be reduced quickly and dependably by dialysis, but this is rarely necessary. For most patients, one or another of the above agents will provide an effective and safe means of control. In the rare patient for whom all of these measures are contraindicated or ineffective, dialysis for control of serum calcium may be helpful, although temporary. For the hypercalcemic patient receiving dialysis for a more conventional indication, the use of a calcium-poor dialysis fluid may provide an additional benefit in control of the serum calcium.

A sequential approach to the treatment of hypercalcemia is crucial, and the individual therapeutic modalities should be employed in sequence. The physician should first establish the effectiveness of a program to preclude adverse effects of complex drugs. Therapeutic response may indicate the pathophysiologic mechanism of hypercalcemia. The time until anticipated response of the calcium level is of some importance in the determination of when to advance to the next level of therapy (Table 6.4).

Table 6.4 Time until response* of hypercalcemia to various agents

Saline and diuretic	6–12 hours
Sulfate	6–12 hours
Phosphate (IV)	6–12 hours
Mithramycin	12–36 hours
Phosphate (oral)	2–4 days
Steroids	3–5 days
Indomethacin	3–5 days
Aspirin	Variable

*Response defined as a decrease in calcium level, but not necessarily to a normal level.

The specific sequence of therapy for hypercalcemia depends on the quantitative calcium level, a quantitative evaluation of the symptoms, the mechanism of hypercalcemia, the type of tumor producing it, and the pattern of metastases if present. Acutely decompensated patients are generally treated with fluids, diuretics, and phosphates, in that order. Resistance of the calcium level is then treated by steroids or mithramycin. In chronically or minimally symptomatic patients, the use of prostaglandin antagonists or a trial of tumor-specific therapy should be employed. A summary of the sequence of therapy is described in Table 6.5.

5.0 Other Disorders of Calcium Metabolism

In addition to the hypercalcemic syndromes, other disorders of calcium metabolism may be observed. Hypocalcemia can develop as a consequence of protein catabolism and inanition, which is a common accompaniment to the cachexia syndrome of cancer. The hypocalcemia is generally preterminal and is not of clinical importance. One consequence of hypocalcemia is the development of secondary clotting abnormalities with bleeding or hemorrhage, but this effect is rare. For the most part, the etiology of hypocalcemia is difficult to assess in the multifactorial preterminal state. Calcium supplements, however, are a common and important aspect of alimentation regimens designed to augment total body mass and immunologic function.

Calcitonin is involved in the normal physiologic mechanism by which calcium levels are regulated in conjunction with parathormone. In patients for whom calcitonin levels are elevated, such as those with medullary tumors of the thyroid, hypocalcemia almost never develops. Furthermore, in the occasional patient with ectopic secretion of calcitonin reported with oat cell carcinoma, hypocalcemia has not been observed.

6.0 Summary

Hypercalcemia represents one of the most common metabolic complications of malignancy and may be observed in the spec-

Table 6.5 Therapeutic sequence for hypercalcemia

	Calcium level	
10–12 mg%	↓ 12–15 mg%	15 mg%
Asymptomatic (genitourinary tract only)	Moderate symptoms (gastrointestinal tract)	Life-threatening (central nervous system)
↓	↓	↓
Indomethacin	Saline	Saline + diuretics
↓	↓	↓
Steroids	Diuretics	Phosphates
	↓	↓
	Phosphates	Mithramycin
	↓	
	Corticosteroids	
	↓	
	Mithramycin	

trum of cancers including epithelial, mesenchymal, and lymphatic tumors. The
pathophysiologic mechanism leading to
hypercalcemia is most commonly associated with direct physical dissolution
of the osseous structure as a consequence
of invasion of the bone, and it is rare that a
tumor-secretory product capable of inducing dissolution of bone can be identified.
The range of clinical presentations of
hypercalcemia emphasizes the need to
monitor calcium frequently, particularly
in patients with bone lesions. A special
clinical circumstance not alluded to in
this chapter is the hypercalcemia that
evolves as a consequence of therapeutic
intervention, particularly in hormone-
sensitive breast cancer. The clinical signs
and symptoms of hypercalcemia may be
subtle or flagrant, but with no direct correlation of the quantitative level of calcium
with the degree of symptomatology secondarily induced.

The many therapeutic approaches to
hypercalcemia involve an increasing
degree of potential complications or secondary effects, but the hypercalcemia
can almost always be controlled by one
method or another with mithramycin, the
final common therapy. The crucial factor
in hypercalcemia, however, is tumor control, and for many of the common tumors
associated with elevated calcium (breast
cancer, prostatic cancer, and multiple
myeloma) effective antitumor therapy is
available. For epidermoid carcinoma,
renal cell carcinoma, and most other tumors, however, the tumor-specific therapy
is limited.

References

Ackerman, N. B., and Winer, N. The differentiation of primary hyperparathyroidism from the hypercalcemia of
malignancy. *Ann. Surg.* 181:225–231,
1975.

Bassett, I. W., and Steckel, R. J. Imaging
techniques in the detection of metastatic disease. *Seminars in Oncology*
4:39–52, 1977.

Bender, R. A., and Hansen, H. Hypercalcemia in bronchogenic carcinoma: a
prospective study of 200 patients.
Ann. Intern. Med. 80:205–208, 1974.

Benson, R. C., Jr.; Riggs, B. L.; Pickard,
B. M. et al. Radioimmunoassay of
parathyroid hormone in hypercalcemic patients with malignant disease. *Ann. Intern. Med.* 56:821–826,
1974.

Brereton, H. D.; Halushka, P. V.; Alex-
ander, R. W. et al. Indomethacin-re-
sponsive hypercalcemia in a patient
with renal cell adenocarcinoma. *N.
Engl. J. Med.* 291:83–85, 1974.

Chakmakjian, Z. H., and Bethune, J. E.
Sodium sulfate treatment of hypercalcemia. *N. Engl. J. Med.* 275:862–
869, 1966.

Flower, R. J. Drugs which inhibit prostaglandin biosynthesis. *Pharmacol.
Rev.* 26:33–67, 1974.

Franklin, R. B., and Tashjian, A. H., Jr.
Intravenous infusion of prostaglandin
E2 raises plasma calcium concentration in the rat. *Endocrinology* 97:140–
143, 1975.

Fulmer, D. H.; Dimich, A. B.; Rothschild,
E. O. et al. Treatment of hypercalcemia—comparison of intravenously
administered phosphate, sulfate,
and hydrocortisone. *Arch. Intern.
Med.* 129:923–930, 1972.

Gordon, G. S.; Cantino, T. J.; Erhardt, L. et
al. Osteolytic sterol in human breast
cancer. *Science* 151:1226–1228,
1966.

Haddad, J. G., Jr.; Couranz, S. J.; and Avioli,
L. V. Circulating phytosterols in normal females, lactating mothers, and
breast cancer patients. *J. Clin. Endocrinol. Metab.* 30:174–180, 1970.

Heath, D. A. Hypercalcemia and malignancy. *Ann. Clin. Biochem.* 13:555–
560, 1976.

Kennedy, B. J. Mithramycin therapy in

advanced testicular neoplasms. *Cancer* 26:755–766, 1970.

Klein, D. C., and Raisz, L. G. Prostaglandins: stimulation of bone resorption in tissue culture. *Endocrinology* 86:1436–1440, 1970.

Lafferty, F. W. Pseudohyperparathyroidism. *Medicine* 45:247–260, 1966.

Levant, J. A.; Walsh, J. H.; and Isenberg, J. L. Stimulation of gastric secretion and gastrin release by single oral doses of calcium carbonate in man. *N. Engl. J. Med.* 289:555–558, 1973.

Lindeman, R. D., and Papper S. Therapy of fluid and electrolyte disorders. *Ann. Intern. Med.* 82:65–70, 1975.

Lindgarde, F., and Zettervall, O. Hypercalcemia and normal ionized serum calcium in a case of myelomatosis. *Ann. Intern.Med.* 78:396–399, 1973.

Mayer, G. P. Habener, J. F.; and Potts, J. T., Jr. Parathyroid hormone secretion in vivo: Demonstration of calcium-independent, nonsuppressible component of secretion. *J. Clin. Invest.* 57:678–683, 1976.

Neelon, F. A. CAMP and calcemia *Ann. Intern. Med.* 86:821–822, 1977.

Mundy, G. R. et al. Evidence for the secretion of an osteoclast stimulating factor in myeloma. *N. Engl. J. Med.* 291:1041–1046, 1974.

Mundy, G. R. et al. Bone-resorbing activity in supernatants from lymphoid cell lines. *N. Engl. J. Med.* 299:867–871, 1974.

Omenn, G. S.; Roth, S. L.; and Baker, W. H. Hyperparathyroidism associated with malignant tumors of non-parathyroid origin. *Cancer* 24:1004–1012, 1969.

Powell, D. et al. Nonparathyroid humoral hypercalcemia in patients with neoplastic diseases. *N. Engl. J. Med.* 289:247–260, 1966.

Robertson, R. P. et al. Plasma prostaglandin E in patients with cancer with and without hypercalcemia. *J. Clin.*

Endocrinol. Metab. 43:1330–1335, 1976.

Seyberth, H. W. et al. Prostaglandins as mediators of hypercalcemia associated with certain types of cancer. *N. Engl. J. Med.* 293:1278–1282, 1975.

Seyberth, H. W. et al. Characterization of the group of patients with the hypercalcemia of cancer who respond to treatment with prostaglandin synthesis inhibitors. *Trans. Assoc. Am. Physicians* 89:92–104, 1976.

Shaw, J. W. et al. Urinary cyclic AMP analyzed as a function of the serum, calcium and parathyroid hormone in the differential diagnosis of hypercalcemia. *J. Clin. Invest.* 59:14–21, 1977.

Silva, O. L., and Becker, K. L. Salmon calcitonin in the treatment of hypercalcemia. *Arch. Intern. Med.* 132:337–339, 1973.

Tashjian, A. H., Jr. Prostaglandins, hypercalcemia, and cancer. *N. Engl. J. Med.* 293:1317–1318, 1975.

Tashjian, A. H., Jr. et al. Evidence that the bone resorption-stimulating factor produced by mouse fibrosarcoma cells is prostaglandin E2—a new model for the hypercalcemia of cancer. *J. Exp. Med.* 136:1329–1343, 1972.

Tashjian, A. H., Jr. et al. Successful treatment of hypercalcemia by indomethacin in mice bearing a prostaglandin-producing fibrosarcoma. *Prostaglandins* 3:515–524, 1973.

Tashjian, A. H., Jr. et al. Hydrocortisone inhibits prostaglandin production by mouse fibrosarcoma cells. *Nature* 258:739, 1975.

Vaughn, C. B., and Vaitkevicius, V. K. The effects of calcitonin in hypercalcemia in patients with malignancy. *Cancer* 34:1268–1271, 1974.

Williams, R. H., ed *Textbook of endocrinology.* 4th ed, p. 312. Philadelphia: W. B. Saunders Co., 1968.

Part III

Oncologic Complications Related to Organ Systems

Chapter 7

Osseous Complications of Malignancy
M. Drew
R. B. Dickson

1.0 Background

Although primary bone tumors are rare, metastatic tumors involving bone are common, and their incidence increase with age. As many as 60 percent of cancer patients will be found to have osseous metastases at autopsy, although only about 30 percent will have had symptoms of osseous metastases while alive. The symptomatic osseous metastases lead to the disabling complications that prevent independent functioning. Early detection and introduction of appropriate therapy depend on awareness of the potential for osseous complications.

Osseous lesions, whether primary or metastatic, create problems for the patient in four ways. First, they commonly cause pain. Second, their ability to destroy or weaken the bone structures can lead to fracture under normal loads and to secondary loss of function. Third, these tumors may interfere with such surrounding structures as spinal cord, peripheral nerve, muscle, or ligament. This interfer-

ence may occur through direct invasion of the lumbar or brachial plexus, by indirect pressure on the spinal cord, or by mechanical collapse and secondary loss of function (see also Chapter 5). A fourth effect of bone metastases is related to medullary cavity involvement. There may be such extensive replacement of bone and marrow by tumor that the normal hematopoietic system is crowded out, leading to leukoerythroblastic changes. All patients with bone metastases have a limited bone marrow reserve.

It is clear that the orthopedic management of these patients depends on general principles of cancer therapy. These principles include early clinical recognition of the problem, comprehensive radiologic evaluation, and multidisciplinary planning of therapy, including specific management of the tumor both systemically by chemotherapy and locally by radiation therapy and/or surgery. The critical orthopedic factor in the treatment of osseous complications of malignancy, which is not part of the treatment of other visceral complications, is the need for external or internal fixation to "carry the load" for the diseased bone during antitumor treatment and osseous healing.

Considerable progress has been made in the past ten years toward both external and internal support systems for bones. Casting materials have improved, although plaster of Paris remains the standby. Removable splints or braces (orthotics) are superior to those available only a few years ago. Internal stabilization of long, weight-bearing bones after pathologic fracture has improved substantially because of both new metallic devices and the use of "bone cement," methylmethacrylate, as a spacer and local support. Prophylactic fixation prior to fracture is used more commonly and has been successful in reducing patient morbidity.

Furthermore, adaptation of joint replacement methods from arthritis surgery has given functional limbs to patients with tumor involvement of hip, knee, and shoulder joints. Segmental resection, coupled with aggressive chemotherapy and radiation of primary bone or soft tissue sarcoma, can spare limbs that previously required amputation. Finally, such experimental orthopedic methods as cadaver transplantation of bones and joints and artificial long bones, particularly the femur and tibia, are developing.

The primary site sources of metastatic bone tumors differ between men and women. For men, in decreasing order of frequency, the primary tumors of the lung, prostate, gastrointestinal tract, and thyroid gland are commonly associated with osseous metastases. For women, the primary tumors of the breast, lung, gastrointestinal tract, and thyroid are the most common tumors metastic to bone. Both breast and prostatic cancer, two hormone-responsive epithelial tumors, develop bone metastases in up to 80 percent of patients (Table 7.1). These account for more than half of osseous metastatic lesions. Although renal lesions have a high frequency of bone metastases, the relative incidence is low compared with that of gastrointestinal cancers.

Bone metastases may be radiologically osteoblastic or osteolytic, but all osseous lesions are a combination of osteolysis and osteoblastic reaction to the tumor.

Table 7.1 Relative incidence and frequency of clinical bone metastases

Primary cancer site	Relative incidence	Frequency of bone metastases
Breast	60%	60%
Prostate		80%
Lung	25%	30%
Gastrointestinal	10%	5%
Renal Cell	3%	25%
Other*	2%	–

*Includes thyroid, melanoma, and lymphoma and other rare or uncommon tumors.

Osteoblastic bone lesions occur with breast, prostate, lung, kidney, and thyroid primary tumors but may occur with tumors from any source.

Tumors commonly producing an osteoblastic bone reaction are breast, prostate, renal cell, lung cancer, and the hematologic malignancies, such as lymphoma. Thyroid and gastrointestinal carcinoma also produce osteoblastic lesions radiographically, as do carcinoid tumors metastatic to bone. The common denominator for most of the osteoblastic- or sclerotic-appearing bone metastases is the slow growth of the lesion, which allows the bone-forming cells to react to the presence of the tumor. Thus, breast, prostatic, and particularly thyroid cancers may implant in the cortical bone and grow slowly. The only tumor that produces little or no osteoblastic reaction is multiple myeloma. One reason for this may be that the tumor is derived from native osseous cells within the marrow cavity and does not seem to elicit an osteoblastic reaction. In fact, there have been fewer than 50 reported cases of osteoblastic multiple myeloma.

Osteoblastic and osteolytic lesions are radiographically and clinically distinct. Osteoblastic lesions less commonly produce pain than do osteolytic lesions. This may be related to the fact that osteoblasts maintain the supporting structure of the bone without expanding the periosteum, which is the primary mechanism for pain production in bone lesions.

Osteoblastic lesions are less frequently associated with pain than osteolytic lesions.

Pathologic fractures are also less common in a bone in which osteoblastic reaction to the tumor is present. It is important, however, to recognize that sclerotic bone, laid down in reaction to tumor, is not deposited along the lines of mechanical stress, as is normal bone deposition to a fracture site, but it encapsulates the tumor resulting in a mechanically compromised bone. Orthopedic management is therefore directed at insuring support, even in the absence of pain.

The spine is the most common site for implantation of osseous metastases, followed in decreasing frequency by the ribs, pelvis, proximal ends of the long bones, sternum, and the cranial vault. The sites of metastases may be influenced by the distribution of blood, although skeletal metastases are more common than would be predicted from the relatively low flow rate of blood to bone. The anatomical distribution of blood may influence tumor emboli to implant in bone. Batson demonstrated that the vertebral venous system, which has no one-way valves, communicates freely with the caval, portal, azygous, and pulmonary venous systems. When intrathoracic or intra-abdominal pressure is increased by coughing, sneezing, or straining at stool, a reversal of blood flow can occur into the venous vertebral system. Thus, the Batson plexus provides a series of passageways by which cancer cells, in addition to the arterial hematogenous route to the bone, can be seeded directly into the bones, bypassing the liver and lungs.

The skeleton is divided structurally and functionally into two overlapping components. The bone marrow cavity functions as a reservoir for hematopoietic stem cells to proliferate and mature. Surrounding the marrow, or medullary cavity, is the bony cortex, which provides the supporting structure for the whole organism. The vascular supply traverses both components of the osseous system, and increases the likelihood of marrow involvement in radiographically demonstrable bone lesions.

Cortical osseous lesions are universally associated with infiltration of medullary bone marrow.

Secondary or metastatic tumors are more common than primary tumors, but the latter affect a younger population and are occasionally radiographically confused with solitary bone metastases. The three common bone tumors are osteogenic sarcoma, Ewing's sarcoma, and chondrosarcoma (Table 7.2). Osteogenic sarcoma, a tumor of young adolescence, is usually a lesion of the extremities. It has been associated in adults with long-standing Paget's disease and as a carcinogenically induced tumor, secondary to radiation in patients with previous breast cancer or with retinoblastoma. Ewing's sarcoma is a primary bone tumor of older adolescence and commonly disseminates to the lungs and lymph nodes. Thus, unlike osteogenic sarcoma, Ewing's tumor is not usually managed by amputation. Both osteogenic sarcoma and Ewing's sarcoma may be manifest as primary extraosseous tumors of the soft tissue, as well as intrinsic tumors of the bone. Chondrosarcoma, unlike the other two tumors, characteristically develops in older people and is commonly found in the appendicular skeleton. These tumors generally grow slowly and recur locally. It is critically important to distinguish primary bone tumors from metastatic bone tumors, and to use radiographic features of the osseous lesion in the determination. Another important tumor in this age group is the benign giant cell tumor of bone which recurs locally, and is only rarely metastatic to other bones or extraosseous sites (Fig. 7.1).

2.0 Diagnosis and evaluations of bone lesions

Osseous lesions may present either synchronously at the time of the primary tumor or metachronously at some interval following detection and treatment of the primary tumor. The principal symptom of metastatic bone tumors is pain, which may be characteristic but is more often nondescript. Typically, the pain, which begins as mild and intermittent, gradually becomes more frequent, more severe, and lasts longer. It is often localized and is usually worse at night. Like the pain of arthritis, it is often activity related and responds to changes in barometric pressure, and may be responsive to such standard antiarthritic remedies as salicylates.

Localized bone pain, in a patient with a known malignancy, must be assumed to be caused by the tumor. Such benign processes as arthritis, Paget's disease, and osteomyelitis, or even incidental nonpathologic fractures, are other diagnostic

Table 7.2 Clinical features of the three common primary bone tumors

Primary bone tumors	Age in years	Location	Primary origin	Metastatic sites
Osteogenic sarcoma	10–30	Metaphysis	Femur, tibia	Lung
Chondrosarcoma	30–50	Variable	Femur, pelvis, ribs	Local
Ewing's sarcoma	4–20	Shaft	Femur, tibia	Lymph nodes, lung, bone, central nervous system (possibly)

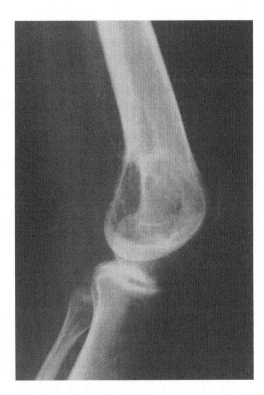

Fig. 7.1 Radiograph of knee of a patient with a giant cell tumor of medial aspect of distal femur with sclerotic margins.

ray demonstrated a solitary nodule with irregular borders presumed to represent cancer. The pulmonary lesion was surgically operable and potentially curable, but the metastatic series showed a solitary lesion of the humerus that was typical for metastases. Open surgical biopsy, however, failed to demonstrate tumor, and the patient underwent exploratory thoracotomy.

Biopsy is necessary for solitary bone lesions, even with prior malignancy, to establish histopathologic confirmation.

---

possibilities. Extraosseous diseases may also cause referred pain; for example, hepatic tumors may cause shoulder pain, and retroperitoneal tumors in the psoas muscle may lead to hip or thigh pain. Postherpetic neuralgia, or shingles, with or without a cutaneous rash, may also mimic bone pain. Finally, bone pain may develop secondary to a tumor-associated process, such as hypertrophic pulmonary osteoarthropathy. The presence of an osseous lesion in a patient with definite or possible malignancy does not by definition mean metastases to the bone. If the bone lesion is solitary, surgical biopsy is mandatory.

Patient A, a 70-year-old man, had chronic pulmonary disease and routine chest x-

The mechanism of pain production by bone lesions is important in planning therapy. The pain may be produced by interruption or stretching of the periosteum, which is replete with multiple nerve plexi over the bone, or the pain may be secondary to a structural defect in the cortex that compresses neural structures. This distinction is important because pain from loss of structural integrity may persist even after effective tumor therapy. In this setting, structural support using braces or other forms of external immobilization may be necessary. An important aspect of bone pain is the consistency of the pain. A sudden alteration of pain often indicates a pathologic fracture complicating a cortical bone lesion.

Patient B, a 55-year-old man with lung cancer, developed a painful solitary bone lesion in the left hip, which was not detectable by standard radiographs although it was evident by bone scan. He was treated with local radiation therapy, but after five fractions had a sudden increase in the intensity of the hip pain. Radiographs demonstrated a fracture of the femoral neck, and surgical placement of an endoprosthesis immediately relieved the pain (Fig.7.2).

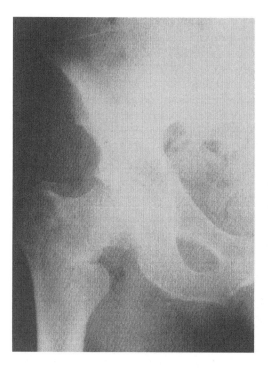

Fig. 7.2 Pathologic fracture through the base of the femoral neck (Patient B).

Acute increase in the intensity of localized pain is indicative of a pathologic fracture.

One unique form of bone pain associated with metastatic lesions is that of diffuse whole-body pain associated with intra-cavitary or intramedullary metastatic tumor. This clinical pattern of pain is unique and often so intense that the patient cannot tolerate even the weight of light clothing or of bed sheets and requires absolute immobility. This type of pain is typical of patients with melanoma, metastatic to bone and bone marrow. The diagnosis may be established by a bone marrow biopsy, even when radiographic studies are normal.

Physical examination is important in localizing the critical lesion and in choos-ing the appropriate orthopedic treatment. Particular attention to areas of localized bone tenderness and to pain associated with motion of joints is indicated. Examination should include the range of active and passive motion of the local area, including joints above and below the suspected lesion. These measurements will provide a basis by which to judge the effectiveness of therapy. Testing for strength and coordination and observing gait and upper-extremity function will help to localize osseous lesions and permit objective determination of progress. Weakness in one muscle or muscle group, such as the quadriceps, suggests either neurological involvement or direct muscle invasion by tumor. Generalized and asymmetrical weakness in an extremity suggests atrophy from the underlying disease or limitation of motion due to pain. Neurologic testing, including sensory and reflex testing, is vital in metastatic lesions of the spine because changes in the neurologic status may signal the onset of spinal cord compression. Observing how patients move, whether they can get on and off examining tables or tie their shoes, often helps decide what ancillary help, such as braces or a walker, may be useful.

The diagnostic evaluation of malignant bone lesions involves radiographic studies designed to evaluate the extent of disease and to define precise sites. The standard radiographic survey or metastatic series can establish the presence of lesions for those patients with pain, if the lesions are advanced and involve more than 50 percent local bone resorption. Tomography of a localized area of pain may be employed to delineate the precise extent of the tumor. Rarely can tomography define a bone lesion when standard radiographs cannot, but it may help to evaluate isolated or solitary lesions identified by bone scanning in such radiologically obscure areas as the sacrum.

The radionuclide scans of bone and

bone marrow are separate studies that use different radionuclides; technetium pyrophosphate localizes within cortical osteoblasts, indium in the marrow reticuloendothelial system. Radionuclide scanning allows detection of disease at an earlier stage than do standard radiographs, and bone lesions can be evaluated within the entire skeletal structure.

Bone scans are more effective than standard radiographs in detection of metastatic lesions.

The superior sensitivity of bone scanning is shown by the appearance of lesions on a scintiscan three to six months before radiographic visualization. The bone scan, while more sensitive than the radiographs, is nonspecific for tumor growth. The radionuclide scan may be inaccurate and may not detect disease when there is minimal osteoblastic response, such as in multiple myeloma. Furthermore, when bone metastases are symmetrical and homogeneous, there is no focus or "hot spot." This occurs occasionally in prostatic or breast cancer when bone becomes homogeneously osteoblastic, and the entire bone skeleton is involved.

The use of radionuclide scanning to monitor patients with known malignancy of the bone is not advocated because the anatomic contour of the lesion is more precisely defined by standard radiographs.

Standard radiographs are more effective than bone scan as a monitor of therapy.

The bone scan may demonstrate persistent or even increased osteoblastic activity with tumor regression representing an osteoblastic healing process (Fig. 7.3).

Another diagnostic procedure, particularly for solitary bone lesions, is arteriography, which defines the precise extent of disease and the tumor vascularity and may be therapeutic by allowing access to perfuse the tumor with fragmented gel foam sponges to induce thrombosis and allow for better control of hemorrhage during an operation.

Closed bone marrow biopsy may be diagnostic for patients with unusual bone pain and can evaluate lesions that are surgically inaccessible. Osseous lesions are almost always multiple and associated with bone marrow invasion, and marrow biopsy is highly pathologic. When the biopsy is performed near the radiographic lesion, the diagnosis may be confirmed for most patients. Even when lesions do not involve the pelvis radiographically, standard iliac crest biopsy may render a diagnosis.

Bone marrow biopsy in standard sites (anterior or posterior iliac crest) may yield diagnostic information even in the absence of specific site involvement.

Biochemical evaluation of bone lesions by serum alkaline phosphatase, calcium, and phosphate determinations, or urinary excretion of hydroxyproline has been erroneously advocated as a diagnostic screen and monitor of bone tumors. These tests are nonspecific and are neither diagnostic nor quantitatively relevant since fluctuations may be related to physiological or other nonmalignant disease processes. They are collectively of little use in monitoring patients with bone metastases.

A summary of the diagnostic procedures for osseous lesions is reviewed in Table 7.3. The most critical procedure is the simple diagnostic radiograph, which defines the lesion in most patients. The ancillary procedures are quantitative assessments and are used only in special clinical circumstances.

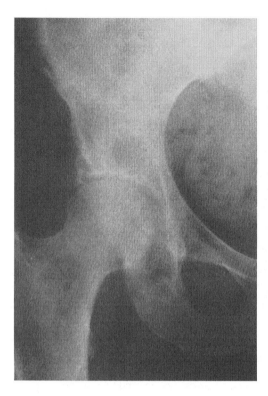
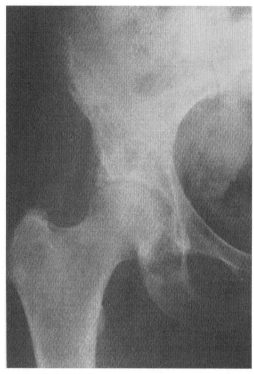

Fig. 7.3 Healing osteoblastic reaction may be indistinguishable from osteoblastic reaction to tumor destruction but the local healing areas are often spherical. Note osteolytic areas (A) with secondary deposition of bone matrix (B).

3.0 General principles in orthopedic management of osseous lesions

The orthopedic management of malignant osseous lesions focuses on the relief of pain secondary to pathologic fracture, the promotion of stability and organ function, and the prevention of secondary osseous complications. Osseous lesions are common sites of metastases and, although not life threatening, may produce major pain requiring palliation. Orthopedic management must be integrated with tumor-specific therapy to increase the palliative effect.

The orthopedic considerations for osseous lesions producing either instability or pain must involve life expectancy and prognosis. The median survival time of pathologic fracture in one large study of metastatic osseous lesions was 37 months; therefore, fixation for pain relief and stability are necessary to maintain the patient's life style. Other critical factors in determining management include the type of primary tumor, the specific site of the osseous lesion, and the local and distant extent of the tumor. The specific therapy for the pathologic fractures involves immobilization and stabilization, reconstruction with either closed or open surgical reduction, and fixation supplemented by local radiation. The tumor-specific therapy, radiation, may either precede or follow the orthopedic procedure.

Internal fixation has been improved by the development of the exothermic cement, methylmethacrylate, which insures

Table 7.3 Diagnostic procedures for malignant bone lesions

Procedure	Purpose
1. Standard radiographic procedures	
Radiographic survey	Detection and monitoring
Radionuclide scan	Detection
Tomography	Delineation of occult lesions
2. Invasive procedures	
Myelography	Detection of spinal cord compression
Arteriography	Delineation of local disease and hemorrhage control
3. Other procedures	
Bone marrow biopsy	Diagnosis of unexplained bone pain or inaccessible bone lesion
Biochemical studies (e.g., alkaline phosphatase)	Nonspecific

the stability of fragments and locks the prosthetic device within the osseous structure. When this is employed as an adjunct to internal fixation, 95 percent of patients who are ambulatory prior to fracture, will regain the ability to walk. Methylmethacrylate does not inhibit the healing of fracture sites, and even for large cortical defects and for periosteal, callous, and new bone formation it will fill the gaps. It is chemically inert, and the toxicity of the monomer and the exothermic reaction is minimal. The substance is introduced into the intramedullary cavity to form a cast, and the internal fixation device is inserted into the cast while the cement is still semisolid. Its solidification reinforces the fixation device to the bone. Structurally inadequate bone may be resected and replaced with methylmethacrylate to bridge the fracture site, thus acting as a permanent spacer and providing stability independent of the metallic fixation device.

Tumor control with radiation therapy is also essential to the local management of the pathologic fracture site. Radiation therapy necessarily affects the osteoblasts

as well as the tumor, and may therefore inhibit healing at local sites. Healing following radiation therapy may not be radiographically evident for more than six months. Unlike radiation, chemotherapeutic drugs, and hormonal therapy in particular, do not interfere with osteoblas-

Table 7.4 Responsiveness of bone metastases to local radiation and systemic therapy

Primary tumor	Response to therapy Radiation	Systemic
Breast	++++	+++
Prostate	++++	+++
Renal	++	−
Lung	++	+
Gastrointestinal	++	+/−
Hematologic	+++	+++

+ = response
− = no response
+/− = equivocal response

tic activity and therefore the use of these forms of systemic therapy may be important. Since bone lesions are rarely solitary, systemic therapy is usually indicated. The response to local radiation or systemic therapy depends on the primary tumor type. All tumors are at least partially responsive to local radiation; systemic therapy affects many but not all metastatic lesions (Table 7.4).

Malignant lesions of the bone, whether metastatic or primary, may be divided into two anatomical groups: (1) metastatic lesions of the appendicular skeleton (long bones) with or without pathologic fracture, and (2) metastatic lesions of the axial skeleton with or without pathologic fractures. Certain orthopedic considerations apply to both groups, and the critical issue is that of surgical or nonsurgical orthopedic treatment. The general aims of treatment are palliation of pain, maintaining reasonable function coupled with local or systemic tumor therapy, and secondarily, promoting healing of the local bone defect.

Current surgical techniques allow fixation either prophylactically or after fracture of virtually all metastatic lesions in the pelvis and long bones. The use of rods, plates, and hip, knee, and shoulder replacements in addition to the use of bone cement are sufficient for most problems. Custom-made devices can be used in special situations. These range from special plates to a complete femur, hemipelvis, and recently, three lumbar vertebrae. Thus, the decision to use aggressive surgical treatment depends on whether nonsurgical techniques can be successful to control the tumor.

4.0 The management of specific osseous metastases

The common sites of osseous metastases are the vertebral column, the ribs, the pelvis, and the proximal long bones. Other common pathologic sites include the calvarium, which rarely causes secondary complications requiring orthopedic intervention. Similarly, pathologic fractures of the ribs infrequently require orthopedic management, and fractures of the humerus are usually treated conservatively with external immobilization and radiation. Orthopedic surgery is predominantly used for lesions of the lower extremity, and the surgical approaches range from fixation with rods and plates to joint replacement.

Appendicular skeletal lesions without fracture. Metastatic lesions to the long bones of the upper or lower extremities are common, generally proximal, and often associated with major morbidity. The lesions of the upper or lower extremities should be treated prophylactically with internal fixation when a lesion is expected to fracture. The decision for internal fixations is based on the degree of cortical involvement for both weight-bearing and non–weight-bearing bones. A 50 percent compromise for cortex and 30 percent compromise for weight-bearing bones are reasonable guides for prophylactic surgical intervention. Protection of the patient with crutches or a walker for partial weight bearing is always recommended in femoral or tibial lesions without internal fixation. Thirty percent of lower extremity weight is alleviated by use of a cane in the opposite hand, and 50 percent may be alleviated with crutches or a walker. This protection should be continued until early bone healing is radiographically evident (usually at least six weeks) and should be accompanied by careful explanation of its reason and probable duration, since a patient's ceasing to comply with these restrictions is the most common reason the conservative nonoperative method of management fails.

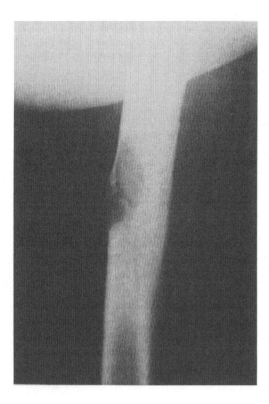

Fig. 7.4 Lytic lesion of the mid-shaft femur (A) with pathologic fracture that developed in Patient C following radiation *therapy and pain relief; internal fixation with Sampson rod (B).*

Patient C, a 76-year-old woman with carcinoma of the breast, presented with pain in the left leg. X-rays showed a lytic lesion of the left femoral shaft occupied about 30 percent of the cross-sectional area. Because of her age and the size of the lesion, radiation therapy and protection with a walker were elected. Two weeks later, walking without her walker at home, she sustained a pathologic fracture (Fig. 7.4) requiring internal fixation with a Sampson rod and cement.

For weight-bearing bones with lesions compromising more than 30 percent of bone cortex, prophylactic internal fixa- **tion prior to radiation is essential. For non–weight-bearing bones (upper extremities) the quantitative bone destruction must involve 50 percent of the cortex.**

Protection is also important in upper extremities. First, patients must be cautioned to restrict use of the extremity and to avoid heavy lifting or sudden loading. A sling, during the day, for patients with humeral lesions, or a removable splint for those with radial or ulnar lesions, is recommended. In addition to protection, pendulum exercises to maintain elbow and shoulder motion at minimal risk are always advisable.

Prophylactic operative fixation of long

bones is usually done by intramedullary fixation with a rod. The Sampson rod, which is very strong and provides excellent proximal and distal fixation, has proven the most useful, but any of the many available devices may be used successfully (Fig. 7.5). Technically, it is important to use the largest device that the individual bone will accommodate. The femoral neck presents special problems in prophylactic fixation. For neck lesions above the intertrochanteric line (an imaginary line between the lips of the greater and less trochanters) multiple pins are best. If the lesion extends into or below the intertrochanter area, fixation with a nail into the femoral head attached to a side plate, a Richards compression screw, an intramedullary device, or a Zickel nail is needed (Fig. 7.6). The introduction of the Ender nail (a flexible device in-

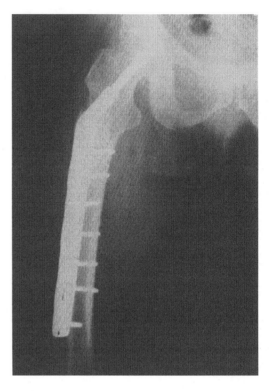

Fig. 7.6 Richards compression screw for pathologic fracture of proximal femur (A); Zickel nail

serted from the medial aspect of the femur and extending into the femoral head), has provided another device useful in both prophylactic and postfracture fixation of femoral lesions from the intertrochanteric line to the lower one-third of the femur. This device is particularly useful because the procedure takes only thirty minutes and blood loss is minimal. For successful fixation, the device selected must extend into bone unaffected by tumor both distally and proximally. Bone cement is rarely needed in prophylactic fixation but may be used.

The primary reason for prophylactic fixation is to decrease morbidity and risk to the patient. Therefore, the surgical procedure required for prophylactic fixation must be compared to that which

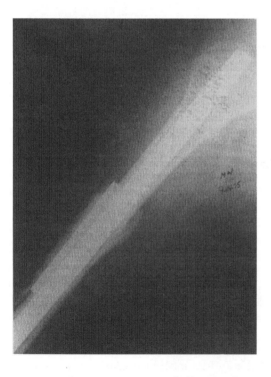

Fig. 7.5 Sampson intramedullary rod supplemented by cement to fill destroyed bone.

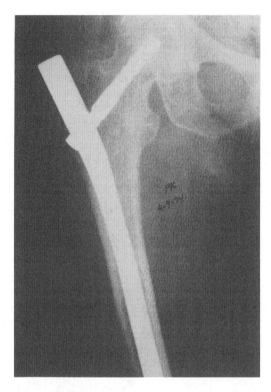

(B) applied for tumor extension inferiorly; and Enders Nail

would be required should fracture occur. If a blind nailing, without opening the area of tumor, or simple pin or nail fixation is needed, the differential for risk between prophylactic and therapeutic surgery is small. If major surgery, such as replacement is necessary for prophylaxis, it is preferable to treat the patient conservatively and to operate only if a fracture does occur or if severe pain or functional limitations are present.

Lesions complicated by pathologic fracture. Pathologic fractures, wherever they occur, are functionally analogous to nonpathologic fractures, and therefore management of the cancer-related fractures is also similar to management of nonpathologic fractures. Pathologic frac-

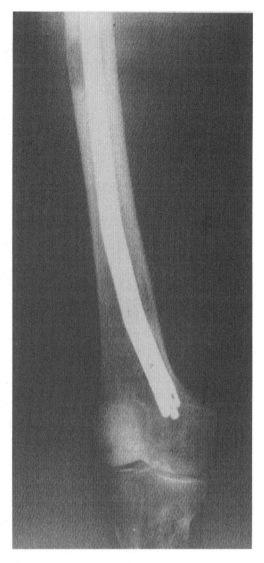

(C) applied prophylactically for a mid-femur lesion.

tures occur, as a rule, in patients who are somewhat systemically debilitated; therefore, the following factors may alter their orthopedic management:

(1) healing of the fracture may be retarded or may not occur at all; (2) bone may be so destroyed in some areas that replacement of whole parts with metal or bone cement is necessary; and (3) there

may be metastases of areas in the same bone or adjacent bone requiring more extensive fixation or replacement. The net effect of the pathologic fracture is to make the surgery for these fractures more radical. The orthopedic surgeons must assume that they are replacing the damaged area of bone rather than supporting it while healing takes place. In this context, methylmethacrylate is a critical element. First, it increases the fixation of metallic implants by filling gaps in bone allowing axial loading without displacement. Second, it can be molded into a bone defect in the cortex after placement of a metal device such as an intramedullary nail or a cortical plate.

As noted previously, local control of the tumor with radiation or with systemic antitumor therapy is always necessary since continued bone destruction will inevitably loosen inserted devices. Antitumor therapy should be started one to two weeks after fracture fixation to allow early soft tissue wound healing to take place. Neither metal nor methylmethacrylate interfere with radiation or chemotherapy.

Postoperative management of physical rehabilitation will vary with individual circumstance, but the use of the extremity is usually possible within days of the operation except where technical problems have prevented adequate fixation. In lower extremities, use of crutches or a cane may continue for several weeks until radiographic follow-up shows that fixation is adequate, and no tumor has recurred.

Fractures of the femoral head and neck. The management of fractures of the head and neck of the femur depends on the extent of bone involvement. Adequate fixation of these fractures requires normal bone in the femoral head itself and little or no bone destruction along the medial side of the femoral neck. In most cases such support is lacking, and fixation of the fracture, if attempted, will be inadequate

and will cause the nail or screw to extrude through the diseased bone requiring surgical revision.

Patient D, a 54-year-old woman with carcinoma of the breast, underwent fixation of a proximal femoral fracture with a Zickel nail (Fig. 7.7). Over the next eight months she walked with a cane but developed severe pain on ambulation. X-rays showed that the nail had protruded superiorly, and the head was moving inward. Proximal femoral replacement with long-stem Bateman prosthesis allowed the patient ambulation free from pain for the three years until her death.

Thus, most fractures at the head and neck of the femur should be treated with surgical replacement. A long stem down the medullary cavity may be used if meta-

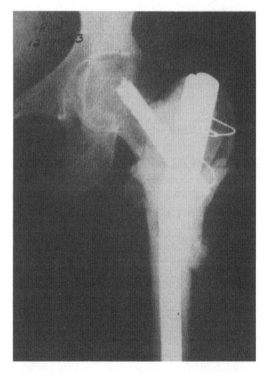

Fig. 7.7(A) Sequential treatment of pathologic fracture of femur: Zickel nail in place.

static disease is present in the shaft, but the stem must extend beyond the distal extent of the lesion.

Most proximal femur fractures associated with metastatic cancer of the femoral head or neck require an endoprosthesis.

Various endoprostheses are available. The Moore prosthesis is the most commonly available device, but the Bateman prosthesis has a high density polyethylene cup between two metal cups and provides a more effective diffusion load over the acetabulum. Fixation of any endoprosthesis should be with cement (Fig. 7.8). Ambulation with crutches is begun within ᵢ 72 hours of surgery and hospital stay averages two weeks.

Total hip arthroplasty, replacing both sides of the hip, is necessary and indicated when there is bone destruction on both pelvic and femoral sides of the joint.

Patient E, a 58-year-old woman with carcinoma of the breast, had received 5000 R to the pelvis over two years for pain control. She was minimally ambulatory on crutches, and radiographs showed extensive destruction of the femur and acetabulum (Fig. 7.9). Total hip replacement was carried out because of persistent pain. Pathology showed no viable tumor but extensive radiation necrosis o, bone. Eighteen months postoperatively the patient was ambulatory on one cane for short distances and on Loftstrand crutches for long distances.

Even with extensive destruction at the

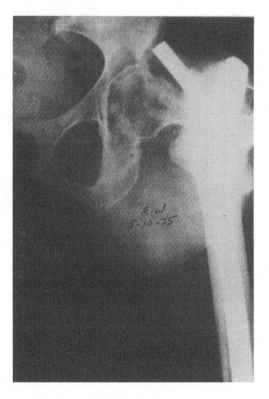

(B) Extension of Zickel nail.

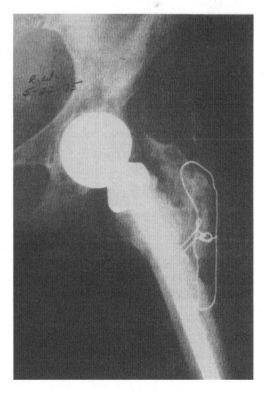

(C) Bateman prosthesis in place.

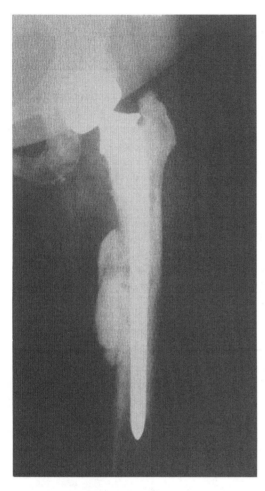

Fig. 7.8 Long-stem Bateman endoprosthesis with cement bridging a medial
femoral control defect and providing fixation for the prosthesis within the medullary cavity necessary because of the diffuse bone involvement.

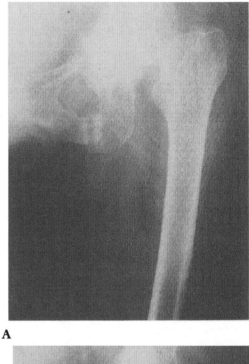

A

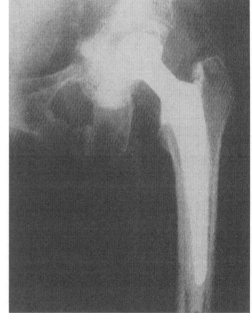

B

pelvic site of the joint, the use of metal
stabilization devices below the cement
with total hip replacement can produce
excellent results.

Patient F, a 45-year-old woman with carcinoma of the breast, was unable to stand
because of pain and weakness. Total hip
replacement with a specially ordered
metal cement retainer fixed to the pelvis
with screws and cement was performed

Fig. 7.9 Pathologic fracture of the femoral
neck with involvement of the acetabulum
(A); the acetabular side is replaced by
a plastic (non–radio-opaque) material indicated by the wire and supplemented
with cement (B).

(Fig. 7.10). The patient was ambulatory with a walker one week postoperatively and at six months with a cane, despite significant peripheral neuropathy unrelated to the procedure.

Such cases as these require careful planning since failure to obtain good anchorage of the acetabular component in the remaining pelvic bone will cause failure of the procedure. Total hip replacement may be employed for cancer patients and is usually indicated if such patients should be candidates in the absence of cancer.

Fractures between the neck of the femur and the shaft at the level of the lesser trochanter are treated in the same way as femoral neck fractures. Replacement of the proximal femur with a long neck prosthesis may be used when there is exten-

sive bone destruction (Fig. 7.11). If the femoral head is not diseased, fixation with a nail plate or Richards compression screw supplemented by cement may be used. Fractures of the femur below the lesser trochanter and above the distal floor of the femur require similar surgical procedures. In the subtrochanteric area, a Zickel nail, Sampson subtrochanteric rod, or Ender nail may be used and all provide excellent fixation (Fig. 7.12). Conservative management of such fractures with cast or cast brace is rare unless surgery is absolutely contraindicated.

Fractures of the distal femur and proximal tibia. Supracondylar fractures of femur or proximal tibia may be managed with cast braces, which have hinges to allow knee motion, if bone involvement

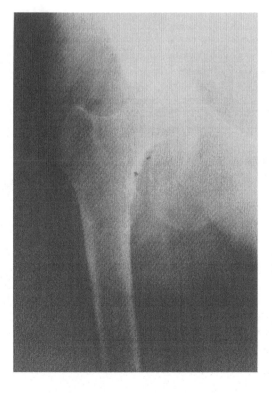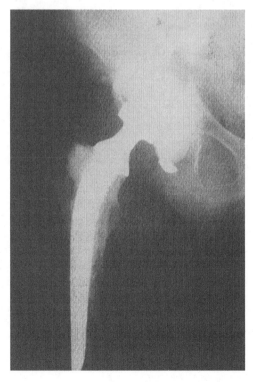

Fig. 7.10 *Metastatic carcinoma predominantly involving the acetabulum and sparing of the femoral head (A); the de-* struction of the medial acetabular wall required total hip replacement with metal cup (B).

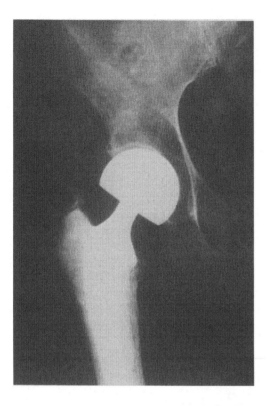

Fig. 7.11 Metastatic breast cancer to proximal femur at the level of the lesser trochanter necessitating long neck prosthesis.

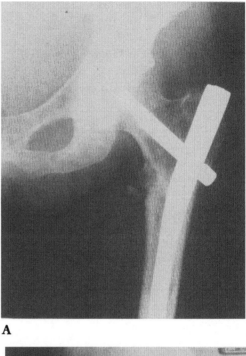

A

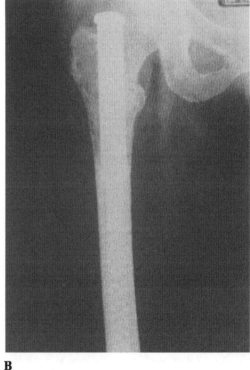

B

by tumor is limited to less than 50 percent of the diameter of the bone. The use of a cast brace allows weight-bearing ambulation and moderately good function, but may interfere with local radiation therapy. A window may be cut in the cast to allow radiation therapy over limited areas. If extensive bone destruction is present, internal fixation is needed. The technique may employ stabilization with rods, cement, and/or mesh (Fig. 7.13). Total knee replacement with a semiconstrained prosthesis may be necessary if subchondral bone is not present to support the articular surface of the knee (Fig. 7.14).

Fractures of the tibia shaft due to metastases are exceedingly rare, and unless extensive destruction is present, these can be conservatively managed by weight-

Fig. 7.12 Pathologic subtrochanteric fracture treated with Zickel nail (A); fracture at more distal level treated with Sampson rod (B).

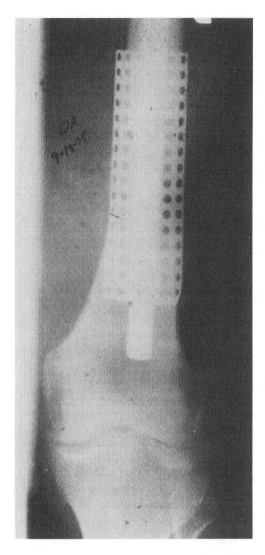

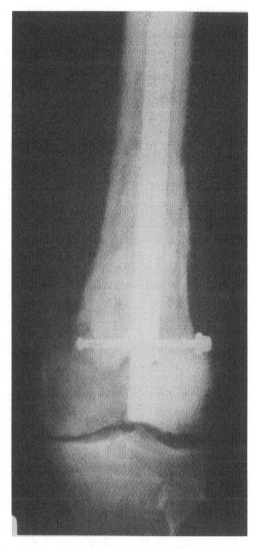

Fig. 7.13 Distal femoral fracture fixed with an intramedullary rod and cement enclosed with stainless steel mesh (A); supracondylar fracture fixed with a rod, cement, and a bolt through cement and rod for rotational stability (B).

bearing casts or cast braces with a window, if necessary, for radiation therapy.

Upper extremity lesions (humerus, clavicle). Since the upper extremity is generally subject to less stress, and temporary loss of the use of one arm does not prevent function for the whole patient, fractures of the clavicle and humerus may be managed without surgical fixation.

Fixation with a rod in the humerus prior to fracture carries little risk and prevents the morbidity of the fracture, but it is seldom necessary. A pathologic fracture of the humerus heals within 8 to 10 weeks, and operative fixation is not necessary.

Fractures of the clavicle are usually treated with a figure-of-eight bandage and local radiotherapy. Such fractures heal within eight weeks. If prior radiation has

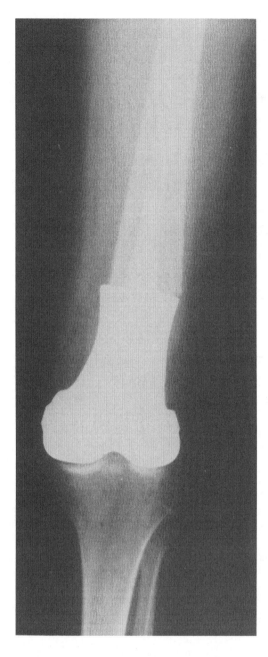

Fig. 7.14 Prosthetic device for knee replacement.

been given to the area, or healing does not take place as expected, excision of the clavicle is the preferred treatment. The clavicle fractures can be pinned if healing

does not take place, but excision is the more satisfactory procedure since it allows immediate use of the arm.

Humeral fractures of the neck and shaft are successfully managed with a sling and swath supplemented by splints and local tumor treatment. If the fracture shows no callous by eight weeks or if gross motion is then felt at the fracture site, replacement of the proximal humerus or internal intramedullary fixation should be carried out.

Patient G, a 56-year-old woman with carcinoma of the breast, sustained a pathologic fracture of the humeral shaft. Treatment included sling, swath, and radiation. No healing occurred, and the patient could not use the arm because of pain and gross instability. Internal fixation with cement and rod was performed, and the patient regained use of her arm within six weeks (Fig. 7.15).

Upper-extremity pathologic fractures may be managed by tumor-specific treatment; operative intervention is necessary only in the absence of radiographic healing.

Fractures of the supracondylar area of the humerus are internally fixed when nonpathologic and should be conservatively treated when pathologic fractures occur. The same principle applies to fractures of the radius and ulna.

Axial Skeletal Lesions. The axial skeleton, including the skull, spine, and pelvis, is the most common site of metastasis to the osseous system. Skull lesions are not clinically important because they do not have significant symptoms. Occasionally, these lesions cause mild or profound headaches and may expand to involve the dura and brain substance or the

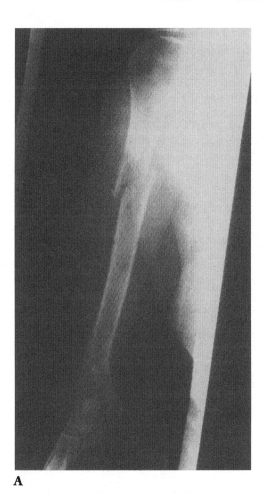

A

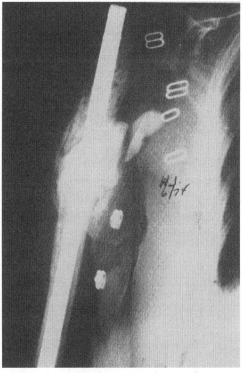

B

Fig. 7.15 Pathologic fracture of the proximal third of the humerus without healing at three months (A); fixation with rod and cement restored stability (B).

contiguous facial bones including the orbit. These effects are uncommon, however, and therapy generally involves radiation to the localized areas if significant symptoms develop.

Spinal and pelvic metastases are, in contrast to skull metastases, often associated with major secondary symptoms. Spinal metastases may be classified into cervical, thoracic, and lumbar lesions; the orthopedic treatment for each is somewhat different. The three major questions evaluating lesions of the spine are: (1) is there an associated neurologic deficit; (2) is the osseous structure of the spine unstable; and (3) is the quality of the bone in and around the tumor lesion adequate?

Lesions of vertebral bones may lead to pain, instability, or neurologic defects, depending upon the vertebral level and the extent of tumor involvement.

A neurologic deficit in patients with spinal metastases must be treated as an oncologic emergency because spinal cord compression is a major complication (see also Chapter 5). Impingement on the cord may be a consequence of epidural tumor or secondary subluxation of the vertebral column. The stability of a laminectomy or a spinal decompression procedure is a major goal and may require structural support by internal fixation.

*Patient H, a 32-year-old woman, had met-
astatic renal carcinoma to many spinal
vertebrae. She presented with progressive
thoracic back pain and developed
marked weakness of the lower extremities
within two days. Myelography demonstrated spinal cord compression, and the
patient underwent a posterior decompression with removal of a large implant of
epidural tumor. The extent of tumor
within the thoracic vertebra mandated
stabilization of the spinal column. Harrington rods with hooks anchored in lamina with supplemental bone cement stabilized the spine (Fig. 7.16). Eight months
later there was neither weakness nor back
pain.*

Surgical decompression is recommended for almost all patients with neu-

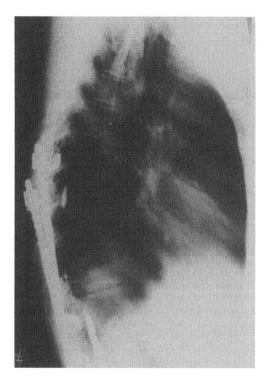

Fig. 7.16 *Stabilization of thoracic spine
with Harrington rods (Patient H) following
extensive decompression.*

rologic symptoms of spinal cord compression, except those for whom neurologic
symptoms and particularly paraplegia is
dense and has been present for more than
five days.

Stability of the spinal column is a crucial
aspect of orthopedic management of
spinal metastases. If the spine is stable,
and subluxation has not appeared and is
not imminent, spinal metastases may
be treated symptomatically. If subluxation
has or will occur, internal or external
orthopedic support during treatment and
healing are essential to avoid neurological
sequelae. The radiographic parameters for
determining stability for vertebral column
metastasis are kyphos angle, pedicle facet
involvement, and degree of vertebral
subluxation. Solitary lesions of the vertebral column or body are always stable
unless collapse develops with an acute
kyphos of more than 70°. Neurologic
changes associated with extreme kyphosis
are produced by traction on the spinal
cord, and external bracing may be applied
to prevent the neurological complications. Pedicle or facet joint involvement
by tumor, particularly if unilateral, is
likely to produce subluxation and must be
braced externally. Scoliosis of more than
15° in the anterior projection across two
vertebrae is almost always secondary
to destruction of the pedicle and facet.

Subluxation of the vertebral body of
more than three millimeters laterally signals instability in spinal column metastasis and requires orthopedic intervention.
In the presence of any of the three radiographic abnormalities associated with
vertebral metastases (increasing kyphosis,
scoliosis, or subluxation), orthopedic
support is mandatory. The goals of therapy
for vertebral metastasis are to relieve pain
and to obviate neurologic deficit. This
distinction is crucial, and for patients in
whom treatment for pain is all that is
indicated, the critical ingredient is relief
of the stress placed on the osseous structure. External support with such devices

as corsets, braces, and body jackets is supplemental to, not a replacement for, bedrest. Palliative treatment of the imminent or acute neurologic complications requires external or operative stabilization. External support may be applied either singularly or in conjunction with internal support, but it must persist until healing is evident. External supports include the Halo-vest or body cast as well as many types of removable supports. Internal supports for the spinal column are generally provided by the Harrington rods with a posterior surgical approach.

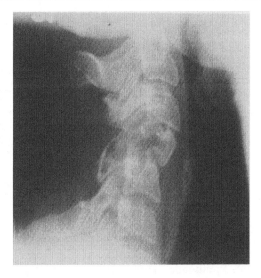

A

Cervical spine lesions. Internal fixation is never required for lesions of the cervical spine unless a decompressive laminectomy is indicated. Internal fixation invariably involves the use of Harrington rods or spinous process wiring of adjacent vertebrae with a cement pack. External fixation of cervical spine lesions is often applied with the halo apparatus. The halo is an elliptical metal ring fixed to the skull by four to six pins imbedded in the outer table of the skull and attached to a metal structure rigidly fixed within a body cast or a plastic vest. The halo apparatus achieves absolute immobilization of the cervical spine and can reduce displacement of cervical vertebrae. With such a device, even grossly unstable cervical lesions may be treated. The only contraindication is the presence of cranial metastasis with the potential danger of perforation of the dura. The apparatus is well tolerated and can be applied with local anesthesia and the pins left in place for up to three months. Patients are invariably capable of walking and are self-sufficient.

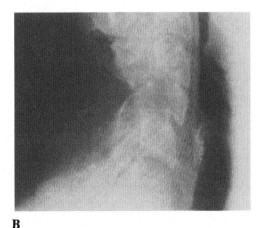

B

Fig. 7.17 *Cervical spine involved with metastatic carcinoma and destruction of C4 with forward subluxation of C3 on C5 (A); reduction maintained in a halo until bone healing was achieved (B).*

Patient I, a 22-year-old woman with disseminated breast cancer, had diffuse involvement of the cervical spine and early subluxation (Fig. 7.17). She was placed in a halo and received local radiation therapy to the cervical spine, which

promptly relieved pain. Within two months, early bone healing was evident, and the halo was replaced by a soft cervical collar.

Another type of cervical stabilization device is the SOMI (sternal- occipital- mandibular-immobilizer), which can be used effectively when the halo is contraindicated because of associated skull lesions. The SOMI is particularly effective in preventing flexion or extension of the cervical spine, which is critical particularly in odontoid lesions (Fig. 7.18). Rigid or soft cervical collars are used for symptomatic treatment and do not effectively immobilize cervical spine. This type of external support should be used rarely for patients with an unstable spine since each support does not prevent neurologic complications.

Thoracic and lumbar spinal lesions. In the thoracic spine, the support from the anterior ribcage usually prevents subluxation; external and internal support are therefore rarely indicated but occasionally necessary (see Patient H). More often, lesions of the thoracic spine are treated symptomatically with local radiation therapy.

Lumbar vertebral lesions are less likely to develop secondary neurologic sequelae since the spinal cord ends at the second lumbar vertebra. Furthermore, although the lumbar spine is subjected to major stress with ambulation and everyday activities, the paraspinous muscle and tendons and the structure of the osseous lumbar vertebrae provide sufficient support. Nonetheless, nerve entrapment may result in serious neurologic deficits and pain; since lumbar metastasis often causes pain, local radiation therapy is commonly used.

Pelvic lesions. Lesions of the pelvis rarely lead to neurologic deficits but lesions of the pubic ramus, ischium, and acetabulum do have major secondary effects and preclude ambulation in some patients. Surgery for these lesions is rarely indicated. Radiation therapy is invariably employed for pain relief. Limited weight bearing using a walker is usually possible except in fractures of the acetabulum, associated muscle weakness, or other

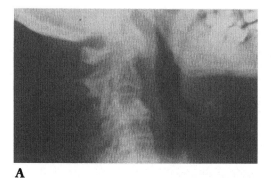

A

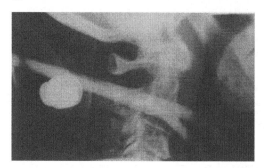

B

Fig. 7.18 Odontoid fracture with forward displacement of C1 on C2 (note malalignment of spinous processes) (A); displacement reduced and maintained in SOMI brace (B).

physical limitations. In acetabular lesions, if the head collapses into the socket either superiorly or medially, total hip replacement may be necessary to relieve pain and promote ambulation.

Amputation in the orthopedic management of metastases. Amputation may be a curative procedure for primary or locally recurrent extremity lesions, either bone or soft tissue sarcoma. Metastatic lesions to the extremities, however, rarely require amputation simply because of the extent or localization of the destructive process.

Patient J, a 52-year-old man, presented with a fibrosarcoma of the maxilla eroding into the maxillary sinus. Surgical exci-

sion and local radiation controlled the
local tumor promptly and completely, but
two years later he developed pain in the
left leg and lytic lesion of the tibial plateau
was observed with radiography (Fig.
7.19). There was no evidence of other distant metastases, but the tumor involved
the joint and supporting structures of
the knee. Amputation was necessary because the knee was unstable, and tumor
margins would have been inadequate
in any operative procedure designed to be
limb sparing.

Amputation as a palliative procedure for bone metastases is required in rare instances.

Palliative amputation in this case was
designed to provide optimal functioning
but not total tumor control. Thus, a disar-
ticulation is not indicated if a shaft amputation is above the disease and capable
of providing an optimal bed for a
prosthesis.

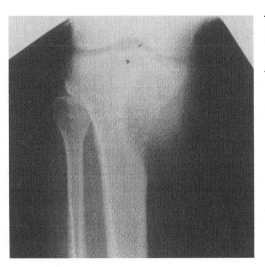

Fig. 7.19 Fibrosarcoma of the proximal
tibia necessitating amputation.

A major complication of amputation is
the development of phantom limb pain.
The sensation of a persistent limb is often
associated with excruciating, narcotic-
resistant, distal extremity pain. The mechanism of the pain is unknown, and therapeutic maneuvers, including nerve block,
transcutaneous nerve stimulation, hypnosis, and acupuncture have had relatively
little impact. The pain often persists for
months but eventually the intensity
recedes.

Aseptic necrosis of the femoral head. In
patients with malignancy, many therapeutic agents have been implicated in the
secondary development of aseptic necrosis of the femoral head. The lesion is specifically associated with the long-term
use of corticosteroids but may also develop
as a consequence of therapeutic radiation
to the hip area. Aseptic necrosis has also
been reported as a delayed complication
of relatively short-term chemotherapy
in Hodgkin's disease and non-Hodgkin's
lymphoma. Hip pain in such patients
is generally due not to the underlying disease, but to the osseous necrosis.

Aseptic necrosis of the femoral head is a therapeutic complication of malignancy and most common in lymphoma.

The management of aseptic necrosis of
the femoral head, secondary to radiation
or chemotherapy, invariably requires
surgery.

*Patient K, a 26-year-old woman, had had
Stage IV Hodgkin's disease for 10 years.
She had received a total of 6000 R to the
inguinal node areas exposing the femoral
heads. In addition, she had received intermittent MOPP chemotherapy. She
developed localized hip pain without radiographic changes when the disease
was in remission, and she had been off*

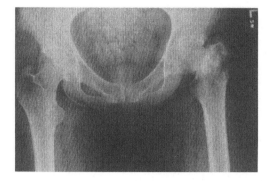

Fig. 7.20 Femoral neck fracture (Patient K) secondary to radiation and chemotherapy; no evidence of malignancy but with total bone necrosis of femoral head.

therapy for at least one year. The hip pain increased until she was unable to walk and radiologic studies revealed femoral head necrosis and femoral neck fracture (Fig. 7.20). Total hip replacement resulted in complete restitution of function.

Conservative management is generally possible for an extended period employing non–weight-bearing measures, but if life expectancy is substantial, and the underlying disease is controlled, early surgical approaches may be applicable.

5.0 Summary

The osseous complications of malignancy are common since the skeletal structure is the most frequent site of metastasis of some of the most common tumors in humans. Osseous metastasis is accompanied by pain, pathologic fracture, myelophthisic anemia, and disturbances of calcium homeostasis. The diversity among secondary effects of bone metastases require multidisciplinary approaches to diagnosis and therapy.

Orthopedic management of such structural defects as pathologic fractures is important to maintain stability and function and to relieve pain in axial and appendicular skeletal lesions. Internal fixation and prosthetic replacement are important considerations in prophylaxis and therapy of both primary and secondary osseous lesions (Table 7.5). Conservative or nonoperative intervention is advis-

Table 7.5 Devices used for fixation of metastatic lesions of bone

Cervical spine	
Stable	Soft collar
	"Philadelphia" collar
Unstable	SOMI brace
	Halo jacket
Dorsolumbar spine	
Stable	Corset
	Brace (Taylor, Norton, Brown, etc.)
	Body jacket (plaster or plastic)
Humerus	Cast
	Intramedullary rods

Table 7.5 *Continued*

Radius and ulna	Plates and screws (A-O) Intramedullary rods
Acetabulum	Total hip replacement
Femoral neck	Multiple pins Richards screw Proximal femoral replacement (Bateman or Moore prosthesis) Total hip replacement
Intertrochanteric area	Richards screw Ender nails Proximal femur replacement
Subtrochanteric	Ender nails Sampson rod Zickel nail Long neck proximal femoral replacement (Bateman, total hip replacement)
Femoral shaft	Intramedullary rods
Knee (distal femur, proximal tibia)	Cast Brace Total knee replacement
Tibia	Cast Intramedullary rod Plate and screws (A-O)

NOTE: Bone cement with or without mesh may be used to supplement any of the above devices.

able for non–weight-bearing and unstressed skeletal structures.

A critical part of the total management of osseous metastasis involves radiation and chemotherapy. Local radiation therapy is essential to promote tumor control and supplements any orthopedic procedure that could be compromised by secondary overgrowth of tumor. Radiation therapy relieves pain in most patients, irrespective of the type of tumor, although some lesions, such as breast and prostate cancer, myeloma, and lymphoma, are exquisitely responsive. A delicate balance must be maintained because radiation therapy affects the healing osteoblast reaction and inhibits tumor expansion. Therefore, effective tumor cell kill can result in loss of structural support and an inability to heal the local lesion.

Chemotherapy, including hormone treatment, is an essential part of the total management of osseous metastasis. These frequently responsive tumors may be controlled in distant sites and prevented from growing and reseeding local bone areas. Osteoblasts are not readily affected, and healing may proceed in the face of tumor cell kill. The healing rate, however, is generally slow.

In addition to the therapeutic role of the orthopedic surgeon and the medical and radiation oncologists, the support services of diagnostic radiology, physical medicine, and rehabilitation are important and essential ingredients in the effective management of osseous metastases.

References

Altman, H. Intermedullary nailing for pathological impending and actual fractures of long bones. *Bull. Hosp. Joint Dis.* B:239–251, 1952.

Bhalla, S. K. Metastatic disease to the spine. *Clin. Orthop.* 73:72, 1970.

Borak, J. Relationship between the clinical and roentgenological findings in bone metastases. *Surg. Gynecol. Obstet.* 75:599–604, 1942.

Bremner, R. A., and Jelliffe, A. M. The management of pathological fracture of the long bones from metastatic cancer. *J. Bone Joint Surg.* 40-B:652–659, 1958.

Carpenter, P. R., et al. Angiographic assessment and control of potential operative hemorrhage with pathological fractures secondary to metastasis. *Clin. Orthop.* 123:6–8, 1977.

Clain, A. Secondary malignant disease of bone. *Br. J. Cancer* 19:15–30, 1965.

Fager, G. A. Management of malignant intraspinal disease. Surg. Clin. North Am. 47:743, 1967.

Fidler, M. Prophylactic internal fixation of secondary neoplastic deposits in long bones. *Br. Med. J.* 1:341–343, 1973.

Francis, K. C. Role of amputation in treatment of metastatic bone cancer. *Clin. Orthop.* 73:61, 1970.

Griessmann, H., and Schuttemeyer, W. *Chirurg* 17–18:316–333, 1947.

Harrington, K. D. et al. Methylmethacrylate as an adjunct in the internal fixation of malignant neoplastic fractures. J. Bone Joint Surg. 54-A:1665–1676, 1972.

Harrington, K. D. et al. Methylmethacrylate as an adjunct in internal fixation of pathologic fractures. *J. Bone Joint Surg.* 54-A:1047–1054, 1976.

Henderson, F. R., and Sheinkop, M. D. Management of osseous metastases. *Seminars in Oncology* 2(4):399–404, 1975.

Hussbau, H., et al. Management of bone metastasis multidisciplinary approach. *Seminars in Oncology* 4(1):93–97, 1977.

Jaffe, H. L. *Tumors and tumorous conditions of the bone and joints.* Philadelphia: Lea and Febiger, 1958.

Marcove, R. C., et al. Cryosurgery in treatment of solitary or multiple bone metastases from renal cell carcinoma. *J. Urol.* 108(4):540–547, 1972.

Michelson, M. R., and Bonfiglio, M. Pathological fractures in the proximal part of the femur treated by Zickel nail fixation. *J. Bone Joint Surg.* 58-A:1067–1070, 1976.

Parrish, F. F., and Murray, J. A. Surgical treatment for secondary neoplastic fractures. *J. Bone Joint Surg.* 52-A:665–686, 1970.

Schurman, D. J., and Amstutz, H. Treatment of neoplastic subtrochanteric fractures. *Clin. Orthop.* 97:108, 1973.

Zickel, R. E., and Mouradian, W. H. Intramedullary fixation of pathological fractures and lesions of the subtrochanteric region of the femur. *J. Bone Joint Surg.* 58-A:1061–1066, 1976.

Chapter 8

Gastrointestinal Complications of Malignancy
R. Reinhold

1.0 Background

Primary gastrointestinal malignancy, particularly colon cancer, is the most common visceral tumor in humans. As in other cancers, the clinical management of intestinal tumors is related to the natural history of that tumor, the stage or extent of disease, and the responsiveness of the tumor to various therapeutic modalities. Tumors within the gastrointestinal system are often occult for long periods and present clinically only after extensive disease is already established. Furthermore, gastrointestinal tumors are generally resistant to therapeutic radiation and chemotherapy. The resistance of gastrointestinal tumors to these modalities is an important consideration in determining a therapeutic approach to the major complications of intra-abdominal malignancy.

The three major gastrointestinal com-plications of malignancy are obstruction, hemorrhage, and perforation with peritonitis. Complications attributable to the accessory gastrointestinal organs, such as the liver, biliary tree, and pancreas as well as peritoneal surfaces, are clinically manifested as ascites, jaundice, and maldigestion. Because the gastrointestinal tract is the primary source of alimentation in humans, the clinical manifestations of gastrointestinal disease are weight loss, inanition, and marasmus (protein depletion).

The three most common gastrointestinal complications of malignancy are bleeding, obstruction, and perforation, all of which are best managed surgically.

In contrast to such visceral systems as the respiratory and genitourinary tracts, complications that evolve within the gastrointestinal tract are generally related to primary as opposed to metastatic malignancy. With the exception of metastasis to the liver, metastatic disease to the gastrointestinal system is uncommon [Table 8.1].

2.0 Gastrointestinal obstruction

The most common gastrointestinal complication of malignancy is obstruction of the intestinal lumen. Obstruction is rarely complete. Symptoms of gastrointestinal obstruction may be intermittent; subtle alterations in bowel habits often reflect colonic lesions, while nausea and vomiting usually reflect upper-gastrointestinal lesions.

Therapeutic management of gastrointestinal obstruction from esophagus to rectum and including the biliary tree generally requires surgical bypass or decompression. Surgery should be undertaken for any patient in whom intubation, either by nasogastric or Miller-Abbott tube, must be maintained to decompress the proximal bowel. Gastrointestinal obstruction is invariably associated with colicky pain and rapid inanition, and in the absence of multiple sites of obstruction, surgical decompression should be performed. The type of surgical procedure varies with the site of obstruction and the extent of tumor (Table 8.2). In general,

Table 8.1 Gastrointestinal complications of primary and metastatic malignancy

Complication	Primary tumor	Metastatic tumors
Obstruction		
Esophageal	Esophagus	Breast
Gastric/duodenal	Stomach/pancreas	Lymphoma
Small bowel	Varied sites (jejunum most common)	Ovary/breast/lung/colon/ melanoma
Colon	Left colon and rectum	Lymphoma
Biliary tree	Bile duct	Pancreas
Hemorrhage	Stomach, right colon	Rare
	Small intestine	Melanoma
Hepatic metastases	Hepatoma	Most common sites: stomach and pancreas, 80% colon, 40% esophagus, 60%
Ascites	Mesothelioma	Hepatic metastasis (e.g., breast, ovary, colon) Serosal implants (ovary) Pseudomyxoma peritonei (bile duct, appendix ovary)

resection is undertaken even in the presence of metastases to prevent contiguous tumor growth into adjacent segments of bowel and therefore potential reobstruction.

Esophageal obstruction. Esophageal obstruction is marked by dysphagia, which frequently progresses over a period of weeks and months. Dysphagia may cause a transition from solid to liquid foods, and finally an inability to handle salivary secretion. Partial obstruction may progress to complete obstruction if a large bolus of solid food is ingested. Recurrent upper respiratory tract infections and cough can develop as a consequence of a disordered swallowing mechanism, with intermittent pulmonary aspiration occurring during periods of somnolence.

An esophageal tumor will on occasion invade the muscular walls and other mediastinal structures such as the trachea, and form a tracheo-esophageal fistula because of the anatomic lack of a defined serosal layer. Management of the esophageal lesion depends on the site of the primary tumor (upper, middle, or lower third). Only 14 percent of patients with esophageal carcinoma are curable with either surgical resection or primary radiation therapy; more than 50 percent of all

Table 8.2 Surgical management of obstruction in the gastrointestinal tract

Site	Options	Objective
Esophagus	Tumor resection: esophagogastrectomy, colon interposition	Cure
	Dilatation/intubation	Palliation
	Cervical esophagostomy	Palliation
Gastric	Partial gastrectomy	Cure
	Bypass: gastrojejunostomy	Palliation
	Gastrostomy	Palliation
Small bowel	Local resection	Cure/palliation
	Local bypass: enteroenterostomy	Cure/palliation
	Complete bypass ileostomy	Cure/palliation
Colon	Local resection	Cure
	Temporary colostomy with or without immediate tumor resection	Palliation
	Cecostomy	Palliation
Biliary tract	Intubation (T-tube with external drainage)	Palliation
	Roux-en-Y and resection of biliary tree or pancreas	Cure
	Choledochojejunostomy or cholecystojejunostomy	Palliation
	Hepatic-enteric anastomosis	Palliation

esophageal cancers are not surgically resectable at the time of presentation. In patients who are technically operable, primary esophagectomy and esophago-gastrostomy is the treatment of choice for maximum palliation, even in the presence of local or distant metastases. The risks of surgery should be carefully considered, however, because surgical mortality is substantial in these patients, owing to technical surgical difficulties, to the general inanition associated with the tumor, and to diseases associated with esophageal cancer, such as alcoholism and chronic lung disease.

For proximal lesions, those above the aortic arch, radiation therapy is the treatment of choice. Surgical treatment requires either colon interposition or, if the tumor cannot be resected, a cervical eso-phagostomy and gastrostomy. Interposition is technically difficult with a high mortality, and the latter is difficult for the patient to manage. For distal lesions, those of the middle and lower third, primary esophago-gastrostomy is necessary. In patients in whom the tumor is not surgically resectable, mechanical intubation of the esophagus by placement of a Souttar's or Celestin's tube may be necessary. The tube is inserted using endoscopy or using gastrostomy and by wedging it through the tumor in the esophageal fistula formation.

Radiation therapy is an alternative form of palliation for esophageal lesions and has achieved a cure rate comparable to surgery, but complete obstruction is rarely alleviated adequately. Radiation therapy may be associated with significant secondary edema and esophagitis. Combined modality therapies employing surgery with preoperative or postoperative radiation have increased the potential for cure while maximizing the duration of palliation. One major complication of combined modality therapy has been the development of stricture formation;

intermittent esophageal dilatation with bougienage is used for such patients.

Esophageal obstruction is maximally palliated by surgery combined with radiation.

The radiographic features of esophageal obstruction are typical for carcinoma and are only infrequently confused with obstruction secondary to achalasia. Occasionally, metastatic disease to the esophagus may produce a radiographic picture of achalasia. When metastases do arise in the esophagus, the primary tumor is generally a breast carcinoma. Invasion of bronchogenic carcinoma to the esophagus is common.

Patient A, a 45-year-old man, presented with a four-month history of weight loss (25 lb) and on close questioning revealed a progressive intolerance of solid foods. At presentation the patient could ingest only eggs and liquids. Barium swallow demonstrated a large distal esophageal lesion with stricture (Fig. 8.1).

Upper-gastrointestinal obstruction (stomach and small intestine) Whereas dysphagia is the most common symptom in esophageal obstruction, obstruction of the stomach, duodenum, and small bowel produces intermittent emesis. Obstruction is the most common symptom of small bowel tumors because of the narrow lumen. It is less common with pancreatic tumors, which may obstruct the biliary tree before the intestinal lumen is compromised, and uncommon also in gastric tumors, where the large lumenal space generally allows for mucosal interruption with bleeding before obstruction develops. For tumors of the pancreas, a gastroenterostomy is generally indicated if the tumor invades the wall of the duodenum. For obstruction secondary to gas-

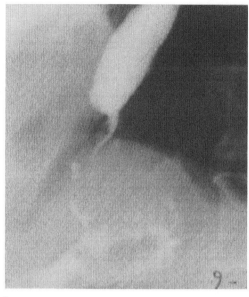

A

Fig. 8.1 Barium swallow demonstrated large irregular lesion at the gastroesophageal junction with irregular interruptions of the mucosal lining (A). The contrasting lesion of the barium swallow (B) demonstrates smooth tapering of the barium column without mucosal interruption secondary to extrinsic compression from mediastinal lymph nodes due to metastatic breast cancer.

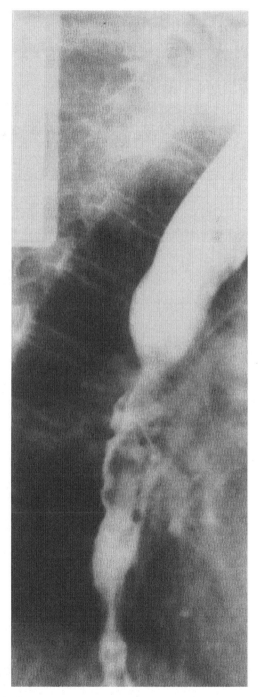

B

tric cancer, surgical resection of the tumor is desirable if it is operable and even if metastasis has occurred; if resection is not technically practical, a gastrojejunostomy to the posterior wall of the stomach may provide adequate bypass and prevent recurrent obstruction.

For gastric tumor obstruction, bypass and tumor resection are indicated if technically possible.

The most common site of obstruction in the upper-gastrointestinal tract is the small bowel. Obstruction is commonly associated with metastatic disease to the small bowel, as primary tumors of the small intestine are extremely rare. The therapeutic dilemma of small bowel obstruction is that the obstructions are often multiple, as metastases are the most common etiology, and therefore either multiple entero-enterostomies or an ileostomy may be necessary to alleviate the obstruction. In most instances, a trial of Miller-Abbott tube decompression should be attempted before resorting to an exploratory laparotomy for decompression.

Small bowel obstruction is most often due to metastases, unlike obstruction of other sites, which is generally due to the primary tumor.

The most common tumors metastatic to the small bowel, causing obstruction, are ovarian, breast, and colon cancers, and occasionally melanoma.

Patient B, a 46-year-old woman, presented with a large pelvic mass, and at laparotomy had a Stage III ovarian carcinoma. She was treated with chemotherapy for four months with regression of all measurable tumor; at laparoscopy, no residual tumor was evident. Six weeks following laparoscopy she developed typical symptoms of small bowel obstruction. In spite of a seven-day course of Miller-Abbott decompressive therapy, her obstruction persisted. At exploratory surgery, the patient was found to have multiple sites of partial small bowel obstruction and nearly complete obstruction of the sigmoid colon. Ileostomy was required for palliation.

Lower-gastrointestinal obstruction (colon and rectum). Primary tumors of the colon and rectum are the most common malignancies of the gastrointestinal tract. Lesions of the descending and sigmoid colon are more frequent than those of the cecum and ascending colon. The clinical manifestations of the left-sided lesions are

obstruction because (1) the stool becomes dehydrated and forms mass and bulk and (2) tumors in the left colon are frequently circumferential, thereby effecting a decrement in lumen size.

Obstructive carcinomas of the left colon have a significantly lower potential for cure than do tumors of the transverse or right colon; this may be due to the late development of obstructive symptoms. Obstruction over a protracted period carries the risk of perforation, particularly at the cecum. As with other sites of gastrointestinal obstruction, surgery is the treatment of choice, and therapy depends upon the site of obstruction and the availability of distal anastomotic sites. Surgical decompression and primary anastomosis for colonic obstruction depend on a careful assessment of the bowel wall, the extent of disease, and the potential for secondary complications at the anastomotic site (Table 8.3). A temporary or permanent colostomy may be necessary if the disease is regionally extensive or if another major morbid disease precludes primary resection and anastomosis. The stoma site for a colostomy is important for patient tolerance and must be carefully planned. Preservation of the sigmoid generally allows for ease of stoma and bowel function management with greater patient acceptabil-

Table 8.3 Surgical principles of decompression of colonic obstruction

1. In the presence of perforation and significant sepsis, decompress without anastomosis.

2. In the presence of long-standing obstruction, decompression permits reconstituting alimentation prior to definitive surgery.

3. Anastomosis should be side-to-side to maximize lumen and minimize reobstruction possibility.

ity. Increased stool consistency permits management by daily irrigation (Fig. 8.2).

Two types of colostomy are used for decompression. The transverse colostomy is created in the right-upper quadrant supra-umbilically, where it is easy to bring the transverse colon to the anterior abdominal wall. In a temporary colostomy, the colon is brought up in loop fashion. In a permanent transverse colostomy, patient management is facilitated if the colon is divided, and the proximal end is brought out in the upper quadrant where it can be easily fitted with an appliance. The distal colon is brought to the left of the mid-line as a mucous fistula and requires no appliance. In a sigmoid colostomy, the stoma is placed in the left-lower quadrant just above the belt line, where a colostomy appliance can be easily fitted without interfering with normal clothing. A sigmoid colostomy is usually performed as an end stoma because it is more difficult to obtain sufficient colon to bring both limbs to the same anatomic site. In addition, the end colostomy permits a tighter seal with ostomy devices. The

mucous fistula, which is created to obviate a blind pouch above the obstruction, can be placed anywhere in the left-lower quadrant. In abdomino-perineal resection, there is no distal mucous fistula. In the Hartman procedure, the distal colon is resected and the rectum oversewn.

A mucous fistula must be created when there is low-lying sigmoid or rectal obstruction, for to close in the sigmoid with distal obstruction would create closed-loop intestinal obstruction. Cecostomy, a temporary drainage procedure to relieve acute obstruction when resection of the distal point of blockage is planned, is not a useful procedure in cancer patients, as the appliances are ill fitting, and the obstruction is often unresectable. Thus, for obstructive right-colon lesions, either right colectomy with end-to-end anastamosis or permanent ileostomy is technically more acceptable than cecostomy.

Patient C, a 62-year-old man, presented with a two-year history of progressive obstipation and three months of tenesmus. Rectal bleeding had not been obvious,

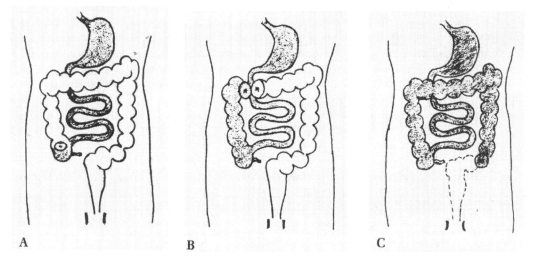

A   B   C

Fig. 8.2 Three types of colon decompression: cecostomy, which should always be a temporary decompressing procedure only (A); transverse colostomy, which is the most common form and is readily manageable (B); and sigmoid colostomy, which is generally an end colostomy with an associated mucous fistula (C).

but the stool was benzidine positive and the hemoglobin 7 gm%. Examination revealed a large (seven-cm) rectal lesion, which was fixed posteriorly and extended anteriorly onto the bladder, lying approximately 5 cm from the anal verge. Abdominal x-rays and barium enema revealed typical features of obstruction (Fig. 8.3). At laparotomy, the tumor was found to be confined to the pelvis, and the bowel was distended. A sigmoid colostomy with distal mucous fistula was performed. Subsequently the patient received pelvic radiation and abdominal perineal resection was planned.

Obstructing lesions of the colon must be bypassed by enterocolostomy or external colostomy with or without a primary initial resection.

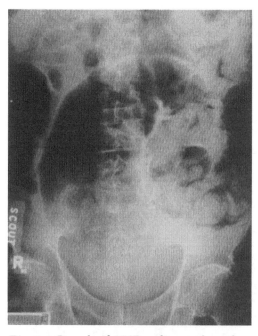

Fig. 8.3 Standard KUB radiograph and barium enema demonstrated obstructive lesion of the rectum with accumulation of enormous fecal material throughout the colon (Patient C).

The choice of primary resection for rectal lesions with anastomosis, or anterior resection, versus an abdomino-perineal resection depends upon the site of tumor; lower lesions (at < 7 cm) require A–P resection to provide tumor-free margins. Alternative therapy (fulguration or radiation) may avoid colostomy, and the decision is based on clinical features of the tumor. Small lesions posteriorly located in the rectal pouch are ideally suited for electrocoagulation.

In contrast to obstruction of the small intestine, obstruction of the colon rarely occurs as a complication of metastasis to the bowel wall. Pelvic tumors (ovary, cervix, bladder) tend to displace rather than compress or invade the sigmoid colon.

Perforation. Perforation of the colon with fecal contamination of the peritoneal space can develop in a variety of circumstances. Local perforation can occur in association with local sepsis in tumors that grow contiguously through the bowel wall. Complete obstruction of the left colon with massive distention of the cecum may lead to perforation.

Perforation secondary to distal obstruction and distention of the proximal colon may result in generalized peritonitis.

The incidence of perforation increases substantially when the cecal diameter exceeds 15 cm. Emergency transverse colostomy is necessary in such patients, as cecostomy is not an optimal procedure.

Patient D, a 62-year-old woman, presented with intermittent abdominal pain and a 12-cm mass on pelvic examination. Barium enema demonstrated a perforated lesion in the left colon (Fig. 8.4), and the patient underwent a diverting colostomy and a primary sigmoid resection without

The third clinical circumstance in which perforation can develop is when the tumor forms the entire thickness of the bowel wall; this problem occurs particularly in lymphomas of the gastrointestinal tract. Radiation therapy causes rapid dissolution of tumor, which results in acute perforation. Primary resection and anastomosis may be attempted in the presence of local sepsis, but the majority of such cases require fecal diversion initially, with or without primary tumor resection.

3.0 Biliary tract complications

Abnormalities within the biliary tree may result in (1) malabsorption of ingested food because of the inability of bile salts to digest fats; (2) jaundice, secondary to deposition of bilirubin in the skin; and (3) the most annoying complication, pruritis, secondary to deposition of bile salts in the skin. Pruritis often requires palliation. The combination of jaundice and pruritis invariably implies obstruction of the biliary tree. Jaundice without pruritis may simply be a manifestation of intrahepatic disease and an inability of the liver's secretory system to handle the increased load of bilirubin.

Pruritis usually follows obstruction of the biliary tree and is due to bile salt deposition, not to increased bilirubin.

The differential diagnosis of biliary tract complications includes common duct stones and hepatocellular disease. Tumors affecting biliary drainage are varied. The most common tumor to cause painless obstructive jaundice is a tumor of the pancreas involving the head although bile duct tumors are also associated with the symptom complex. In rare instances metastatic tumors can produce jaundice and biliary pruritus, particularly in breast

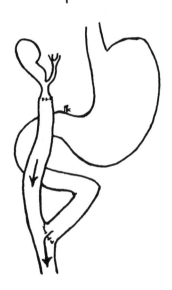

A

B

Fig. 8.4 Surgical decompression of the biliary tree may be accomplished by a cholecystojejunostomy (A) or by a choledochojejunostomy employing a rous-en-Y (B). The former procedure is more likely to be associated with recurrent jaundice.

anastomosis. Four weeks postoperatively, a colostomy closure was performed.

Local colonic perforation commonly occurs as a consequence of tumor growth through the bowel wall.

---

cancer or as a consequence of lymphomatous infiltration of the retroperitoneum with extension into the porta hepatis.

Patient E, a 62-year-old woman, had breast cancer in 1968 and developed multiple bone lesions in 1975. She developed progressive itching over two months, and just prior to admission was noted to have developed dark urine and light stools. On examination she was deeply jaundiced and had multiple excoriations. She was treated with local radiation therapy to the porta hepatis area after ultrasonography demonstrated enlarged nodes in the retroperitoneum. The tumor receded, and the patient's condition improved dramatically.

Another major complication of biliary obstruction is ascending cholangitis, which commonly develops in association with primary bile duct tumors. Controversy exists regarding the relationship of sclerosing cholangitis to bile duct carcinoma.

Almost invariably, surgery is the optimal therapy for biliary obstruction. The procedures employed depend upon the primary tumor, its resectability, and the extent of the local tumor. In the elderly and gravely ill, the simplest immediate procedure is external drainage by insertion of a T-tube. For most patients, however, internal diversion is preferable because it avoids the difficulties encountered with external collection devices.

Surgical procedures used to alleviate biliary obstruction are the choledochojejunostomy or the choledochoduodenostomy, although the latter is often difficult because of tumor size and position (Fig. 8.5). For patients in whom a bypass procedure is successful, the decrease in jaundice occurs over two to four weeks, while pruritus generally recedes within days. Cholecystojejunostomy, using the gallbladder as the anastomotic site, may be

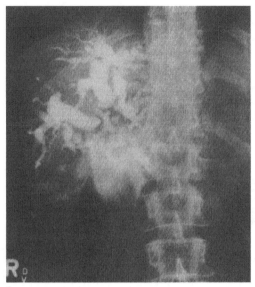

A

Fig. 8.5 Dilated biliary radicles demonstrated by transcutaneous hepatic cholangiography (A). Insertion of needle with catheter results in decompression of the biliary radicles (B, C).

complicated by the reappearance of jaundice secondary to tumor encroachment on the cystic duct.

Biliary diversions result in gradual decrease in jaundice, and relapse implies an inadequate bypass or extension of the tumor.

In patients with extensive local tumor precluding adequate drainage or access to an anastomosis by the gallbladder or extrahepatic biliary tree, the Longmeyer procedure, Hepaticojejunostomy, may be employed. Medical therapy with cholestyramine may be used for patients who have partial biliary obstruction. The rationale for using this drug is that cholestyramine binds bile salts, thus preventing reabsorption and bile salt deposition in the skin.

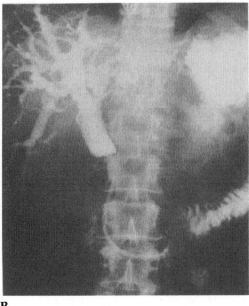

B

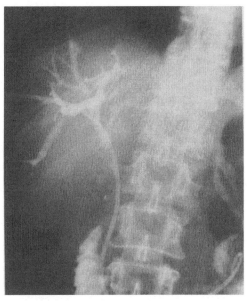

C

4.0 Hemorrhage in the gastrointestinal tract

Gastrointestinal hemorrhage associated with malignancy of the gastrointestinal tract (e.g., carcinoma of the cecum) is generally indolent and is commonly detected by occult blood in the stool. Two-thirds of all patients with gastric cancer have anemia, but only 10 percent present with hematemesis. Tumors most commonly presenting with gastrointestinal bleeding are cancers of the stomach, cecum, and rectum. The differential diagnosis to be considered for cancer patients who have internal gastrointestinal bleeding includes coagulopathies related to the malignancy, such as thrombocytopenia, and incidental diseases, such as aspirin-induced gastritis and polyposis with secondary colonic hemorrhage. The external bleeding associated with rectal tumors is rarely exsanguinating and because of its bright red color is often confused with local hemorrhoidal bleeding.

The most common cause of anemia in patients with malignancy is gastrointestinal blood loss (iron deficiency).

Metastatic tumors that cause hemorrhage in the bowel are unusual, as the tumors generally implant on the serosal surface. In an occasional patient, however, mucosal interruption may result in occult but significant bleeding.

Patient F, a 77-year-old woman, presented with right-lower quadrant pain and anemia (hematocrit 22 percent). Occult blood was detected and the patient had noted intermittent melena. Barium enema was equivocal, but colonoscopy defined a lesion of the hepatic flexure.

Patient G, a 45-year-old woman with malignant melanoma known to be metastatic to various cutaneous sites, presented with a chronic anemia that had all the typical features of iron deficiency, includ-

ing a 4 + benzidine-positive stool. The patient underwent gastroscopy, colonoscopy, and an upper-and lower-GI series, but no lesion was found. She subsequently underwent laparotomy because of a transfusion requirement of three units of packed cells per week. At operation, recurrent melonoma with two jejunal lesions, which had eroded through the mucosa, were resected completely, and no further bleeding ensued.

Surgery is the primary therapy for gastrointestinal hemorrhage, although local radiation has been used for both gastric and rectal lesions. In low rectal lesions fulguration may be employed, but primary resection is generally necessary to definitively control bleeding, whether or not the mucosal lesion is associated with metastases.

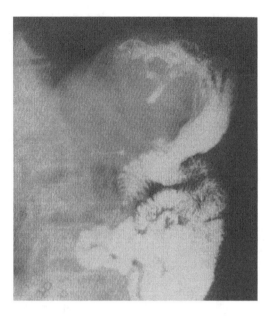

Fig. 8.6 Upper-GI series demonstrating leiomyosarcoma of the stomach with typical features of superficial ulceration.

Patient H, a 69-year-old woman, presented with early satiety and anemia. An upper-GI series demonstrated a lesion of the cardia (Fig. 8.6) with typical radiographic features of leiomyosarcoma. At operation the liver was found to be extensively replaced by tumor. Partial gastrectomy was performed to control bleeding in spite of the presence of the liver metastases.

Resection of the primary tumor is often necessary to palliate local symptoms in spite of the presence of metastases.

In the patient presenting with metastases synchronous with discovery of an asymptomatic primary tumor, therapy should be directed at the metastases, as prognosis is determined by the presence of secondary disease.

5.0 Hepatic metastases

The liver filters the portal circulation from the gastrointestinal tract. Therefore, it is

not surprising that the liver is a major implantation site of metastases from gastrointestinal tumors. In some patients the liver may be the only site of metastasis; only rarely is a solitary metastatic lesion within the liver observed. The secondary effects of such metastases are jaundice, ascites, portal hypertension, hepatomegaly, and painful distention of Glisson's capsule. Hepatic metastases are often associated with fever, which may result from the liver's inability to detoxify endotoxin released from the bowel, or from tumor necrosis. Anorexia and an altered nutritional state are also common accompaniments of hepatic metastases.

Hepatic metastases cause a variety of clinical manifestations (pain, fever, altered nutrition), but rarely produce hepatic coma.

The therapeutic management of hepatic metastases generally involves systemic chemotherapy. It is unfortunate that chemotherapy is relatively ineffective for the vast majority of tumors that metastasize to the liver, and is particularly unsuccessful in colon cancer. Even in those patients who have chemotherapy-responsive tumors, hepatic metastases are often resistant to treatment. A number of local therapeutic procedures have therefore evolved in an attempt to improve responses. Hepatic resection of metastases should only be undertaken in patients with solitary lesions.

Patient I, a 55-year-old woman, had had a primary rectal carcinoma and was well for three years. Routine follow-up examination revealed an elevation of the alkaline phosphatase. Liver scan demonstrated a large solitary lesion of the right dome of the liver, which was confirmed by angiography. The patient underwent an 80 percent resection of the liver (extended right hepatectomy), for no other evidence of intra-abdominal disease was found at surgery. On postoperative day two, the liver enzymes rose to maximum levels (SGOT 200, LDH 1500) and the bilirubin reached 3 mg%, but all returned to normal by day seven. The plasma carcinoembryonic antigen fell from 128 ng-ml to 80 ng-ml by the tenth postoperative day.

The other surgical procedure involved in the treatment of hepatic metastases is dearterialization, or interrupting the arterial supply to the tumor by ligation of the hepatic artery. The same goal can be achieved by infusing substances that cause embolization within the tumor. Infarction of the tumor is associated with necrosis of normal liver tissue as well, but the resulting ischemic hepatitis is short lived, and the blood supply to the normal liver is regenerated over six weeks. These procedures are palliative and may yield short-term control in 25 to 50 percent of patients.

Another local modality is the infusion of chemotherapeutic agents, either by the surgical placement of a hepatic artery catheter or by the transcutaneous placement of a hepatic artery catheter under radiologic guidance. The rationale for chemotherapy with a catheter infusion is that the higher dose provided by directly bathing the tumor may allow for a substantially higher intracellular drug dose and a higher likelihood of response. In institutions where hepatic artery infusion is performed with expertise, the response rate for agents such as 5-fluorouracil may approach 60 percent.

Finally, in patients with end-stage disease or in whom the primary symptom related to liver metastases is pain, radiation to the liver may provide excellent palliation. In such patients, 2500 rad may be delivered (maximum hepatic tolerance to avoid radiation hepatitis) over 10 to 14 days. Although hepatic radiation causes gastrointestinal side effects, enlargement of the liver leads to displacement of the gastrointestinal tract, so that radiation exposure to the bowel is minimal. The median survival of patients treated by hepatic irradiation is five months.

In patients who have hepatic metastases synchronous with discovery of the primary tumor, one of the therapeutic modalities for the metastases must be considered, particularly if the primary tumor is asymptomatic.

Patient J, a 59-year-old woman, presented with iron deficiency anemia and right-shoulder pain secondary to massive hepatic metastases from an asymptomatic cecal carcinoma. She was treated with hepatic infusion of 5-fluorouracil, which resulted in dramatic regression of liver size and a decrease in plasma carcinoembryonic antigen from 3700 ng-l to 1400 ng-ml. Three months after the infusion, a

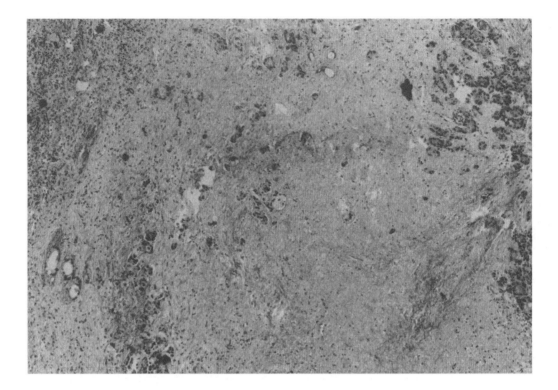

Fig. 8.7 Liver biopsy specimen (Patient J) demonstrating necrosis and fibrosis of the tumor following infusion chemotherapy.

right hemicolectomy was carried out for a Duke's C lesion. Liver biopsy showed necrosis and fibrosis as well as tumor (Fig. 8.7).

It is critical that the symptomatic disease be treated first and that a sufficient time interval elapse before treating the asymptomatic primary lesion.

Metastases determine prognosis in the presence of an asymptomatic primary tumor; therefore, initial therapy should be directed at the metastases.

6.0 Ascites

Ascites is observed in 5 to 50 percent of patients with malignancy. While occur-ring in few patients with breast or lung cancers, ascites is common in patients with ovarian tumors. Ascites frequently occurs as a consequence of multiple tumor implants along the peritoneal surfaces and exudation of a high-protein content fluid. Ascites also develops in association with hepatic metastases, which lead to increased portal pressure and secondary transudation of serous fluid. In both circumstances, the therapy is palliative. Patients who have pain from abdominal distension, inanition resulting from protein loss into the ascitic fluid, or compression of intra-abdominal viscera with early satiety can be managed by periodic paracentesis (see also Chapter 13).

Two forms of ascites unique to cancer patients are: (1) chylous ascites secondary to interruption of the cisterna chyli by retroperitoneal malignancy, particularly lymphoma, and (2) pseudomyxoma peritonei. The latter produces a gelatinous material exuded throughout the abdominal cavity in association with a mucocele of the appendix or bile duct, or with ovarian cystic and mucin-secreting carcinomas. Management of these forms of ascites often involves surgery or repeated paracentesis. Because the prognosis for ascites-producing tumors may be measured in years in spite of the extent of tumor, and therapeutic efforts should be vigorous.

7.0 Anorexia, maldigestion, and malabsorption

Anorexia, maldigestion, and malabsorption commonly accompany cancer, and can lead to weight loss and marasmus, causing immunosuppression and intolerance to therapy. The mechanism of anorexia is unknown; maldigestion may result from an insufficiency of enteric enzymes, particularly the exocrine function of the pancreas and the biliary tree, and malabsorption results from abnormalities within the bowel wall, surgical therapy such as short bowel syndrome, or radiation enteritis.

The end result of these complications is often a vicious circle of events that results in deterioration of the patient's condition. Methods of alimentation, both enteral and parenteral, may interrupt the circle and promote tumor responsiveness to therapeutic modalities. The specific management of nutritional complications of malignancy is discussed in Chapter 14. Both enteral (oral supplements) and intravenous hyperalimentation may reverse and possibly prevent nutritional loss. Assisted alimentation can augment the patient's ability to endure tumor-specific therapy, but the use of hyperalimentation to sustain life for a patient with an incurable and untreatable tumor should be avoided. Hyperalimentation is contraindicated in the patient with end-stage, pre-terminal, symptomatic cancer.

8.0 Gastrointestinal pain syndromes

Abdominal distress associated with obstruction of the gastrointestinal tract generally presents early as colicky pain. Relief of obstruction and secondary bowel distention can be effectively achieved by tube drainage or surgery. Three additional pain syndromes related to gastrointestinal malignancy are unusual but characteristic and recalcitrant to therapy, because surgery is not feasible and other tumor-specific therapies are generally ineffective. These syndromes are hepatic pain secondary to massive distention of the liver; retroperitoneal pain secondary to pancreatic carcinoma infiltrating the paraspinal musculature; and pelvic pain secondary to rectal, bladder, or cervical cancers that invade the presacral plexus.

Hepatic metastases may cause abdominal pain by either of two methods. First, individual lesions may implant on the liver surface and undergo necrosis, producing distention and inflammation of the peritoneal surface along with pain. Second, metastatic lesions may lead to massive liver replacement with tumor and progressive distention of the Glisson's envelope. For the most part, tumors within the liver parenchyma, such as hepatomas and carcinoid tumors, are resistant to systemic therapy. Carcinoid tumor is the most common metastatic tumor to lead to a protracted clinical course with massive liver distention. In such instances the use of hepatic irradiation of up to 3000 R over two or three weeks may lead to significant pain reduction.

Pancreatic carcinoma typically invades the retroperitoneal space and the neural structures. The resulting pain is similar to chronic low-back pain secondary to arthritic disease of the lumbar spine. It is unusual, however, for patients with pancreatic carcinoma to have a long history of back pain prior to detection of the tumor. Radiation therapy may temporarily ameliorate the pain, but the tumor invariably becomes resistant to irradiation. Neuro-surgical procedures are ineffective, and the use of celiac nerve block has been of only transient benefit.

The most difficult of the gastrointestinal pain syndromes is pelvic pain and tenes-mus, a persistent, painful sensation of the need to defecate. This syndrome is the major disabling complication of colorec-tal carcinoma and is caused by extension of the tumor into the rectal cul-de-sac. Often associated with partial obstruction, this pain syndrome may also occur in conjunction with other pelvic tumors, but is most characteristic of rectal cancer. Although colostomy may relieve the ob-struction and divert the fecal stream, the syndrome does not abate completely and may require lumbar cordotomy. Fre-quently, pelvic or perineal pain develops in patients who have had previous sur-gery for rectal cancer in the absence of a definitively palpable mass or who have disease detectable by biopsy.

Patient K, a 72-year-old woman, com-plained of pelvic discomfort, which had been associated with an intermittent in-ability to defecate for 12 months. She had had a sigmoid carcinoma resected five years previously. Complete evaluation, including bone scan and sigmoidoscopy, revealed no evidence of tumor. Plasma carcinoembryonic antigen level was ele-vated, at 11.5 ng-ml. The patient under-went exploratory laparotomy; although no tumor was visible, biopsies of the retroce-cal space demonstrated nests of carci-noma cells.

The development of pelvic pain in pa-tients with a previous history of colon or rectal cancer is presumptive evidence of tumor recurrence even in the absence of a palpable mass.

Recurrent gastrointestinal cancer is some-times not detectable clinically because of occult localization of the tumor and its growth in linear sheets with secondary scar tissue, as opposed to its coalescence into a solid mass. Furthermore, pelvic irradiation is a commonly used therapy, and as a result, recurrent tumor cells may be imbedded in fibrous tissue. Pelvic pain in patients not having previously received radiation therapy may be treated with irradiation. Response is variable and often transient, and neurosurgical procedures may be necessary, but in the absence of a unilateral pain syndrome, the neurosurgical success is limited.

9.0 Gastrointestinal complications re-lated to drugs and electrolyte abnormali-ties

Drug therapy and electrolyte imbal-ance can produce metabolic disturbances that result in constipation, emesis, and diarrhea. For patients receiving narcotic analgesics for abdominal pain, secondary constipation may cause accentuation of the pain and may produce an increased need for narcotics. Thus, a continuing cycle of pain and narcosis may develop. In patients receiving narcotics, it is often necessary concomitantly to employ stool softeners and mild cathartics to maintain the fecal stream flow. Another drug-related gastrointestinal complication is bleeding that can develop from salicylate-induced gastritis. Many analgesic preparations contain salicylates, which may induce disorders of platelet function and increase the potential for mucosal bleeding, partic-ularly in patients with thrombocytopenia.

The types of drugs most particularly associated with gastrointestinal complica-tions in malignancy are the cytotoxic chemotherapeutic agents (see Chapter 18). The nausea and vomiting induced by these drugs develops predominantly as a consequence of stimulation of the emetic center in the central nervous system. The pattern of vomiting varies according to the drug or combination of drugs used. For example, cyclophosphamide induces vomiting, particularly in conjunction with Adriamycin, approximately 4 to 5 hours following intravenous injection and lasts an additional 8 to 12 hours; in contrast, nitrogen mustards induce vomiting approximately 45 minutes following injection, and the vomiting lasts approximately 4 to 5 hours. Dacarbazine (DTIC) is associated with profound emesis that recedes as the drug is injected on a daily schedule, a phenomenon referred to as tachyphylaxis. In most if not all situations, chemotherapy-induced vomiting is transient and acute and, as it is related to a basic central nervous system stimulatory effect, may be suppressed by sedation.

The antimetabolites—5-fluorouracil, cytosine arabinoside, and methotrexate in particular—induce vomiting often in association with diarrhea, particularly for the fluoridated pyrimidine, and are related mechanistically to a direct effect on the colonic mucosa. All such effects are dose related and may be minimized by dose adjustment. The schedule of drug administration may accentuate or minimize the drug effect. For example, 5-fluorouracil may be administered at higher doses without gastrointestinal toxicity when given by a continuous infusion. In contrast, methotrexate, if administered by continuous infusion, promotes adverse gastrointestinal effects.

The chemotherapeutic agents that are natural products (i.e., plant alkaloids) induce gastrointestinal complications primarily as a consequence of a neurogenic paralysis of the bowel, producing paralytic ileus.

Patient L, a 55-year-old woman with renal cell carcinoma, was treated with a single dose of vincristine. She had had no prior gastrointestinal symptoms, but over the course of one week was unable to have a bowel movement and developed abdominal distention unassociated with colic. Examination revealed absent bowel

sounds, and the rectal ampulla was filled with solid stool. Abdominal x-ray demonstrated a massively dilated large bowel with fecal impaction.

For patients in whom acute abdominal distention develops secondary to paralytic ileus, the clinical picture may be attributed to obstructive lesions; patients rarely require laparotomy for disimpaction. For the most part, the periwinkle alkaloid's effect on the bowel is dose related, but occasionally an idiosyncratic reaction develops from extreme sensitivity to the drug.

Electrolyte abnormalities that induce secondary gastrointestinal effects in malignancy are hypercalcemia and hypokalemia. In both instances constipation is a prominent symptom, and particularly with hypercalcemia anorexia, nausea, and vomiting are often present. Hypokalemia may be caused by excessive diarrhea or vomiting, but if the mechanism of hypokalemia is, for example, diuretic urinary loss, then secondary constipation may occur. Correction of the electrolyte abnormality results in rapid reversal of the syndrome.

10.0 Special tumors of the gastrointestinal tract

The three tumors of the gastrointestinal tract that produce specific gastrointestinal symptoms are carcinoid tumors, islet cell tumors of the pancreas, and lymphomas.

Carcinoid tumors can originate throughout the bowel from the stomach to the rectum. They appear to be more common in the distal colon and are clinically indistinguishable from other intestinal tumors. The carcinoid syndrome develops in a small proportion of patients with hepatic metastases. For such patients, gastrointestinal complications may include hypermotility of the bowel, crampy abdominal pain, explosive diarrhea, and malabsorption. In addition, cutaneous flushing may occur. The syndrome may be managed by metabolic inhibitors of the mediators or by specific treatment of the hepatic metastases. Arterial embolization or ligation may also abort the syndrome temporarily.

The nonbeta cells of the pancreas islets have been implicated as mediators of the Zollinger-Ellison syndrome, the pancreatic cholera syndrome, and the diabetes and dermatitis syndrome associated with secretion of gastrin, vasoactive intestinal peptide, and glucagon, respectively. For the most part, these pancreatic tumors remain occult and are associated with a long clinical history of ulceration, malabsorption, or dermatitis. The tumors may be difficult to identify even at operation, are commonly multicentric, and often recur or are metastatic to the liver. Therapeutic management requires resection of the primary tumor because metabolic antagonists of the mediator substance are ineffective.

The management of gastrointestinal lymphoma is different from the therapy of gastrointestinal carcinoma. The most common lymphomas to affect the gastrointestinal tract are lymphosarcoma, histiocytic lymphoma, and Hodgkin's disease. These tumors are rarely clinically apparent although they are commonly observed at postmortem examination. There is an increased incidence of gastrointestinal involvement in patients whose lymphoma originated in Waldeyer's ring.

Gastrointestinal lymphoma derived within the wall of the gastrointestinal tract is a primary malignant process; secondary lymphoma may arise from retroperitoneal disease and invade and extend into the bowel. In addition a unique abdominal lymphoma is associated with alpha chain disease. This "alpha chain lymphoma" commonly causes malabsorption; the lymphomas as a group generally present with intermittent obstruction of the gastrointestinal tract.

Lymphoma is exquisitely responsive both to radiation therapy and to chemotherapy, and is thus essentially curable by those modalities. Therefore, the role of surgery in lymphoma of the bowel should be limited to documenting the diagnosis and removing any solitary lesions at the time of laparotomy. Major organ resection, bypass procedures such as ileostomy, or other morbid surgical procedures are not necessary as debulking methods unless the lesion forms the wall of the bowel.

11.0 Summary

The gastrointestinal complications of malignancy are generally related to primary tumors and less commonly to secondary metastases. The major gastrointestinal complications are obstruction, hemorrhage, and pain, all of which are most effectively managed by surgical intervention. The critical function of the gastrointestinal tract in alimentation necessitates an awareness of both enteral and intravenous hyperalimentation as primary therapeutic modalities for patients with extra-abdominal or intra-abdominal malignancy. The resistance of intra-abdominal tumors to radiation therapy and chemotherapy highlights the importance of the surgical management of gastrointestinal complications, but the medical considerations are crucial.

References

Eras, P., and Sherlock, P. Hepatic coma secondary to metastatic liver disease. *Ann. Intern. Med.* 74:581–583, 1971.

Foster, J. H. Survival after liver resection for cancer. *Cancer* 25:493–502, 1970.

Hudgkins, P. T., and Meoz, R. T. Radiation therapy for obstructive jaundice secondary to tumor malignancy. *Int. J. Radiat. Biol.* 1:1195–1198, 1976.

Longmire, W. P., Jr., and Tomplins, R. K. Lesions of the segmental and lobar hepatic ducts. *Ann. Surg.* 182:478–493, 1975.

Klatskin, G. Adenocarcinoma of the hepatic duct at its bifurcation within the porta hepatis: an unusual tumor with distinctive clinical and pathological features. *Am. J. Med.* 38:241–256, 1965.

Kurtz, R. C.;Sherlock, P.; and Winawer, S. J. Esophageal varices. *Arch. Intern. Med.* 134:50–51, 1974.

McDermott, W. V., Jr.; Greenberger, N. J.; Isselbacher, K. J.; and Wever, A. L. Major hepatic resection: diagnostic techniques and metabolic problems. *Surgery* 54:56–66, 1963.

McDermott, W. V., Jr.; Paris, A. L.; Clouse, M. E.; and Meissner, W. A. Dearterialization of the liver for metastatic cancer. *Ann. Surg.* 187:38–46, 1978.

Taylor, I. Cytotoxic perfusion for colorectal liver metastases. *Br. J. Surg.* 65:109–114, 1978.

Chapter 9

Pulmonary Complications of Malignancy
J. Lokich

1.0 Background

The lungs are a common site of metastasis; in addition, they house the most common primary tumor in men, bronchogenic carcinoma. Clinical detection of pulmonary lesions is simplified because of the accessibility of the lungs to routine radiologic examination. Cough, dyspnea, and chest pain often accompany primary pulmonary pathology, but the development of pulmonary symptomatology usually implies advanced disease. It is common, however, to observe extensive malignancy without any pulmonary symptomatology (Fig. 9.1), although reserve function with exercise may elicit some symptons.

Malignant disease in the chest is manifest in a variety of radiographic patterns, which can be categorized as discrete coin lesions, endobronchial lesions, interstitial infiltrations, lymphangitic infiltrations, and alveolar consolidation. Anatomically the lungs may be viewed in parts: (1) the mediastinum and its contents, (2) the pleural surfaces, and (3) the pulmonary parenchyma. Tumor involvement of the mediastinum may lead to a variety of clinical manifestations, including superior vena cava syndrome, dysphagia, or tracheal compression with stridor. All three complications rarely occur together. Primary or secondary pulmonary tumors may result in intractable pleural effusions or pleuritic pain. Parenchymal lesions may be asymptomatic or can result in secondary lobular collapse, consolidation with infection, cough, and dyspnea. The pulmonary complications of malignant disease are diversified, and the secondary effects of therapy compound the complexity of the diagnostic approach.

2.0 Differential diagnosis of pulmonary pathology

A variety of symptoms may be produced

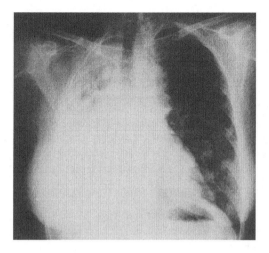

Fig. 9.1 Chest radiograph demonstrating multiple pulmonary metastases in both lesions in a patient with acinic cell carcinoma of the salivary gland. Patient was completely asymptomatic in spite of extensive pulmonary disease for five years.

by thoracic tumors, and patients may present with multiple symptoms and physical signs (Table 9.1). Some symptoms are characteristic of specific anatomic lesions; for example, hoarseness signals recurrent laryngeal nerve compression, and singultus (hiccups) indicates phrenic nerve stimulation. Weakness, lethargy, and somnolence may be secondary to metabolic or paraendocrine effects of the tumor, and all are generally ominous.

The primary pulmonary symptom is dyspnea. Dyspnea can be qualitatively and quantitatively characterized by the limitations and complications experienced by the patient. It may result from simple fatigue due to generalized muscle wasting. Dyspnea generally occurs at pO_2 levels of less than 50 mm Hg, but the patient may experience exercise-induced dyspnea in spite of resting pO_2 levels as high as 80 mm Hg, because of an inability to compensate for the increased oxygen requirement. Dyspnea does not invariably occur with pulmonary cancer and may not be

experienced even by patients with extensive tumor involvement. Alternatively, the development of dyspnea in spite of a relatively normal lung radiograph suggests occult diffusion block or arteriovenous shunt, which may result in decreased arterial oxygenation.

Patterns of breathing and dyspnea may be useful in localizing pulmonary lesions and establishing a diagnosis.

Two common breathing patterns are orthopnea, dyspnea relieved by an upright position, and platypnea, dyspnea relieved by a reclining position. Orthopnea generally results from cardiac failure with increased fluid in the lower lung fields. The upright posture allows oxygenation of the arterial supply to the upper lobes. In platypnea, the reclining posture allows improved perfusion of the upper lobes because the pulmonary artery resistance is less.

Patient A, who had a mesothelioma in the left lower lobe, experienced only minimal dyspnea. One week prior to admission he developed unilateral leg edema, and one day prior to admission had acute, increasing dyspnea and right chest discomfort. A lung scan demonstrated decreased perfusion in the right-lower lobe although ventilation was inadequate. A chest x-ray showed no abnormality of the right lower lobe. The patient noted that the dyspnea was relieved when he was in a reclining position. Because of the tumor in the patient's left lower lobe and a pulmonary embolism in the right lower lobe, ventilation of these lobes was inadequate. Perfusion of the upper lobes was facilitated by the patient's assuming a reclining position, which permitted perfusion of the well-ventilated upper lobes.

Pulmonary lesions can be categorized according to diagnosis or etiology: (1)

Table 9.1 Symptoms produced by pulmonary tumors

Symptom	Comment
Cough	Intrabronchial tumor, extrinsic bronchial compression, secondary inflammatory reaction pneumonitis
Chest pain	Invasion of intercostal nerves, contiguous growth onto pleural surface
Dyspnea	Generally attributed to decreased blood flow or shunting, not directly to tumor volume.
Orthopnea	Upright posture promotes ease of breathing related to increased ventilation capacity, typical of congestive heart failure.
Platypnea	Reclined posture promotes ease of breathing related to increased perfusion capability, typical of lower lobe disease.
Other forms of dyspnea	Flexed posture promotes ease of breathing related to decreased pain in pericardial inflammation. On-side reclining position, related to improved ventilation or perfusion.
Hoarseness	Vocal cord paralysis secondary to mediastinal tumor destruction of recurrent laryngeal nerve or hypothyroidism secondary to thyroid radiation.
Stridor	Impingement on the large airway, represents need for emergency tracheostomy.
Other	Includes secondary symptoms of paraneoplastic syndromes, dysphagia, palpitations, referred shoulder pain, singultus (hiccups), fever.

therapy-induced (e.g., radiation pneumonitis), (2) infections (including bacterial, viral, and fungal), (3) vascular (e.g., pulmonary emboli), and (4) neoplastic. The clinical and radiographic features of a pulmonary lesion may establish a diagnosis without histologic confirmation. Pulmonary lesions can also be categorized by the anatomic distribution and radiographic appearance of the lesions(s): (1) circumscribed or "coin lesions"; (2) diffuse or localized alveolar infiltrate; and (3) interstitial or lymphangitic infiltrate.

The lungs are exquisitely sensitive to radiation therapy and, at doses beyond 1500 to 2000 rad, an inflammatory reaction in the lungs is uniformly observed. Radiation pneumonitis is clinically important, however, in only a small proportion of patients and develops in direct proportion to the dose rate or fraction delivered per unit time. Patients may develop either of two types of radiation pneumonitis six weeks to 18 months following radiation therapy. Acute pneumonitis is characterized by cough, sputum production, and fever, often in association with dyspnea. Radiographically, a localized interstitial infiltrate confined to the radiation portal develops. This type of radiation pneumonitis is responsive to corticosteroid therapy. The second clinical syndrome is a chronic, progressive pulmonary fibrosis that may or may not be associated with a previous acute radiation pneumonitis. Few clinical symptoms are associated with the interstitial fibrosis, although dyspnea may develop if the volume of lung irradiated is large. Radiographically, the lung tissue within the radiation portal is replaced by dense fibrous tissue.

Pulmonary infections and, in particular, opportunistic infections are common in the compromised host. As some infections are potentially remediable with specific therapy, treatment for pulmonary infections is important. The most common radiographic manifestation of pulmonary infection is interstitial infiltration. All the various pneumonities including *Pneumocystis carinii*, viral infection (cytomegalic inclusion disease), fungal infection, and the common bacterial pathogens may produce an interstitial process. In contrast, neoplasia, particularly solid tumor neoplasia, almost invariably produces a nodular pattern radiographically and therefore is easily distinguishable from infection. One exception is the pulmonary involvement associated with lymphomas, especially non-Hodgkin's lymphoma, in which an alveolar interstitial pattern is common.

Tuberculosis has been emphasized in the literature as an opportunistic infection because tumor therapy may decrease host defenses and promote dissemination of infection in patients previously exposed to occult tuberculosis. Cavitation of nodular lesions in the lung is not necessarily evidence of tuberculosis, as cavitation may be observed in growing or regressing malignancies, possibly related to a limitation of blood supply or to central necrosis (Fig. 9.2). Although tuberculosis is exceedingly uncommon today, prophylactic, single-agent antituberculosis therapy is often used for patients undergoing therapy with corticosteroids.

3.0 Diagnostic procedures in pulmonary evaluation

The diagnostic methods used to evaluate pulmonary lesions are directed at establishing the etiology and delineating the extent of disease. Radiologic procedures and monitoring also characterize the natural or biologic evolution of the neoplastic disease by quantitatively measuring growth rates of discrete nodules. Nonradiologic procedures quantify tumor burden and may be therapeutic as well. For example, thoracentesis for pleural effusion or bronchoscopy for an obstructed primary or secondary bronchus provide palliation as well as diagnostic information; their therapeutic effects are a major reason for their application. General diagnostic procedures are outlined in Table 9.2.

Radiologic procedures. Radioisotope scanning of the lung has limited application in the evaluation of pulmonary lesions because scans generally identify lesions that are visible by standard radiography and do not distinguish inflammatory from neoplastic lesions. For example, nonspecific or unrelated pulmonary problems, such as pulmonary arterial thrombosis, chronic obstructive pulmonary disease, and pleural effusion, all may appear as identical abnormalities on a standard scan.

Three radionuclide scanning agents are employed for separate diagnostic applications. The technetium (^{99m}Tc)-labeled macro-aggregated albumin scan is primarily used to evaluate pulmonary arterial

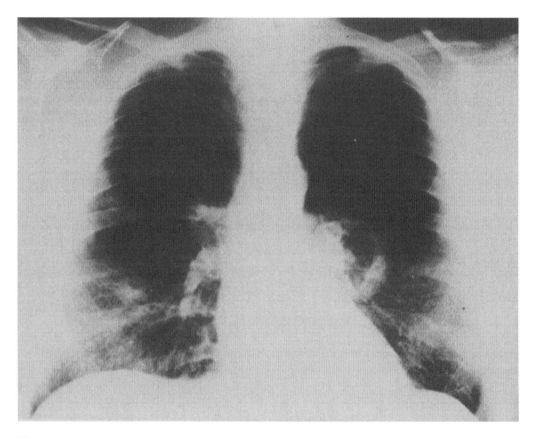

Fig. 9.2 Tomographic chest radiograph demonstrating central cavitation of the primary pulmonary carcinoma with markedly thickened wall.

blood flow. Abnormalities of the ^{99m}Tc scan often indicate one of many disease processes that affect the pulmonary vasculature, including reflex arterial constriction secondary to hypoxic pneumonitis. Because intrapulmonary tumors generally resemble nonneoplastic disease on a ^{99m}Tc scan, the diagnostic potential of such scans is limited. Gallium (^{97}Ga) scanning was developed with the expectation that ^{97}Ga would localize within the tumors and therefore be tumor specific. Tumors as well as inflammatory lesions, however, accumulate the radioisotope. The tumors most likely to do so are melanoma and lymphoma, particularly diffuse histiocytic lymphoma. Occasionally the ^{97}Ga scan is a useful diagnostic tool in the presence of normal chest radiographs.

Patient B, known to have diffuse histiocytic lymphoma, presented with progressive dyspnea and a normal chest radiograph. Gallium scanning demonstrated diffuse pulmonary uptake (Fig. 9.3), and the patient therefore underwent an open-lung biopsy. On histologic analysis, the lung demonstrated diffuse interstitial infiltration with histiocytes and a nonspecific inflammatory pattern.

In this case, the ^{97}Ga scan was useful in detecting subclinical disease, although the lung biopsy did not identify a pathologic process. It did, however, eliminate lymphoma as the cause of the pulmonary symptoms. The possibility that ^{97}Ga scanning may reveal pulmonary bleomycin

Table 9.2 Diagnostic procedures in the evaluation of pulmonary complications of malignancy

I. *Radiologic procedures*
    A. Nuclide scans
       1. Gallium
       2. Technesium-albumin
       3. Bleomycin-cobalt
    B. Tomography
    C. Transcutaneous biopsy (needle)
    D. Fluoroscopy
    E. Angiography
II. *Surgical procedures*
    A. Bronchoscopy
    B. Mediastinoscopy
    C. Transbronchial biopsy
    D. Mini-thoracotomy (Chamberlain procedure)
III. *Pulmonary function tests*
    A. Lung volumes
    B. Diffusing capacity
    C. Arterial blood gases
IV. *Other*
    A. Tumor markers
    B. Sputum cytology

toxicity has been proposed, but the confirmatory biopsy studies are inconclusive.

The third type of radionuclide scanning procedure involves the labeling of chemotherapeutic agents with radioisotopes. The most recent application of this method has been the use of cobalt-labeled bleomycin, but its use is currently limited while studies are continuing.

Tomography is the use of multiple, sequential x-rays employing the laminography technique at one-centimeter intervals from anterior to posterior. Tomography may be useful in identifying parenchymal lesions that are difficult to visualize with standard radiographs; in fact, it has become standard practice in many institutions for routine staging of patients who are likely to develop pulmonary metastases, such as those with osteogenic sarcoma, malignant melanoma, and Hodgkin's disease. Tomography has failed, however, to demonstrate significant value for routine screening, particularly in the cost-benefit analysis. It rarely, if ever, reveals occult nodular lesions in a patient whose standard chest x-ray is

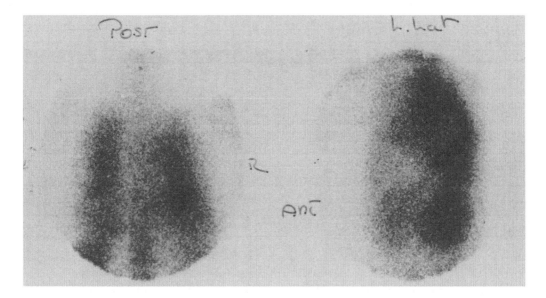

Fig. 9.3 Normal chest radiograph was observed in spite of a gallium scan that demonstrated homogeneous distribution and uptake throughout both lung fields.

normal. On the other hand, if lesions are present on the chest x-ray, tomography may define the lesions more precisely. The more important application of tomography is the evaluation of patients with a solitary metastasis to determine whether the lesion is in fact solitary and whether the opposite lung is free of disease. In this setting, a tomographic evaluation is a therapeutic guide, because solitary lesions are commonly treated surgically while multiple bilateral lesions are treated differently.

Tomography rarely identifies occult pulmonary lesions in patients with normal standard radiographs.

Another major application of tomography is the evaluation of airway patency. In patients with mediastinal lesions, the tracheal air column may be difficult to visualize on standard chest radiographs. Therefore, mid-line laminographs of both the PA and lateral positions may be useful in precisely outlining the airway (Fig. 9.4).

Tomography is useful for quantitating pulmonary lesions and evaluating the patency of the tracheal airway.

The use of the transcutaneous needle biopsy in obtaining specimens for pathologic examination has become standard procedure. Discrete lesions almost anywhere in the pulmonary fields can be identified with a biopsy using fluoroscopy. A needle is inserted directly through the skin and the lung to the lesion, and the lesion is aspirated for cytologic examination. The specimen obtained is analyzed cytologically, in a fashion similar to sputum or cervical smears. Thus, neither the architectural features of the cells nor the invasive quality of the tumor can be discerned. The transcutaneous biopsy is useful and safe for circumscribed peripheral lesions.

Needle biopsy should not generally be performed on a pulmonary nodule that is to be surgically excised by thoracotomy, because the lesion may be an operable primary carcinoma or a solitary metastasis. The morbidity of the transthoracic biopsy, although minimal, is unnecessary if tho-

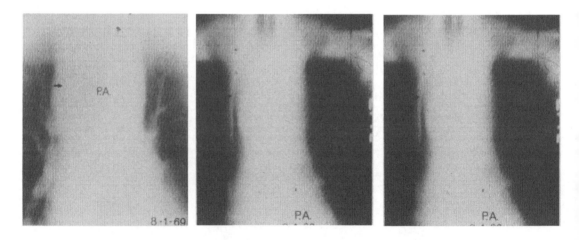

Fig. 9.4 Radiographic tomograms of the mediastinum demonstrate displacement of the trachea and compromise of the air column caliber.

racotomy is planned, and tumor seeding may also occur. Needle biopsy is not helpful for benign lesions and lymphomas, particularly Hodgkin's disease, because if present, malignant cells are difficult to identify in the specimen obtained.

Patient C, a 40-year-old patient with Stage II Hodgkin's disease for two years, presented with a discrete nodule in the lingula. Needle biopsy provided inadequate tissue samples, and a major pneumothorax required tube drainage. At thoracotomy a wedge resection of the single nodule was performed; histologic examination identified the nodule as Hodgkin's disease.

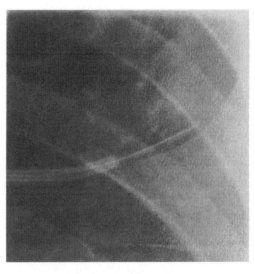

Fig. 9.5 *Magnified portion of chest radiograph demonstrating bronchial catheter with intraluminal brush for biopsy.*

The transbronchial needle aspiration is performed for proximal or parahilar pulmonary lesions in proximity to the mediastinum (Fig. 9.5). With this method, the diffuse interstitial infiltrate may be successfully diagnosed in up to 75 percent of patients. The potential complications of the transbronchial needle biopsy are relatively minor, but for patients with underlying pulmonary disease, the possibility of a pneumothorax presents a major problem, as it may critically compromise the already compromised host. Furthermore, thrombocytopenia and neutropenia commonly coexist in such patients, so that hemorrhage and secondary infection are also significant hazards of the procedure.

Transthoracic needle biopsy is applied to discrete lesions and should not be employed for patients with severe chronic obstructive pulmonary disease or for patients in whom thoracotomy is necessary.

Fluoroscopy is extremely useful in the evaluation of pulmonary lesions, for it can (1) distinguish pleural-based or osseous lesions from parenchymal ones, (2) identify pulsations in vascular lesions, (3) evaluate diaphragmatic and pericardial motion, and (4) identify calcifications within discrete lesions. The simplicity of fluoroscopy mandates that this radiologic precedure be part of the routine evaluation of all patients with pulmonary lesions.

Arteriography is rarely used to evaluate pulmonary lesions, but it is useful in delineating lesions contiguous with the heart and great vessels. Pulmonary tumors do not receive arterial blood flow from the pulmonary artery but from the systemic circulation.

Surgical procedures. Fiberoptic bronchoscopy permits evaluation of all of the major bronchi to approximately the fourth order of bronchial branching, allows direct visualization of endobronchial lesions, and provides access for biopsy specimens. In addition, fiberoptic bronchoscopy can obtain for cytologic examination brushings from the bronchial epithelium distal to the site of visualization. An important and too often neglected aspect of bronchoscopy is its therapeutic application for patients with acute or chronic obstruction. Reexpansion of the lung even after long periods of collapse may be possible with bronchoscopy if infection has not destroyed its elasticity and the integrity of the pulmonary structure.

Bronchoscopy is the procedure of choice therapeutically and diagnostically for patients with lobular collapse.

Mediastinoscopy employs a rigid scope that is introduced either through the superclavicular fossa or in a parasternal incision into the mediastinum for direct visualization of the mediastinal lymph nodes. Biopsy material may be obtained through the scope directly from the pathologic nodes observed if the scope is introduced from the supraclavicular fossa or directly anterior to the suprasternal notch. Observation is limited to the depth of the tracheal bifurcation and carina. Mediastinoscopy should be performed primarily for patients with a radiologically abnormal mediastinum for whom: (1) the diagnostic considerations include such nonmalignant disease as sarcoid; (2) the suspected diagnosis is an illness, such as Hodgkin's disease, which does not require thoracotomy for therapy or diagnosis; and (3) surgery for a primary bronchogenic carcinoma would be influenced substantially. For example, a T_3 lung lesion with occult lymph node involvement in the mediastinum would be considered inoperable if mediastinal node metastases were confirmed; a thoracotomy would therefore be deferred.

The mini-thoracotomy, or Chamberlain procedure, is designed to obtain maximal diagnostic information when the therapeutic potential for a thoracotomy is mini-

mal, as for patients with benign fungal infection or established metastatic disease. Another advantage of the Chamberlain procedure is that for patients with diffuse interstitial disease or major pulmonary compromise, diagnostic information is obtained in a setting of controlled pulmonary function with a closed ventilation system, and a postoperative chest tube allows for continued control of pulmonary function.

The non-Chamberlain thoracotomy should rarely be used when the suspicion for advanced primary malignancy or metastatic disease from extrathoracic sites is high, or when the disease may be benign. Any pulmonary abnormality should be observed over time before surgical thoracotomy is undertaken.

Patient D, a 77-year-old woman, presented with colon cancer and a solitary pulmonary nodule. Six months later, four nodules were observed, and the tumor's doubling time was found to be 30 days. In this case the lung nodules were chronologically related to the colon lesion, and the growth rate precluded thoracotomy.

Patient E, a 30-year-old man with metastatic pulmonary nodules from embryonal carcinoma of the testis, had an excellent regression of the nodules with chemotherapy (Fig. 9.6). The lesions persisted at six months, and the patient underwent thoracotomy with removal of all lesions. Histologic examination revealed benign teratoma, which represented a transition from or maturation of his earlier lesions.

Pulmonary nodules require an observation period prethoracotomy if suspicion is high for benign or incurable metastatic disease.

Pulmonary function tests. With few exceptions, pulmonary function tests are

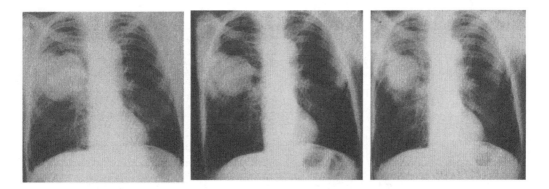

Fig. 9.6 Sequential radiographs of mass lesion in the right thorax that had been present for two years and that responded *dramatically to chemotherapy after which excision was accomplished.*

of limited value in diagnosing pulmonary lesions. They are, however, useful guides for therapeutic procedures and a means of quantifying the tumor's effect on physiologic pulmonary function. Lung volume determinants are affected by a variety of pathologic processes, including radiation therapy, and are therefore uniformly nonspecific. Diffusing capacity may be subclinically affected in patients with lymphangitic extension of tumor or a nonspecific interstitial pneumonitis. This may be the singular abnormality observed, and therefore, diffusing capacity can be a sequential monitor of the effectiveness of treatment when radiographic studies are inadequate. Pulmonary function tests are important for patients with chronic obstructive pulmonary disease since they can determine the patient's ability to undergo thoracotomy. Like pulmonary function tests, arterial blood gases also may reflect a physiologic effect of the tumor that is not apparent from radiographs, and serial monitoring of blood gases is useful in evaluating the effectiveness of treatment, particularly when the tumor causes major arterio-venous shunting of blood and secondary hypoxia.

Other diagnostic procedures. A variety

of additional diagnostic and therapeutic procedures may be used to evaluate patients with pulmonary abnormalities. Tumor markers, such as human chorionic gonadotropin, carcinoembryonic antigen, and a great many tumor-associated antigens or secretory products may be helpful. In addition, assays of immunologic response to fungal and viral infections may be useful.

Sputum cytology is positive in only a very small proportion of patients; cytologic diagnosis of primary bronchogenic lesions by sputum cytology does not exceed 20 percent despite the frequency of advanced disease and involvement of the bronchus. Class III and IV specimens may be obtained from patients with a number of nonspecific inflammatory lesions, including those with chronic lung disease. Occasionally, patients with metastatic lesions to the lungs from extrathoracic sites will yield a positive sputum cytology that is diagnostic for that tumor type. Some opportunistic infections may be confirmed by sputum evaluation. Several histochemical stains, such as the silver stain for *Pneumocystis carinii* infection, can be employed in evaluating the sputum specimen as well.

Because diagnostic pulmonary procedures have attendant risks, the patient with a pulmonary lesion or complication of malignancy requires that the surgeon, radiologist, pathologist, and oncology subspecialist be methodical and meticulous in diagnostic and therapeutic management.

4.0. Pulmonary parenchymal lesions

The pulmonary parenchyma comprises the alveoli and the bronchial and vascular structures including veins, arteries, and lymphatic channels. Primary tumors of the lung can be derived from any of the parenchymal structures, but primary bronchogenic carcinoma is classified histopathologically into four categories: (1) adenocarcinoma; (2) epidermoid or squamous cell carcinoma; (3) undifferentiated carcinoma, large or small cell; and (4) unusual variants including giant cell tumor, mixed tumor, carcinoid tumor, and bronchoalveolar tumor. The anatomic derivation of each tumor has been established, with the exception of the oat cell carcinoma, which remains controversial. Current theory proposes that the oat cell, carcinoid, and bronchial adenoma are all related and derive from the Kulchitsky cell. Pathologic differences among the three relate directly to their malignant potential. Metastatic tumors from extrathoracic sites may be indistinguishable pathologically as well as clinically from primary tumors of the lung, and it is common for lung tumors to be evaluated by a search for the primary tumor (see Chapter 20).

The categories of pulmonary parenchymal lesions are summarized in Table 9.3. The groups are based on radiographic characteristics and include such associated secondary features as lung collapse, infection, serous effusion, and adenopathy. The interstitial parenchymal pattern represents a unique and difficult diagnostic dilemma and is discussed separately.

Table 9.3 Neoplastic lesions of the pulmonary parenchyma

Parenchymal nodule ("coin lesion")

Interstitial pattern

Lymphangitic patterns

Lobe collapse
  Endobronchial lesion
  Extrinsic bronchial compression

Superior sulcus (Pancoast) tumor

The "coin" lesion is the most common lesion observed radiographically and can be detected at a size of 5 mm or smaller on chest radiographs. Alternatively, a lesion may reach a size of 10 cm or more without producing obvious clinical symptoms and may escape detection. A common clinical concept is that large lesions, particularly large, slowly growing, solitary lesions, most often represent metastatic or secondary lesions because primary lung cancer generally disseminates early and grows rapidly.

Patient F, a 69-year-old man, had a 15-cm mass discovered on routine chest examination. Retrospective evaluation of the chest x-rays revealed that the lesion had been present two years previously but was not observed (Fig. 9.7). The mass was resected successfully, and the pathologic analysis revealed mucin-secreting adenocarcinoma. Subsequently a primary tumor of the pancreas was identified.

In addition to size, other important radiographic considerations for pulmonary coin lesions are the shape, growth rate, and whether the lesion is solitary or multiple. Nodules in the peripheral lung field are most commonly adenocarcinoma. Proximal lesions closer to the mediastinum and hilum are generally primary epidermoid cancers. Parenchymal lesions

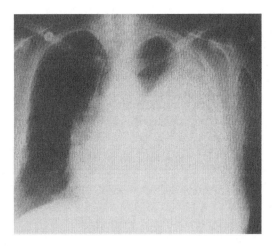 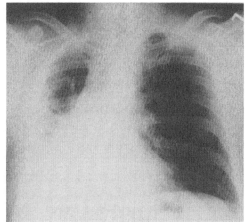

Fig. 9.7 *Chest radiographs indicate pleural effusion (A) with shift of the mediastinum to the contralateral side; lobar collapse* *with effusion (B) is reflected in decreased volume of the lung and shift of the mediastinum to the ipsilateral side.*

observed in association with the mediastinum or hilum enlargement are undifferentiated or squamous tumors and rarely, if ever, represent metastatic lesions. This may be because extrathoracic tumors metastasize by either a lymphatic or a hematogenous route and therefore would not be observed in both the pulmonary parenchyma and the hilar nodes. Therefore, mediastinal lesions without parenchymal lesions are usually metastatic in origin or represent lymphoma. Pleural-based tumors are either mesothelioma or metastases to the pleura from primary tumors of the ovary or breast.

Pulmonary parenchymal lesions are generally spherical. Carcinomas arising in previous inflammatory fibrosis, so-called "scar carcinoma," or in patients with distorted parenchyma secondary to chronic lung disease may develop irregular contours, and close examination of the lung radiographs often reveals dendritic extension at the edge of the pulmonary nodule. Multiple lesions are most often metastases, as it is rare for primary lung tumors to metastasize to other sites in the lung or to the contralateral lung. It is important, however, to rule out the possibility of multiple primary tumors, which develop in approximately 10 percent of patients and may be synchronous in a substantial proportion. The concept of multiple primary tumors is valid when one considers that there are 18 segments to the lung, all of which are exposed in a uniform fashion to the carcinogenic effects of smoking.

The determination of growth rate is one of the most crucial aspects of the evaluation of lung nodules, especially metastatic nodules from extrathoracic sites. Rapid growth is characteristic of testicular tumors and melanoma; slowly growing metastatic lesions include sarcoma and colon and renal cell tumors. The method of growth rate determination and the application of doubling times as a measure of growth rate to principles of therapeutic and diagnostic intervention are discussed in a subsequent section of this chapter.

Pulmonary nodules must be evaluated for size, number, location, shape, and growth rate.

The interstitial pattern should be distinguished from the lymphagitic pattern in the radiographic studies of pulmonary lesions. The latter almost invariably begins in the peripheral lung fields and is radiographically characterized by Kerly B lines. Lymphangitic lesions, furthermore, are invariably neoplastic and almost always represent carcinoma metastatic from the breast, stomach, or other sites.

Interstitial patterns of pulmonary infiltrate must be distinguished from lymphangitic infiltration.

In contrast, interstitial infiltration may be radiographically localized to a single area or may be diffuse and commonly perihilar in distribution. A localized interstitial infiltrate is characteristic of infections, and although intraparenchymal malignancy may be interstitial in distribution, the pattern occurs almost exclusively with lymphomas. Lymphatic metastases are rarely responsive to therapy and are harbingers of death, although occasional patients have prolonged survival.

Lobar collapse can result either from endobronchial obstruction or extrinsic compression of the bronchus. Radiographic evaluation guides therapy; principal radiographic signs of lobar collapse are a decrease in lung volume and a shift of the mediastinum to the side of the collapse.

Lobar collapse is distinguished from parenchymal or pleural disease by decreased volume and ipsilateral mediastinal shift.

In contrast, radiographic opacity secondary to tumor replacement or fluid is associated with shift of the mediastinum to the contralateral lung field.

Patient G, a 64-year-old woman with chronic obstructive pulmonary disease presented with lobar collapse of the left lung, which reexpanded with radiation therapy to the hilum (Fig. 9.8). Six months later the patient developed recurrent dyspnea, and radiographs demonstrated a mediastinal shift to the right side. Chest tube drainage yielded blood fluid and promoted reexpansion of the left lung.

The superior sulcus tumor is a special anatomic category of bronchogenic carcinoma with a unique natural history. The superior sulcus lies at the apex of the right or left lungs and is continuous with the posterior flare of the rib as it sweeps away from the vertebral column. Tumors developing in this area are characterized by a propensity for local invasion of the os-

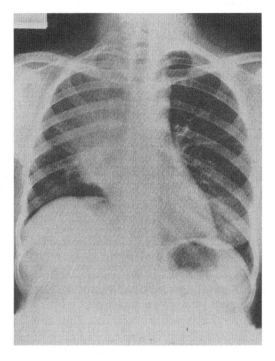

Fig. 9.8 Chest radiograph (Patient G) demonstrating collapse of the right-upper lobe with shift of the mediastinum to the right.

seous structures, the intercostal nerves, and the sympathetic nerves, thus producing pain and Horner's syndrome. Histopathologically this tumor is almost never undifferentiated, nor is it an adenocarcinoma; it is more commonly a low-grade squamous cell carcinoma. The superior sulcus tumor frequently remains localized without extrathoracic dissemination and may have a protracted natural history.

Pancoast (superior sulcus) tumor should be suspected in patients with shoulder pain.

Treatment has focused on maximizing local therapy and has included radiation therapy preoperatively and surgery for removal of contiguous involvement of bone.

Patient H, a 64-year-old chronic smoker, developed persistent shoulder pain that was diagnosed initially as bursitis and treated with local cortisone injections. Chest x-rays demonstrated opacification at the apex of the left lung (Fig. 9.9). Ra-

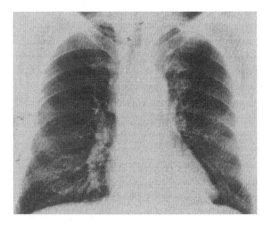

Fig. 9.9 Chest radiograph (Patient H) demonstrates a lesion in the superior sulcus at the medial border of the apex of the right lung.

diation therapy was administered followed by surgical exploration and resection for an epidermoid carcinoma without node involvement.

5.0. Mediastinal lesions

The mediastinum is a primary drainage site for intrapulmonic lesions, and metastases to the mediastinum may result in major compromise of normal mediastinal structures such as the trachea, esophagus, vena cava and great vessels, and heart. With the exception of tracheal obstruction, all the effects of mediastinal tumor have been previously reviewed (see Chapters 2, 3, and 8).

Tracheal obstruction occurs most commonly with lesions developing in either the superior or posterior mediastinum, with lymphoma, or with primary lung cancer. Because the trachea is flexible, lymphomas commonly cause impingement and collapse of the tracheal wall. In contrast, carcinomas within the mediastinum often directly invade the trachea and esophagus.

Tracheal compression is an oncologic emergency requiring radiation therapy, but treatment should be preceded by tracheostomy if the lesion is high and by corticosteroids if the lesion is in the lower mediastinum.

In patients with pericardial disease and low-tracheal obstruction, emergency radiation therapy and corticosteroids are the procedures of choice. In higher lesions derived from the larynx or thyroid, emergency tracheostomy is indicated before therapy is undertaken.

Patient I, a 72-year-old man, presented with one and one-half years of progressive hoarseness and intermittent pneumonia presumed to be aspiration pneumonitis. At admission an emergency tracheostomy was performed, and a T₄ lesion of the larynx was discovered to be invading the peritracheal tissues. Subsequent radiation therapy was delivered to the entire trachea, but regression was minimal, and the patient maintained a chronic tracheostomy.

Mediastinal lesions are complex diagnostic and therapeutic problems. They can lead to critical airway obstruction and vascular catastrophes and can promote fistula formation between viscera, which in turn can lead to perforation or chronic infection.

6.0 Pleural lesions

Pleural effusions are a common manifestation of primary and metastatic lesions of the lung as well as primary tumors of the pleura. Effusions can also develop as secondary phenomena of intra-abdominal tumor (Meigs' syndrome), abdominal inflammation (pancreatitis), intrathoracic infection (empyema), or congestive heart failure. Pleural fluid production may be a consequence of transudation that occurs secondary to high intrapulmonic pressure or decreased oncotic pressure, or it may be a direct exudative process resulting from the secretion of a high-protein fluid from pleural tumor implants or infection. A rare form of pleural effusion is the chylous effusion that is associated with interruption of the thoracic duct.

Thoracentesis may yield useful information for identifying malignant cells, but in the absence of positive cytologic material, the protein and biochemical features of the fluid are not diagnostically important. A cautionary note concerning cytologic evaluation is pertinent. Mesothelial cells are often confused with malignant cells because they have large nuclei, are often phagocytic, and may demonstrate multiple mitosis. In this context a pleural biopsy is complementary to cytologic study in specifically identifying tumor that may have implanted on the pleural surface.

The primary tumor of the pleural surface is mesothelioma. These tumors may present in the absence of an identifiable mass within the lung, or with cytologically positive fluid and no identifiable tumor outside the thoracic cavity. Mesotheliomas are responsive to chemotherapy, and therefore efforts at diagnosis should be vigorous.

Patient J, a 35-year-old woman, presented with a progressive history of shortness of breath over the two months prior to admission and had had a 12-year intensive exposure to asbestos. Mass lesions were identifiable on the pleural surface, and biopsy confirmed mesothelioma. The patient was treated with chemotherapy and had major regression of the tumor (Fig. 9.10).

A pleural effusion that is definitely malignant (i.e., cytologically positive) is categorically incurable, and the diagnostic method for establishing the extent of disease or source of the tumor should therefore be restricted with local (intracavitary) therapy administered as necessary for palliation. A cytologically negative pleural effusion should be evaluated for other possible etiologies. The development of an increasing pleural effusion following therapy may be an inflammatory reaction representing response to an antitumor effect. The major considerations of local (intracavitary) therapy versus systemic therapy depend in large measure on the tumor of origin and the mechanism of fluid production (see also Chapter 13).

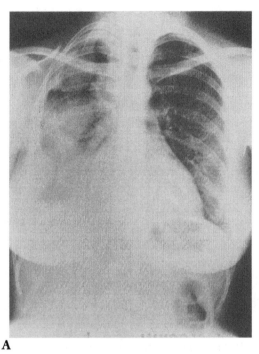

A

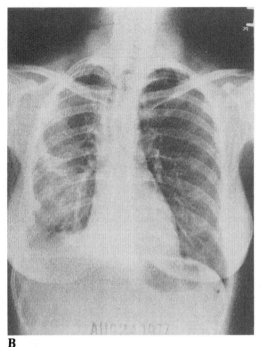

B

Fig. 9.10 Chest radiograph (Patient J) with large pleural lesions in the right lung field (A) that regress dramatically over four months following chemotherapy (B).

7.0 Secondary systemic effects of pulmonary lesions

Pulmonary lesions may be associated with a large variety of extrathoracic manifestations, particularly the systemic paraneoplastic syndromes secondary to ectopic hormone production, which are characteristic of oat cell carcinoma but are also associated with epidermoid tumors of the lung (see Chapters 6 and 19).

Another secondary effect of pulmonary lesions is hypertrophic pulmonary osteoarthropathy (HPO). This syndrome comprises the triad of clubbed digits, periarticular pain, and a pulmonary lesion. Hypertrophic pulmonary osteoarthropathy may be associated with primary malignancies in the lung as well as with metastatic lesions. For example, metastatic connective tissue sarcomas commonly produce HPO. Mesothelioma is the most common primary tumor to produce HPO, but HPO can result from all histopathologic types of malignancy, including Hodgkin's disease. The pathophysiology of HPO has recently been suggested to be related to pleural contact with reflex sympathetic response in the perioseal tissues.

8.0 Therapy for pulmonary complications

Therapy for pulmonary complications of malignancy relates to the etiology of the pulmonary lesion: whether it is primary or metastatic, solitary or multiple, diffuse or localized, and most importantly, whether it is responsive to a potential therapy. The tumor-specific modalities are surgery, radiation therapy, and chemotherapy, as opposed to non–tumor-specific therapy such as antimicrobial agents, corticosteroids, or pleural sclerosing agents. Local therapy (i.e., surgery or radiation) is appropriate for local complications except in those instances where the local therapy has a high morbidity or low potential for response. For example, in the superior vena cava syndrome, surgery is contraindicated because of its morbidity. Additionally, the primary therapy for oat cell carcinoma even in the presence of confined local disease is systemic chemotherapy, because the tumor invariably metastasizes outside the chest and is exquisitely sensitive to multiple drugs. General guides to therapy in pulmonary complications are listed in Table 9.4.

Coin lesions present special diagnostic as well as therapeutic problems. The diagnosis for a coin lesion is determined by the clinical considerations of prior malignancy, disease-free interval, and associated symptoms and sites of disease. For patients with breast or colon cancer, for example, the development of a lung nodule may represent a new primary tumor

of the lung in more than one-half of the cases. In contrast, for patients with Hodgkin's disease, a pulmonary nodule almost invariably represents Hodgkin's disease and not a new primary tumor.

Growth rates. An important aspect of coin lung lesions is the growth rate. Joseph and co-workers developed a mathematical system for evaluating growth rates of spherical nodules by determining the tumor cell doubling time in relation to tumor diameter observed over a specific time interval (1971). The mechanics of determining tumor growth rate are simplistic and involve plotting tumor nodule diameter against time on semi-logarithmic paper. The slope of the line connecting two observation points represents the tumor growth rate and is translated into a specific doubling time by projecting the interval of time over which the growth rate line crosses the doubling time line (Fig. 9.11). Doubling times may differ among individual coin lesions in a single patient and may vary among patients according to tumor type and a multiplicity of unknown factors. Tumors with a short doubling time are associated with rapid

Table 9.4 Therapies for pulmonary complications of malignancy

Lesion or complication	Principal treatment	Comment
Coin lesion	Wedge or lobe resection	Monitor growth rate for a minimum of one month
Lobar collapse	Bronchoscopy	Radiation therapy to treat endobronchial or extra-bronchial compression
Mediastinal compression	Radiation	Pretreatment tracheostomy for high lesions
Tracheal compression	Tracheostomy	Radiation therapy to encompass all sites of disease
Pleural effusion	Tube drainage	Intrapleural irritant

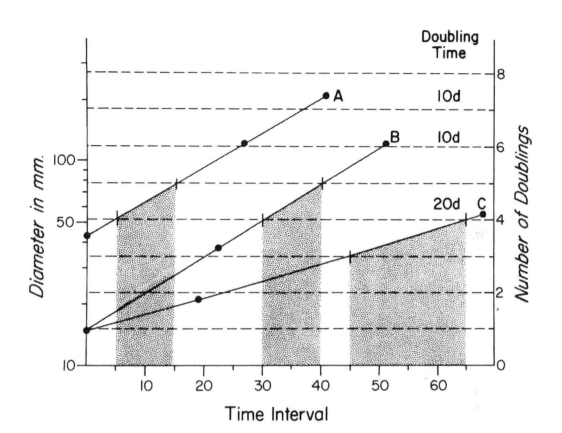

Fig. 9.11 *Growth rate analysis of three tumors A, B, and C. A represents a large tumor with a growth rate comparable to the smaller tumor, B, and more rapid than tumor C, which is comparable in size to B.*

growth and short patient survival, and surgical resection does not add substantially to patient survival for tumors with a doubling time of less than 40 days.

Solitary pulmonary nodules should be monitored without therapy for a minimum of six weeks to establish the growth rate.

This quantitative evaluation of biologic activity of the tumor correlates with the disease-free interval and is applicable regardless of the primary tissue of origin (i.e., melanoma, sarcoma, or carcinoma).

In addition to prior malignancy and growth rate, the presence of solitary or multiple lesions should be calculated into the therapeutic formula. Multiple lesions generally imply a greater potential for dissemination; localized pulmonary resection is therefore less likely to be valuable over the long term.

Lobar collapse, another common pulmonary complication, is generally managed by bronchoscopy followed by local radiation therapy to the site of obstruction. In almost all tumors an antitumor effect sufficient to allow reexpansion is possible and attempted regardless of the duration of collapse. Infection distal to the obstructed branches frequently develops and may delay or even prevent reexpansion because of irretrievable damage to the supporting stroma of the pulmonary parenchyma. Such therapeutic maneuvers must be considered palliative, because a collapsed lung segment generally implies advanced-stage proximal tumor. If bronchoscopy is successful in alleviating obstruction and allowing reexpansion of the lung, radiation therapy should also be administered for prophylaxis against reobstruction.

Mediastinal compression of the trachea may result in critical respiratory compromise. The degree of respiratory inadequacy is related to the fourth power of the radius (r) of the air column, so that small changes in r can result in large changes in air exchange. Radiation therapy may be associated with an initial edema phase and therefore may initially accentuate the respiratory compromise, so that surgical prophylaxis in the form of tracheostomy

may be useful as a primary or preradiation therapy procedure and may be employed even in the presence of tumor surrounding and encasing the lower trachea. At times surgery may involve dissecting the tumor and forcing an endobronchial tube through the mass.

The interstitial infiltrate is the most difficult pulmonary complication of malignancy both therapeutically and diagnostically. The differential diagnosis is often critical, for disease-specific therapy can be life saving. This therapy is also potentially morbid, so that establishing a diagnosis not only permits specific therapy but obviates unnecessary side effects. In spite of aggressive invasive approaches, however, the specific diagnosis often remains obscure, and the potential etiologic causes must be considered in the clinical context to establish empiric therapy (Table 9.5). This is difficult because

Table 9.5 Differential diagnosis and specific therapy of the interstitial infiltrate for patients with malignancy

Diagnosis	Specific therapy	Morbidity of therapy
Infection		
Pneumocystis	Trimethoprim Sulfamethoxazole	Minimal
Fungus	Amphotericin 5-fluorocytosine	Renal, central nervous system
Viral	Cytosine arabinoside (cytarabine) Adenine arabinoside	Marrow suppression
Therapy-Associated		
Bleomycin	None available	—
Oxygen	None available	—
Radiation	Corticosteroids	—
Neoplasia	Tumor-specific chemotherapy	Immune and marrow suppression
Others	—	—
Congestive heart failure		
Pulmonary emboli		
Sarcoidosis		

the nonspecific pathology is observed in an often multifactorial clinical setting.

Patient K, a 25-year-old man with non-Hodgkin's lymphoma, presented with a large mediastinal mass and hilar extension. A complete regression of tumor was achieved with combination chemotherapy that included bleomycin. After completing a maximum cumulative dose of bleomycin, the patient received radiation to the mantle field. Three months later he presented with acute onset of fever (102°), cough, and a chest radiograph demonstrating a left-upper lobe infiltrate. Antibiotics failed to control the lesion, and the interstitial process increased. This patient required intubation and positive pressure oxygen to maintain a pO_2 of 50 mm Hg. At this time an open-lung biopsy was performed, and the pathologic diagnosis was interstitial inflammatory reaction.

An open lung biopsy is often performed to define an appropriate therapeutic course. A treatable infectious cause, which can only be *Pneumocystis carinii* and fungal infection, is identified in less than 10 percent of patients who undergo biopsy, and in many patients the process will regress spontaneously.

Lung biopsy for an interstitial infiltrate will not yield a specific diagnosis to guide therapy in more than 50 percent of patients.

The other potentially reversible pulmonary problems, such as congestive heart failure and pulmonary embolism, do not require a lung biopsy. Therefore, empiric therapy is often used for patients with interstitial infiltrate, and a biopsy is deferred. The empiric therapy is based on the clinical estimate of the severity of the process and its impact both on the patient and on the patient's ability to tolerate the treatment. The therapy chosen should be individually designed, but the physician must consider inclusion of therapy for the most treatable (reversible) diseases.

9.0 Summary

Pulmonary complications of malignancy are common, and the most critical issue in their evaluation is the diagnosis of the various categories of parenchymal, pleural, and mediastinal lesions. Categories of radiographic lesions range from isolated nodules to diffuse infiltration, and each requires a specific therapy based on the clinical probabilities. The principles of the management of lung complications require establishing the treatability and reversibility of a disease process in relation to the diagnostic benefit and the adverse effects of the procedure.

References

Cahan, W. G., and Castro, E. B. Significance of a solitary lung shadow in patients with breast cancer. *Ann. Surg.* 181:137–143, 1975.

Chernow, B., and Sahn, S. A. Carcinomatous involvement of the pleura; an analysis of 96 patients. *Am. J. Med.* 63:695–702, 1977.

Fedlman, N. T.; Pennington, J. E.; and Ehrie, M. G. Transbronchial lung biopsy in the compromised host. *JAMA* 238:1377–1379, 1977.

Felson, B., and Wiot, J. F. Some less familiar roentgen manifestations of carcinoma of the lung. *Semin. Roentgenol.* 12:187–206, 1977.

Joseph, W. L.; Morton, D. L.; and Adkins, P. C. Prognostic significance of tumor doubling time in evaluating operability in pulmonary metastatic disease. *J. Thorac. Cardiovasc. Surg.* 61:23–31, 1971.

Landman, S.; Burgener, F. A.; and Lim, G. H. K. Comparison of bronchial brushing and percutaneous needle aspiration biopsy in the diagnosis of malignant lung lesions. *Radiology* 115:275–278, 1975.

Leff, A.; Hopewell, P. C.; and Costello, J. Pleural effusion from malignancy. *Ann. Intern. Med.* 88:532–537, 1978.

Li, F. P.; Lokich, J.; Lapey, J.; Neptune, W. B.; and Wilkins, E. W., Jr. Familial mesothelioma after intense asbestos exposure at home. *JAMA* 240:467, 1978.

Mountain, C. F.; Khalil, K. G.; Hermes, K. E.; and Frazier, O. H. The contribution of surgery to the management of carcinomatous pulmonary metastases. *Cancer* 41:833–840, 1978.

Muhm, J. R.; Brown, L. R.; and Crowe, J. K. Use of computed tomography in the detection of pulmonary nodules. *Mayo Clin. Proc.* 52:345–348, 1977.

Reeder, M. M., and Reed, J. C. Solitary pulmonary nodule (topics in radiology) *JAMA* 231:1079–1081, 1975.

Zavala, D. C.; Rossi, N. P.; and Bedell, G. N. Bronchial brush biopsy; a valuable diagnostic technique in the presurgical evaluation of indeterminate lung densities. *J. Soc. Thorac. Surg. & Thorac. Surg. Assoc.* 13:519–527, 1972.

Chapter 10

Renal Complications of Malignancy

J. Lokich

1.0 Background

In contrast to most of the visceral complications of malignancy, the secondary genitourinary manifestations of cancer are more commonly due to distant effects from the tumor or the therapy rather than from direct involvement of the kidneys with tumor. Tumors rarely metastasize to the kidneys in spite of high blood flow through these paired organs. Tumor involvement of the ureters, however, occurs commonly as a consequence of pelvic or retroperitoneal metastases. Lymphomas and testicular and ovarian tumors involve retroperitoneal nodes, displace the ureters, and occasionally invade the ureteral wall. Prostatic, bladder, and uterine cancers grow by contiguous extension through and along the ureteral wall. The genitourinary complications of malignancy may therefore be manifestations of either primary tumors of the genitourinary tract or secondary metastases from contiguous or distant tumors.

The clinical manifestation of cancer-related abnormalities of the genitourinary tract cover a broad spectrum of clinical problems (Table 10.1). Obstruction is the most common extrarenal genitourinary complication and develops most frequently in the urethral bladder neck but also along the long course of the ureters within the retroperitoneum. Glomerular and tubular function may be compromised as a consequence of the nephrotoxicity of many cytotoxic drugs and of the antibiotics used to manage secondary infections in malignancy. The nephrotic syndrome is a specific glomerular disease and has been described as a paraneoplastic manifestation of malignancy occasionally preceding the identification of tumor. Although renal infiltration by tumor metastatic to the kidneys is unusual, parenchymal involvement by multiple myeloma or amyloid is common in these neoplasms, and hypercalcemia and hypokalemia may result in tubular dysfunction and azotemia.

Table 10.1 Abnormalities of renal function associated with malignancy

Renal lesion	Common associations
Obstruction	Ureteral and urethral sites due to tumor, metabolic products (uric acid), and drugs
Glomerular/tubular function	Nephrotoxicity of cytotoxic drugs, antibiotics, and radiation
Renal infiltration	Tumor, amyloid, multiple myeloma (protein)
Renal metabolic injury	Hypercalcemia, hypokalemia
Nephrotic syndrome	Immune complexes, renal vein thrombosis, amyloidosis
Infection	Pyelonephritis, ureteritis, cystica, cystitis, urethritis

Clinical abnormalities of the genitourinary tract are generally reversible, although supportive measures, including dialysis, may be necessary to maintain the patient during the azotemic period. For patients with end-stage, disseminated cancer unresponsive to therapy, however, the development of renal failure may justify conservative therapy and observation. The primary clinical effects of renal failure are acute electrolyte disturbances. Other secondary manifestations of renal failure, such as hematologic gastrointestinal and neurologic complications, are rarely noted because the renal failure is acute. Bilateral renal obstruction generally heralds a preterminal state and is associated with resistant tumor. Kidney pain is also uncommon as a malignant complication but may develop as a consequence of secondary infection such as pyelitis or perinephric abscess formation.

2.0 Obstruction of urine flow

Many clinical circumstances exist in which complications of malignant disease result in obstructive uropathy (Table 10.2). Distal ureteral obstruction may develop as a consequence of uterine, bladder, ovary, and prostate cancers, although the latter most commonly results in bladder neck obstruction. Extension of the tumor within the pelvis entraps the ureters, and the clinical syndrome of renal failure may not be associated with easily

Table 10.2 Mechanisms and causes for obstruction of urine flow

1. Intrarenal (tubular) obstruction
   Uric acid crystals
   Methotrexate crystals
   Myeloma light-chain proteins

2. Ureter renal pelvis to pelvic brim
   Retroperitoneal adenopathy
   Ureteral carcinoma

3. Ureter pelvic brim to bladder orifice
   Bladder cancer
   Cervical cancer
   Prostatic cancer

4. Urethral obstruction
   Prostatic cancer
   Rectal cancer
   Cervix and vaginal-vulvar cancer
   Urethral and penile cancer

palpable tumor. These tumors commonly extend in bands along tissue planes and do not form mass lesions. Ovarian cancer is the exception, with pelvic and mesenteric mass lesions resulting in malignant ascites and ureteral obstruction. Examination with pelvic ultrasound is useful in identifying the pelvic tumor and the extent of disease (Fig. 10.1).

Proximal ureteral obstruction in the retroperitoneum is uncommon in spite of ureteral displacement by metastases or primary tumors in the retroperitoneum. Tumors metastatic to the retroperitoneal lymph nodes, such as lymphomas or testicular tumors, generally do not invade the ureter and therefore do not interrupt urine flow. Thus, in spite of much retroperitoneal disease with marked distortion of the ureteral pathway, hydronephrosis is not present, and renal function as measured by creatinine clearance is normal (Fig. 10.2).

Intraluminal obstruction may develop within the renal parenchymal collecting system, in the renal pelvis, or along the

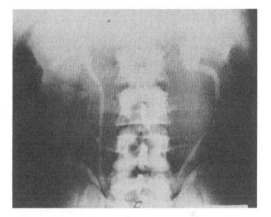

Fig. 10.2 Intravenous pyelogram demonstrating lateral displacement of the left ureter by retroperitoneal lymph nodes in a patient with lymphoma. (Note that medial displacement of ureters is never secondary to retroperitoneal adenopathy.)

course of the ureter as a consequence of either primary tumors of these sites or more commonly as a result of metabolic products of the tumor, such as myeloma proteins and uric acid, or chemotherapeutic agents, especially methotrexate. Renal cell carcinoma is rarely associated with obstruction.

Secondary clinical effects of urinary tract obstruction are progressive deterioration in renal function and superimposed infection with pyelonephritis. Patients with borderline renal function as a consequence of other morbid diseases such as chronic nephrosclerosis or diabetic nephropathy have a limited renal functional reserve so that obstruction secondary to malignancy may result in accelerated renal failure.

Intrarenal obstruction. Intrarenal obstruction develops as a consequence of uric acid deposition, methotrexate crystal formation, or the deposition of myeloma proteins. Uric acid, a degradation product of DNA, is formed as a by-product of cell death. Generally the metabolism and

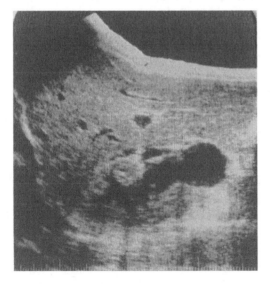

Fig. 10.1 Ultrasonic evaluation of the retroperitoneum demonstrating in prone sagittal section dilated renal calyces.

excretion of uric acid maintain the plasma levels relatively constant despite physiologic cell death. In the presence of tumors, however, the accelerated cell cycle of tumors may elevate uric acid levels. With cytotoxic therapy and acute destruction of a major tumor cell population, uric acid production may exceed the excretory capacity dramatically, and uric acid levels greater than 20 mg/dl may be observed. The most common tumors associated with excess uric acid excretion secondary to therapy are acute lymphocytic leukemia and the non-Hodgkin's lymphomas. Hyperuricemia may also occur in the myelogenous leukemias, but is distinctly unusual in Hodgkin's disease and all of the more slowly responding solid or nonhematologic tumors.

The pathogenesis of uric acid nephropathy is related to a decrease in solubility of uric acid in an acid solution. Therefore, therapy and prophylaxis against uric acid uropathy involves maintaining an alkaline urine to promote solubility. In addition, maximal hydration further dilutes the uric acid concentration. Finally, the use of a xanthine oxidase inhibitor, such as allopurinol, promotes the accumulation of xanthine and hypoxanthine, the precursors of uric acid, thereby preventing uric acid excretion. No clinical evidence currently indicates that uric acid has a direct glomerular or nephrotoxic effect.

Patient A, a 29-year-old man with acute lymphocytic leukemia and a white blood cell count of 200,000 cells per centimeter, was initiated on a combination chemotherapy program of anthracycline, Adriamycin, and cytosine arabinoside (cytarabine). Within 36 hours the white blood count had fallen to less than 30,000 cells per cm, and the patient had a blood urea nitrogen of 80 mg%. Allopurinol and hydration as well as alkalinization had been part of the pretreatment regimen, but were initiated only two hours prior to chemotherapy. Over the next three days, the blood urea nitrogen gradually fell to normal as did the uric acid, and the patient achieved normal renal function.

It is probable that the lymph cell diseases predispose to the development of uric acid nephropathy because of the frequency with which intermitotic death of the malignant cell occurs. The rapid reversibility of uric acid nephropathy does not, however, warrant a cavalier approach to the possiblity of secondary development of nephropathy in patients with highly proliferative tumors and a large tumor burden, particularly for patients with borderline renal function. Therefore, hydration, alkalinization, and allopurinal should be instituted at least six hours prior to initiation of any cytotoxic regimen for such patients. The therapy employed after the development of uric acid nephropathy may necessitate accelerated diuresis employing osmotic agents such as mannitol and fluid solutions.

Uric acid nephropathy occurs almost exclusively with lymphatic diseases and rarely (if ever) with solid tumors.

Methotrexate nephropathy is similar to uric acid nephropathy, although it occurs in different circumstances. Methotrexate, like uric acid, has a pK' less than the pH of urine, and precipitation of crystals at the usual urinary pH is therefore promoted in the renal tubular structure. Acute renal failure may develop in association with chronic low-dose methotrexate therapy (0.5 mg/kg), although it is much more common when high-dose methotrexate (>200 mg/kg) with citrovorum rescue programs are employed. Like uric acid nephropathy, methotrexate nephropathy occurs within 24 to 36 hours after exposure and is invariably transient, but high blood levels of methotrexate are prolonged as a consequence of renal failure. Secondary bone marrow suppression, stomatitis, and dermatitis develop because of the prolonged exposure of these tissues to cytotoxic drug levels. Methotrexate is therefore rarely employed for patients with marginal renal function, and all patients must be evaluated by intravenous pyelography and creatinine clearance. The therapy for the development of renal failure secondary to methotrexate is similar to that for uric acid nephropathy (i.e., hydration and alkalization). Both peritoneal dialysis and hemodialysis are of minor benefit unless liver dysfunction precludes adequate metabolism of the circulating methotrexate. Therapy directed at the "rescue" of the normal cells exposed to the antifolate effect of methotrexate is critical, and "super rescue" must be initiated promptly. Citrovorum rescue is necessary to provide the end product of the methotrexate block and to permit DNA synthesis, thereby prohibiting marrow suppression and other complications of excessive methotrexate.

Patient B, a 39-year-old man with non-Hodgkin's lymphoma, received 5 g of methotrexate by bolus injection. Twenty-four hours later the BUN had risen from 20 to 40 mg% (creatinine 1.0 to 2.4 mg%), and urinary output was <500 cc per 24 hours. Serum methotrexate level was 5.0 x 10/−³ ng/ml, and by day five, the white blood count had fallen to <1000 cells-mm³. Peritoneal dialysis was initiated, but no decrease in the serum methotrexate levels was achieved. By day 10, the renal failure had abated, but the patient died of secondary infection with severe stomatitis and peritonitis.

Methotrexate-induced renal failure is basically due to intrarenal obstruction, but the effect is transient. Therapy is directed at rescue of the marrow and epithelium from cytotoxic effects.

Myeloma kidney represents a form of intrarenal obstruction that develops as a consequence of a deposition of light chains within the tubules. In multiple myeloma the renal lesion is often multifactorial in that one or more ancillary complications affect renal function, including hypercalcemia, infection, and amyloid within the kidney.

Occult or clinically unrecognized multiple myeloma is a common cause of spontaneous renal failure in the elderly.

The therapies for myeloma of the kidney invariably involve specific treatment for the systemic disease, although renal radiation has been employed on the assumption that plasma cells have infiltrated the renal parenchyma. Acute renal failure in myeloma patients can also be caused by intravenous pyelogram radiocontrast material. Renal failure develops as a result of the dehydration and osmotic effect of the dye in a setting of marginal renal function. Thus, renal evaluation should be performed using radionuclide and ultrasonic scanning rather than contrast pyelography for patients with multiple myeloma.

Ureteral obstruction secondary to pelvic or retroperitoneal disease. Ureteral obstruction can develop anywhere along the course of the ureter. As indicated previously, it is unusual for lymphoma or retroperitoneal adenopathy to cause obstruction, because these tumors generally do not invade the ureter but rather displace it. Prostatic and cervical cancer may nonetheless metastasize to the retroperitoneum and cause secondary renal failure by obstruction.

Patient C, an 83-year-old man with known prostatic cancer for eight years, developed right hip pain. On intravenous pye-

logram he was found to have a complete obstruction of the right kidney (Fig. 10.3). Local radiation therapy was employed to the right flank at the tumor site, and over eight weeks, the creatinine decreased from 8.0 to 1.2 mg%.

If the tumor is resistant or the obstruction has been present for a long time, the success of radiation therapy in relieving obstruction is diminished. Furthermore, prior radiation for the primary tumor may preclude retreatment because of the limited tolerance of normal tissues.

Patient D, a 45-year-old woman, had Stage II carcinoma of the cervix treated with radiation. Two years later, she developed diffuse peritoneal and pelvic recurrence and obstruction to the right kidney (Fig. 10.4). She had received pelvic radiation therapy to maximal levels of tolerance; she therefore underwent surgery to evalu-

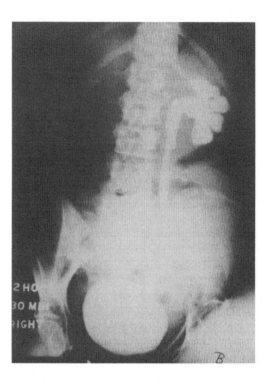

Fig. 10.4 Intravenous pyelogram demonstrating obstructed ureter secondary to carcinoma of the cervix (Patient D).

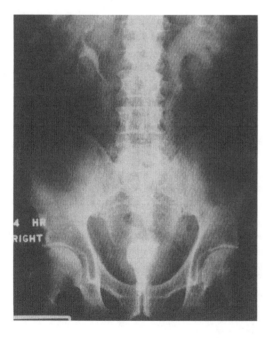

Fig. 10.3 Intravenous pyelogram demonstrating obstructed ureter secondary to prostatic cancer (Patient C).

ate the possibility of ureteral implantation. At operation she was found to have a large, inoperable tumor encasing the right ureter and extending along the posterior gutter.

Tumors that invade the local retroperitoneum and pelvis (bladder, prostate, cervix) are generally responsive to radiation therapy, but eventually become resistant. Systemic chemotherapy is not effective for the majority of these tumors, and patients often require surgical intervention to alleviate the obstruction.

Urethral obstruction. Prostatic and bladder cancers often obstruct the urethra. Primary tumors of the urethra and penis also can cause obstruction, but such tumors are rare. The most common cause of urethral obstruction is benign prostatic hypertrophy, which occurs frequently in the elderly population prone to developing malignancy. Therapy for benign prostatic hypertrophy is generally transurethral resection (TUR); but for patients with contraindications to the morbidity of surgery, shrinkage of the prostate may be induced with estrogen therapy.

Patient E, a 72-year-old man, was receiving therapy for acute myelogenous leukemia when he developed prostatism. Physical examination revealed a large, boggy prostate gland. He had hematuria in association with severe thrombocytopenia due to leukemia. Because of the concomitant presence of thrombocytopenia, estrogen therapy was introduced in an attempt to shrink the prostate and preclude the necessity of TUR. The patient's prostatism promptly abated, and his leukemia went into remission; he survived an additional eight months without return of local symptoms.

In patients with disseminated cancer, TUR and its attendant complications may be avoided by the use of estrogen therapy.

Bladder neck obstruction commonly results from prostatic disease, but contiguous extension of other pelvic tumors may produce an identical syndrome. Primary urethral tumors are a rare cause of urethral obstruction, as are rectal, vaginal, and vulvar cancers. These uncommon causes of obstruction may mimic the clinical syndrome of bladder neck outlet blockage.

Patient F, a 60-year-old man, had rectal carcinoma treated by an abdominal peritoneal resection. Five years later the patient developed urinary symptoms but on examination was thought to have a normal prostate. He was treated by periodic curettage and dilatation for presumed urethral stricture, which was documented by x-ray. Because of the persistence of intermittent urinary symptoms over 18 months, the patient underwent an exploratory operation. A urethral biopsy demonstrated adenocarcinoma consistent with his previous rectal cancer. He received local radiation therapy and had partial relief of his symptoms.

Therapies for urinary tract obstruction. Obstructive uropathy is generally painful, and with the exception of bladder neck obstruction, symptoms other than decreasing urinary output are minimal. Thus, the diagnosis of obstruction along the urinary tract depends upon radiologic studies, including intravenous pyelography, retrograde pyelography, renal scanning, and the noninvasive method of ultrasonography. The echogram can define the obstruction site, identify the impact of hydronephrosis on the kidneys, and delineate the specific type and size of the obstruction.

Treatment of obstructive uropathy may involve radiation and chemotherapy, depending on the type of malignancy, but surgical therapy is almost invariably required eventually. The decision to undertake therapy must be determined in the context of the expectation for disease control beyond the site of urinary obstruction. For patients with another irreversible, morbid disease or with diffuse extraabdominal malignant lesions, and for elderly patients with rapidly growing tumors, the development of obstruction may be a compassionate process allowing the patient to proceed to renal failure and secondary uremic coma. On the other hand, in patients with slowly-growing tumors or for whom therapy may reasonably be expected to promote longevity, surgical decompression to allow for the maintenance of maximum functioning glomerular units is important.

Surgical decompression should be undertaken if the obstructing tumor is localized and if other disease sites can be expected to respond to systemic or radiation therapy.

Radiation therapy is not an effective means of alleviating urinary tract obstruction unless such radioresponsive tumors as the lymphomas are causing the obstruction. Even for relatively responsive tumors, ureteral obstruction will almost invariably require surgical decompression. In those instances in which radiation is employed successfully, as for Patient C, renal function may return to baseline. Although it is likely that the duration of obstruction contributes to deteriorating renal function, no specific period has been established beyond which renal function is irretrievable. Complications of obstruction, such as infection, may contribute to the progressive loss of glomerular units.

Local radiotherapy rarely promotes relief of urinary obstruction secondary to tumor, and renal recovery may decrease with duration of obstruction.

Four basic surgical methods are used to relieve obstruction (Table 10.3). Ureteral stints are placed prior to or at the time of ureteral catheterization and are primarily for patients with direct intralumenal obstruction of the ureters. The placement of the stint requires manipulation of the tumor, and frequently the stint is expelled, requiring replacement at time intervals. For patients with bilateral obstructive disease, a unilateral stint may be used to permit drainage and the development of renal function; however, stints should be placed in both ureters to promote drainage and prevent local infection.

Nephrostomy may be employed with obstruction distal to the renal pelvis. The

Table 10.3 Surgical management of urinary tract obstruction

Ureteral obstruction
  Ureteral stints
  Nephrostomy
  Ileal loop

Bladder neck obstruction
  Suprapubic cystostomy
  Transureteral resection

transcutaneous approach to nephrostomy obviates a major surgical procedure but is generally employed as a temporizing measure to improve renal function while evaluating the effect of systemic or radiation therapy on other tumor sites. This surgical procedure is associated with major morbidity and should be used only for patients who have reasonable life expectancy and quality of life. Suprapubic cystostomy is employed for patients with bladder neck obstruction from bladder or prostate tumor and is also a temporary procedure. An ileal "loop" may be created using a portion of the small bowel to provide a conduit and reservoir from the kidney to the anterior abdominal wall; the ileal loop is the definitive bypass procedure in the urinary tract. Reobstruction within the urinary tract is not problematic, as the non-functional loop of ileum is not retroperitoneal, and the tumor does not therefore compromise the ureters. The loop is more of a conduit than a reservoir because urine flows constantly, and there is no cutaneous sphincter effect.

3.0 Drug-induced renal injury

The renal toxicity of a wide spectrum of medications, including antibiotics and cytotoxic chemotherapeutic agents, has been increasingly identified. Characteristically, drug-related nephropathy is acute in onset, predominantly dose related, and almost invariably reversible. By precisely monitoring renal function, adjusting the medication dosage, and judiciously managing the patient during the period of renal compromise, renal failure can be either prevented or effectively treated. For patients with marginal or compromised renal function or for those with glomerular sclerosis, pyelonephritis, or chronic glomerular nephritis, the use of nephrotoxic drugs is contraindicated; at the very least severe restrictions should be imposed on dosages to prevent exacerbation or potentiation of the renal failure.

The number of cytotoxic drugs that induce renal failure has been increasing (Table 10.4). Methotrexate differs from the other drugs commonly associated with renal failure in that it leads to obstruction whereas *cis*-platinum, the nitrosoureas, cyclophosphamide, and mitomycin C all appear to have a direct toxic effect on the epithelium or glomerular tissue. Cis-platinum is an especially effective drug in the treatment of testicular and epidermoid tumors, and the associated renal failure may be either a cumulative effect with prolonged use of the drug, or may develop acutely.

Patient G, a 50-year-old man with esophageal cancer, presented four months after surgery with multiple pulmonary nodules. He was treated with a five-day course of bleomycin followed on day six by a bolus injection of cis-platinum 120 mg/M². The latter was accompanied by expanded hydration to eight liters for 24 hours. On day 11, the serum creatinine was 4.4 mg% and by day 12 had risen to 13 mg% with decreased urinary output and all the characteristic urinary changes of acute tubular necrosis. On day 21 the patient died of renal failure without sepsis.

Table 10.4 Cytotoxic drugs inducing renal failure

Drug	Mechanism	Comment
Methotrexate	Tubular sludging and direct glomerulo-tubular injury	Preventable by alkalization and hydration
Cis-platinum	Acute tubular necrosis	Cumulative, acute dose-related tubular necrosis prophylactically treated with hydration diuresis
Nitrosourea (Streptozotocin)	Tubulo-interstitial nephritis	Frequent proteinuria (>40%) but acute renal failure uncommon
Cyclophosphamide	Direct irritant of bladder mucosa	Hemorrhagic effect may result in significant blood loss
Mitomycin C	Glomerulo-tubular injury	Rare (<10%), associated with dose
Other drugs 6-Mercaptopurine	Unclear	Rare (<10%), not clinically significant
L-Asparaginase	Unclear	

Acute renal failure associated with *cis*-platinum is typical of heavy metal poisoning. The renal effect may be eliminated completely by sufficient pretreatment hydration; with higher doses of the drug, mannitol diuresis is essential.

Streptozotocin, a nitrosourea, is frequently associated with proteinuria but rarely with acute renal failure. Mitomycin C rarely induces renal damage, but its effects appear to be dose related. Cyclophosphamide has only rarely been associated with renal injury but commonly induces a hemorrhagic cystitis related to a local irritating effect of one of the degradation metabolic products of the drug. The actual incidence of cyclophosphamide-induced hemorrhagic cystitis is relatively low and appears to be more frequent in patients receiving high doses of intravenous therapy. Clinical points of importance are that hemorrhagic cystitis can be potentiated by local radiation therapy and that cystitis can develop up to one year following discontinuance of cyclophosphamide therapy.

Cyclophosphamide-induced hemorrhagic cystitis can develop at any time following use or discontinuance of the drug.

Extreme hemorrhage may require cystectomy, but in less acute circumstances control may be achieved by administering systemic corticosteroids or by bladder instillation of steroids or sclerosing solution.

Several antibiotics used in treating the infectious complications of malignancy have been associated with nephrotoxicity due to their direct effects on the glomerulus and on tubular function. The anthracycline antibiotics, especially gentamicin and its analogs, are prone to induce renal damage, and thus require specific monitoring of blood levels. The antifungal agent amphotericin B is similarly associ-ated with renal toxicity. Combined antibiotics may potentiate renal damage, particularly in a complex clinical setting of multiple nephrotoxic insults and borderline renal function.

Patient H, a 45-year-old man with acute myelogenous leukemia, was initiated on treatment employing Adriamycin and cytosine arabinoside (cytarabine). Seven days following induction of therapy, the patient had pancytopenia and developed a fever to 102°. He was placed on therapy with gentamicin and cephalosporin and five days later had a BUN of 100 and a urinary output of less than 500 cc per 24 hours. The patient was initiated on hemodialysis with rapid resolution of his azotemia. His fever persisted, but after 14 days the blood urea nitrogen had returned to normal, and the patient had entered complete bone marrow remission from the leukemia.

The combination of cephalosporin and gentamicin has been suspected as particularly nephrotoxic, but clinical circumstances often dictate their use. The important issue in cancer management is that reversible renal dysfunction must be treated aggressively, particularly if the tumor can be successfully managed.

Monitoring patients who have neoplastic disease and infection requires close attention to blood levels of potentially nephrotoxic drugs. In addition, the interaction of chemotherapeutic agents with potentially nephrotoxic antibiotics must be monitored clinically. Recent data suggest, for example, that gentamicin renal toxicity is accentuated by the antitumor drug *cis*-platinum.

4.0 Metabolic renal injury

Renal complications secondary to abnormal serum concentrations of electrolytes are especially common in malignant disease. The three categories of electrolyte disturbance are hypercalcemia, hypokalemia, and hyponatremia. The first two are direct causes of tubular dysfunction and can lead to azotemia; the last is a secondary complication of inappropriate antidiuretic hormone secretion that develops without impairing renal function.

Hypercalcemia, in addition to predisposing to the development of nephrolithiasis and ureteral stone formation, may induce an acute insult to the tubular epithelium and cause secondary aminoaciduria and a Fanconi-type syndrome. As a consequence of hypercalcemia, the patient may develop polyuria with a solute diuresis and secondary dehydration. Principal guidelines for therapy of hypercalcemic nephropathy are to control the hypercalcemia with steroids or diuretics and hydration (see Chapter 6), and to avoid ancillary renal insults from chemotherapeutic agents or sepsis.

In the presence of hypercalcemia, nephropathic drugs should be avoided.

Hypokalemia occurs in association with malignant disease as a consequence of Cushing's syndrome, as a paraneoplastic manifestation of cancer, or in association with protracted vomiting, diarrhea, or diuretic abuse. Hypokalemia also may be observed in association with hypercalcemia as a consequence of solute diuresis and, in some instances, with acute leukemia in conjunction with a muramidase-induced renal lesion, although the latter is controversial as a mechanism of renal injury. Therapy for hypokalemic nephropathy is to restore body potassium while carefully monitoring serum electrolyte levels. The potassium loss induced by Cushing's syndrome may require inordinate doses of spironolactone. Hypokalemia secondary to gastrointestinal loss

may necessitate correction of the primary disturbances, such as removal of a pancreatic tumor releasing intestinal vasoactive peptides. Electrolyte disturbances inducing azotemia are not associated with decreased urine output, and with correction of the electrolyte imbalance, the azotemia promptly abates. The singular exception is the patient with chronic hypercalcemia. A chronic elevation of serum calcium levels may lead to hypercalciuria and nephrolithiasis as well as calculus formation.

Disturbances in phosphate metabolism can occur independently of the calcium mechanism and are particularly important in patients who have sudden dissolution of tumor with release of phosphates that are chemical constituents of DNA. The increased circulating phosphates may bind and precipitate calcium, leading to hypocalcemia. The secondary hypocalcemia may result in tetany and clotting abnormalities as a consequence of decreased levels of cofactor.

5.0 Parenchymal (glomerular) renal injury

Two types of glomerular injuries associated with malignancy can be distinguished, the nephrotic syndrome and radiation nephritis. The nephrotic syndrome in cancer may occur as a consequence of immune complex disease or as a secondary manifestation of amyloidosis or renal vein thrombosis. Immune complex disease has been implicated with tumor antigens identified with lung cancer, colon cancer (carcino embryonicnitrogen-like substance) and in the lymphomas, particularly Hodgkin's disease. The lymphomas, in fact, are more frequently associated with nephrosis than are the solid tumors. Treatment of the primary tumor results in rapid resolution of the nephrotic syndrome.

Patient I, a 59-year-old man, presented with right axillary adenopathy and was found to have proteinuria of more than 15 g/24 hours. In addition, a mediastinal mass was observed on x-ray. He had a biopsy revealing Hodgkin's disease; radiation therapy and nitrogen mustard were administered, producing complete dissolution of the tumor and rapid reversal of the nephrotic syndrome.

Radiation nephritis develops as a result of radiation to the kidneys in patients with retroperitoneal adenopathy due to lymphoma or testicular cancer, and in patients who have received radiotherapy for pancreatic carcinoma. This renal complication occurs after radiation to the entire kidney structure bilaterally; the dosage must exceed 3500 rad. A symptom-free period of 12 to 24 months may elapse before the patient develops progressive renal failure and hypertension.

Proteinuria, especially massive (>2 g/24 hours) proteinuria, requires evaluation for renal vein thrombosis or obstruction of the inferior vena cava. This level of proteinuria may develop with or without the other components of the nephrotic syndrome although edema, either generalized or dependent, commonly occurs. Two unusual tumors, hepatoma and renal carcinoma, commonly invade the venus plexus of the retroperitoneum and may cause an acute Budd-Chiari syndrome in association with massive proteinuria. Only rarely do metastatic tumors result in this clinical syndrome.

Invasion or infiltration of the renal parenchyma is a distinctly unusual occurrence in malignant disease, although it occurs commonly in patients with leukemia and lymphoma and is seen at postmortem examination in patients with solid tumors. Even in these circumstances, functional impairment of the kidney is unusual. Because of the renal function reserve and the unlikely event of bilateral metastases to the kidneys, primary and metastatic tumors to the kidneys are extremely rare causes of renal impairment.

6.0 Infections of the genitourinary tract

Like the lungs and gastrointestinal tract, the genitourinary tract is one of the most common sources of infection in patients with neoplastic disease. Granulocytopenia occurs as a consequence of therapeutic modalities in the presence of obstruction, and interruption of mucosal integrity of the genitourinary tract contributes substantially to the high incidence of kidney infections. Sequestered infection is the major clinical concern for patients developing obstruction, and pyelitis and perinephric abscess can be continuing sources of bacteria in the systemic circulation. Treatment for a genitourinary infection involves relief of the obstruction as well as appropriate antibiotic therapy (see Chapter 16).

7.0 Summary

The renal manifestations are diverse and common complications of neoplastic disease. Infection, obstruction, electrolyte abnormality, and nephrotoxic therapies such as radiation, cytotoxic drugs, and antibiotics may each contribute to potentially irreversible renal dysfunction. In some instances renal failure may be managed by correction of electrolyte disturbances or by treatment of the tumor; more commonly, a simple supportive measure for transient renal failure may be applied. Obstruction, however, almost always requires surgical intervention to prevent infection and promote renal function. The use of either peritoneal dialysis or hemodialysis to maintain patients with advanced metastatic disease is reasonable only for the patient with a potentially treatable tumor whose renal failure may be a transient development and for whom control of the cancer is a reasonable expectation.

References

Afzal, M. et al. Hypouricemia and proximal renal tubular dysfunction in acute myeloid leukemia. *Br. Med. J.*. 5934:775–777,1974.

Aptekar, R. Bladder toxicity with chronic oral cyclophosphamide treatment in non-malignant disease. *Arthritis Rheum.* 16:361–467, 1973.

Bryan, C. Acute renal failure in multiple myeloma. *Am. J. Med.* 44:128–133, 1968.

Editorial. Hyperuricemic acute renal failure. *Lancet* 1266–1267, 22 June 1974.

Frei, E., III et al: Renal complications of neoplastic disease. *J. Chronic Dis.* 16:757–776, 1963.

Ghosh, L. et al. The nephrotic syndrome: a prodome to lymphoma. *Ann. Intern. Med.* 72:379–382, 1970.

Kaplan, B. S. Glomerular injury in patients with neoplasia. *Annu. Rev. Med.* 27:117–125, 1976.

Lee, J. C. The association of cancer and the nephrotic syndrome. *Ann. Intern. Med.* 64:41–51, 1968.

Liu, K. et al. Renal toxicity in man treated with mitomycin C. *Cancer* 28:1314–1320, 1971.

Loughridge, L. Nephrotic syndrome in malignant disease of nonrenal origin. *Lancet* 1:256–259, 1971.

Luxton, R. W. Radiation nephritis. *Q. J. Med.* 22:215–242, 1953.

McCurdy, D. M. et al. Renal tubular acidosis due to amphoteracin B. *N. Engl. J. Med.* 278:124–131, 1968.

Mir, M. A. et al. Hypokalemia in acute myeloid leukemia. *Ann. Intern. Med.* 82:54–57, 1975.

Myerowitz, R. L. et al. Nephrotoxic and cytoproliferative effects of streptozotocin. *Cancer* 38:1550–1555, 1976.

Pitman, S. et al. The pathogenesis of methotrexate nephropathy. *Clin. Res.* 24:380A, 1976.

Plager, J. E. Association of renal injury with combined cephalothin-gentamicin therapy among patients severely ill with malignant disease. *Cancer* 37:1937–1943, 1976.

Richmond, J. et al. Renal lesions associated with malignant lymphoma. *Am. J. Med.* 32:184–207, 1962.

Routledge, R. C. et al. Hodgkin's disease complicated by the nephrotic syndrome. *Cancer* 38:1735–1740, 1976.

Sadoff, L. Nephrotoxicity of streptozotocin (NCS-85998). *CCR* 54:457–459, 1970.

Shrom, S. H. Formalin treatment for intractable hemorrhagic cystitis: a literature review. *Cancer* 38:1785–1789, 1976.

Talley, R. W. et al. Clinical evaluation of toxic effects of CPDD—phase I clinical study. *CCR* 57:465–471, 1973.

Zlotnick, A. Renal pathologic findings associated with monoclonal gammopathies. *Arch. Intern. Med.* 135:40–45, 1975.

Chapter 11

Hematologic Complications of Malignancy
M. Bern

1.0 Background

The hematologic aspects of malignancy are diverse and involve the formed elements including the red cells, white cells, platelets, and plasma proteins. Primary hematologic malignancies represent a relatively small proportion of the hematologic manifestations of neoplastic disease. On the other hand, secondary hematologic manifestations of malignant disease are exceedingly common.

The formed elements can be affected by a variety of pathologic mechanisms associated with the malignancy and by therapy directed at the tumor. Radiotherapy and chemotherapy may have a formidable impact on the formed elements, particularly on the white blood cells and platelets. The secondary effects are associated with major morbidity and occasional mortality. The hematologic manifestations of malignancy include coagulation disorders, which can cause either excessive clotting and excessive bleeding or the combined abnormality of excessive clotting leading to consumption and, secondarily, to excessive bleeding.

The management of hematologic complications involves establishing a specific pathophysiology or etiology of the disorder. Even though the causes of many hematologic complications are only partially explained, their early detection can lead to effective therapy. Successful therapy can improve the quality of the patient's life and avoid life-threatening effects. These hematologic complications do not necessarily represent advanced progressive disease; some are associated with early cancers and relatively small tumor burdens. Specific treatment of the manifestation may require supportive therapy while the depleted cell stores are reconstituted, or palliation until tumor control is established. With the exception of complications secondary to chemotherapy, radiation therapy, and surgery, the hematologic manifestations of cancer are generally best managed by controlling the primary tumor.

2.0 Coagulation and fibrinolysis

Among the most frequently described and in many ways best understood hematologic sequelae are alterations of the coagulation system. The homeostasis of coagulation depends on a balance between clot formation and clot lysis. The proteins and phospholipids needed to generate a clot are each balanced by inhibitors that buffer their activity. The intrinsic pathway (Factors VIII, IX, XI, and XII along with prekallikrein) and the extrinsic pathway (Tissue factor and Factor VII) turn on the common pathway (Factors I, II, V, and X) to form a fibrin clot. Platelets contribute to hemostasis by forming the initial platelet plug and contribute phospholipids, powerful cofactors in the pathway leading to clot formation.

The inhibitors of these systems include the physiologic effects of blood flow and of reticuloendothelial clearance of the activated substances, and the chemical and physical effects of antithrombin I (fibrin), antithrombin III (the principal neutralizer of thrombin), alpha$_2$ macroglobulins, and specific inhibitors of each factor. Depletion of inhibition of any of these inhibitors will potentiate clot formation. The fibrinolytic system also opposes the tendency to form clots. Plasminogen activator acts upon plasminogen to form plasmin, which dissolves by hydrolysis the fibrin in the clot. These elements also have inhibitors that act as buffers against overactivity. If the fibrinolytic inhibitors are depleted, overwhelming clot lysis and a secondary hemorrhagic diathesis can occur.

Aside from the uncommon finding of dysfibrinogenemia occurring with hepatoma or deficiencies of Factors I, II, V, VII, IX, and X associated with displacement of liver parenchyma by primary or metastatic cancer of the liver, alterations occur in the homeostatic balance in cancer patients that may push the system toward more thrombosis or more fibrinolysis. The spectrum of manifestations of these acquired coagulopathies ranges from multiple thrombosis in veins and arteries to diffuse hemorrhage. Both situations can be equally morbid or even life threatening.

Increased tendency of cancer patients to form clots. A distinction should be drawn between the diagnosis of "accelerated coagulation" and "hypercoagulability." The latter implies a "primed pump" of greater than normal concentrations of procoagulants ready to activate a cascade. The former exists when the coagulation system is already operating. Patients who are "primed" are those for whom further stimuli would easily induce local or systemic thrombi.

Accelerated coagulation or hypercoagulation can occur concomitantly with malignant disease, and are manifested by acclerated kinetic tests or elevated levels of procoagulants.

Patients who have already suffered such pathologic stimuli and have accelerated coagulation are in the process of forming either micro- or macro-thrombi, at times associated with secondary fibrinolysis. These distinctions can be made by determining several laboratory parameters. The patient prone to hypercoagulation may have elevated levels of fibrinogen; Factors II, VII, VIII, IX, X, and XI; platelet counts; and increased antiplasmins such as alpha$_1$-antitrypsin and alpha$_2$ macroglobulins. The assays of coagulation kinetics will be normal. In contrast, patients with accelerated coagulation will have alterations in the functional or kinetic parameters: acceleration of the whole blood clotting time, silicone to glass clotting time ratio, plasma recalcification time, thromboplastin generation time, and thromboelastogram, as well as a reduction of antithrombin III. Decreases in in vitro and in vivo heparin tolerance may occur. If the process is flagrant and diffuse, consumptive coagulopathy will ensue with reduction of coagulation Factors I, II, V, and VIII, along with elevation of fibrin monomers or fibrinopeptides A and B. The patient will have secondary activation and consumption of plasminogen and plasmin, and will release fibrinogen and fibrin degradation products (FDP/fdp). Adenosine diphosphate-induced platelet aggregation may also be accelerated in vitro. If high concentration of FDP/fdp are present, platelet aggregation will be inhibited.

Disseminated intravascular coagulation represents an extension of the hypercoagulable state manifested as microthrombosis and bleeding.

No single neoplastic determinant exists that can predict which coagulopathy will occur. Studies searching for prognostic signs among the coagulation tests have not been rewarding, and specific prognostications for cancer patients based on these abnormalities are not possible. It seems, however, that four assays may be useful. First, hyperfibrinogenemia is an important finding, as many patients with hyperfibrinogenemia develop venous or arterial thrombi. Second, circulating FDP may have selective importance in ovarian tumors. Of 32 women who were found to have malignant ovarian tumors, 23 (72 percent) had preoperative elevations of FDP (0.5 to 30 mgm%), while only 6 of 131 with benign ovarian tumors had elevations of FDP (from trace to less than 2.0 mgm%). Other reasonable explanations for the slightly raised FDP existed in those 6 women. Third, low levels of the platelet adenine nucleotides, ADP and ATP, in patients with gastric carcinoma,

carry a dire prognosis; patients with low platelet concentrations of ADP and ATP died within 14 days of their diagnostic laparotomy. Fourth, depletion of antithrombin III implies release of esterase enzymes such as thrombin and trypsin. This may be due to intravascular extension of thrombogenic tumors or local release of the esterase, as in pancreatic carcinoma.

Carcinoma and thrombophlebitis. Episodic thrombosis and thromboembolism can be a major problem for patients suffering from carcinoma of the pancreas, lung, stomach, prostate, and breast. Other less frequently encountered diseases associated with thromboemboli are cancers of the gallbladder, bile ducts, and squamous cell carcinomas. This complication can precede recognition of the tumor by many months and, when coexistent with the tumor, should be interpreted as a grave prognostic sign. As many as 56 percent of patients with carcinoma of the body or tail of the pancreas may have one thrombosis, and up to 31 percent will have widely disseminated venous thrombi. The thrombophlebitis that develops tends to be resistant to heparin, especially in those for whom the pretreatment antithrombin III is very low. It is also often poorly controlled by warfarin therapy. The phlebitis is usually migratory and often involves unusual sites such as arms and breasts in addition to the classical sites of legs and pelvis. Death from pulmonary embolus is common.

Patient A, a 58-year-old man, presented with bilateral distal leg thrombophlebitis and malignant ascites due to carcinoma of the pancreas. On admission the prothrombin time was 9.5 sec (control 11.5 sec); the partial thromboplastin time was 24 sec (control 33 sec); the platelet count was 480,000; and the fibrinogen level was 480 mgm%. The silicone to glass clotting time ratio was 1:2, and the antithrombin

III was 8.0 sec (control >18 sec). Fibrin monomers were negative, but the FDPs were 40 mgm%.

The patient's phlebitis was partially controlled with infusions of 96,000 units of heparin per 24 hours. This very large dose was able to prolong the partial thromboplastin time only to 50 sec. Lesser doses were ineffective. After the patient was started on oral anticoagulants, his thrombosis returned within four days, again involving the legs, arms, and abdominal wall veins. He died 20 days after admission from a massive pulmonary embolus.

Phlebitis is a common intravascular consequence, and is often partially resistant to heparin.

Hyperfibrinogenemia is an important antemortem indication for potential thrombosis. Patients with carcinoma and coexistent fibrinogen levels of more than 400 mgm% are often found at autopsy to have thrombi in the pulmonary arteries, inferior vena cava, iliac veins, and portal veins. Many have multiple thrombi. On the other hand, only 0.96 percent of patients with normal antemortem fibrinogen values have such thrombi at autopsy.

Carcinoma and arterial thrombi. Arterial thrombi can develop in patients with carcinoma and often occur in unusual sites. Cryoglobulinemia or cryofibrinogenemia associated with carcinoma may cause small vessel thrombosis in fingers, toes, ears, or the nose on exposure to cold. Occasionally, patients will succumb to major arterial occlusions. The mechanisms are different than those described for venous thrombi even though the laboratory changes are similar.

Patient B, a 62-year-old man with exten- sive, recurrent carcinoma of the urinary bladder, developed congestive heart failure and cold legs. He died within three days despite heparin administration and appropriate medical management. Postmortem examination demonstrated a complete occlusion of the distal aorta by thrombus with minimal atherosclerosis. The bladder carcinoma had intravascular extensions, but had not extended to the aorta.

Mucin-producing carcinomas, often with intravascular extensions, are frequently complicated by thrombosis such as that described here. The extracts of these cancers have procoagulant activity that can replace partial deficiencies of plasma Factors VII, VIII, IX, X, or XI. The cell lysates can substitute for the phospholipid activating substances in the prothrombin time, the partial thromboplastin time, and the thromboplastin generation time.

Arterial thrombosis or embolism may develop in the absence of vascular invasion by the tumor.

When the tumor penetrates the intravascular space, it can activate coagulation by functioning as tissue factor. If severe, this action will cause systemic acceleration of coagulation. This effect is confirmed by the observation that the plasma fibrinogen in patients with carcinoma has been found to contain up to 11 percent soluble fibrin. The antithrombin III levels are usually very low. This suggests that conversion of prothrombin to thrombin and thrombin acting on fibrinogen is an ongoing process. Indeed, fibrinogen and platelets also have been reputed to interact directly with tumors, without involvement of the coagulation system. It is therefore not surprising to find deposits of intravascular fibrin at postmortem examination in the visceral capillary bed. Patients with intravascular fibrin formation more often tend to develop other venous or arterial occlusions around intravenous or intra-arterial lines.

Patient C, a 38-year-old woman with lung carcinoma, developed acute superior vena cava occlusion 48 hours after an intravenous subclavian line was placed for hyperalimentation. The patient's prothrombin time was 9.8 sec (control 11.5 sec) and the partial thromboplastin time was 28 sec (control 33 sec) The antithrombin III was 8.5 sec (control > 18.5 sec) and fibrin monomers were present. The line was removed, and heparin therapy was initiated. Effective tumoricidal chemotherapy was initiated. The clotting parameters returned to normal as the tumor regressed.

Treatment of the primary tumor is often the most effective therapy for the thrombophlebitis. Most cancers associated with coagulopathies, however, are resistant to therapy. Selective treatment directed toward alteration of the coagulation process may still significantly improve the patient's clinical status. Large studies comparing no anticoagulant therapy with selective antithrombotic therapy have not been conducted. Nevertheless, agents that suppress platelet aggregation or anticoagulants can be useful for selected patients. Patients with venous thrombotic

---

Therapy for clotting or bleeding in cancer patients should involve treatment of the tumor as well as the coagulopathy.

---

disease can be helped by administering heparin and then warafin to therapeutic levels. Patients with flagrant thrombosis or disseminated intravascular coagulation benefit from treatment with heparin. All the while, attempts should be made to control the tumor by surgery, radiation, or chemotherapy.

Diffuse intravascular coagulation and cancer. In some cases stimulation toward coagulation is so intense as to cause diffuse intravascular coagulation (DIC). This may be manifested initially as organ failure due to multiple microthrombi of nutrient arteries, followed by a hemorrhagic diathesis with defibrination, consumption of platelets and labile Factors V and VIII, release of FDP, accumulation of fibrin monomers, utilization of antithrombin III, and secondary fibrinolysis. DIC may develop acutely or take the form of a chronic consumptive coagulopathy. It has been described in patients with carcinomas of the stomach, lung, breast, prostate, bronchi, colon, pancreas, gallbladder, ovary, and kidney, as well as rhabdomyosarcomas and melanomas. Recognition of chronic DIC has been recorded to precede the clinical evidence of ovarian carcinoma by 10 months.

Patients with carcinoma should not be expected to present with the classical "textbook" findings of DIC. For example, patients with carcinoma may chronically have elevated fibrinogen levels, and a fall of fibrinogen level to 200 mgm% from 400 mgm% may therefore be significant. As the tumor can activate the extrinsic pathway by acting as the tissue factor, there may be little reduction of Factor VIII but profound reduction of Factor VII. In the early stages fibrin monomers in the circulation may prove diagnostic even with low titers of FDP. Schistocytes are often present. The patients with low-grade DIC may benefit most from heparin therapy.

DIC may be biochemically atypical with normal fibrinogen and Factor VIII.

Patient D, a 54-year-old man with known

recurrent carcinoma of the stomach, presented with acquired easy bruisability,
epistaxis, and hemoptysis. He was afebrile
with a hemoglobin of 10.5 gm%. Venipuncture sites continued to bleed in spite
of applied pressure. The platelet count
was 22,000/mm³, with a 30-min bleeding
time. Plasma fibrinogen was 35 mgm%.
The prothrombin time was 42.5 sec (control 11.5 sec), the partial thromboplastin
time was 110 sec (control 33 sec), and the
thrombin time without incubation was
32 sec (control 15 sec). The thrombin time
extended to 65 sec (control 17 sec) after
45 minutes incubation at 37°C. Factor VIII
level was 24% by function assay. The
FDPs were 120 μgm% by the tanned red
cell hemagglutination inhibition assay
(control <4.4 μgm%.) Fibrin monomers
were present, and schistocytes were found
on the peripheral smear. The coagulopathy was diagnosed as due to DIC, presumably from the thromboplastic effects of
the tumor. There was no evidence of sepsis
and no hypotension. Heparin therapy
was initiated with 4000-unit loading dose
given intravenously, followed by a constant infusion of 1000 units per hour. This
regimen further prolonged the thrombin
time, prothrombin time, and partial
thromboplastin time. Nevertheless, the
bleeding subsided. The platelet count
improved to 79,000 after 48 hours. The
fibrinogen was 108mm%, and the Factor
VIII was 120% after 72 hours of therapy.
The FDPs fell to 20 μgm%. The heparin
was continued for five days at 1000 units
per hour. Thereafter, the dose was reduced
to 500 units per hour and was given for
five days. There was no recurrence of
clinical or laboratory evidence of DIC.
Chemotherapy for the carcinoma was then
initiated, and the herapin was discontinued.

Carcinoma and marantic endocarditis.
Marantic endocarditis is often considered
a manifestation of accelerated coagulation
even though the exact mechanism of the
lesion's evolution is unknown. The marantic lesion is associated in a nonspecific
way with advanced carcinomas. The
valve murmurs or distal emboli of marantic lesions may be the first evidence of
carcinoma. Other forms of hypercoagulability such as thrombophlebitis may be
coexistent. Patients have presented for
medical care of acute cardiac arrhythmia
due to coronary artery marantic embolus,
only to be found to have advanced
carcinoma.

Patient E, a 42-year-old man, was admitted for the evaluation of epigastric pain,
splenomegaly, and displacement of the
duodenum. The patient had no evidence
of prior cardiac disease. On the third
hospital day he suffered an acute attack
of ventricular fibrillation for which resus-
citation efforts failed. Postmortem examination demonstrated a bulky carcinoma
arising from the stomach. The aortic cusps
were thickened with attached pedunculated marantic lesions (Fig. 11.1). The left
coronary artery was occluded by an embolus from the marantic vegetation.

Marantic endocarditis is characterized
by a fibrin and platelet mass attached
to the heart valves. The lesions are most
often left sided and are generally attached
to previously damaged valves. The diagnosis of marantic endocarditis should
be considered for any patient with known
carcinoma presenting with embolic phenomena. Occasionally, the echocardiogram strongly suggests the diagnosis.
Laboratory assays selected to search for
the signs of accelerated coagulation or
hypercoagulability may offer supportive,
but not diagnostic, data. The best form
of therapy is unknown; in fact, it is not
known whether any therapy delays further
propagation of the marantic lesion. Therapy can be selected, however, based upon
the most aberrant of the hypercoagulable

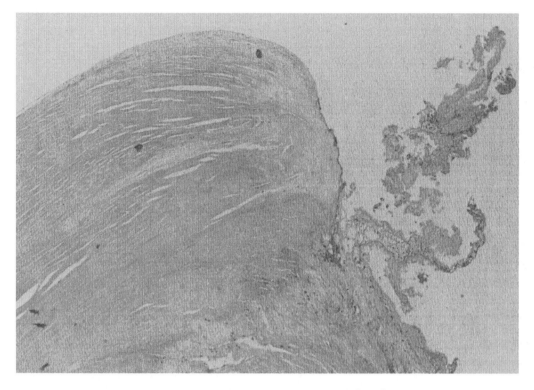

Fig. 11.1 Microscopic view of vegetations on the edge of the heart valve (Patient E) associated with a marantic endocarditis.

parameters: if chronic DIC is present, heparin therapy is employed; if accelerated platelet aggregation is present, aspirin or low molecular-weight dextran is prescribed to disrupt platelet function.

Patient F, a 68-year-old woman with metastatic endometrial carcinoma, presented with evolving neurologic deficits first involving speech, then right-sided paresis, then paralysis of the right side, and, finally, a semicoma. She had new congestive heart failure and elevations of the blood urea nitrogen and creatinine. Aortic outflow murmurs were heard on admission, but disappeared one hour later. The prothrombin time was 17.5 sec (control 13 sec). The partial thromboplastin time was normal. The fibrinogen level was 200 mgm%, and the platelet count was 48,000. Factor VII was 30% of normal, and Factor VIII was 21% of normal. The peripheral smear revealed schistocytes. Fibrin monomers and FDP were elevated, and the antithrombin III was decreased. She was diagnosed as having chronic DIC complicated by marantic endocarditis, and heparin therapy was initiated. The platelet count rose to 285,000; the fibrinogen rose to 450 mgm%. The schistocytes, monomers, and FDPs disappeared. The neurologic deficit had rapid partial resolution. The heart failure and renal failure resolved. No new cardiac murmurs nor embolic episodes appeared. The patient was started on cytotoxic agents to control the endometrial tumor.

Marantic endocarditis may be caused by

local fibrin coagulation on the heart valves or by accelerated platelet aggregation.

Coagulant activity in malignant ascites. The recirculation of ascitic fluid back into the systemic circulation through a peritoneal-venous shunt has been associated with intravascular coagulation abnormalities related to thromboplastic material within the fluid. Malignant ascites has free fibrinogen, elevated antithrombin III, elevated antitrypsin activity and FDPs, which range from 400 to 4,500 μgm% as compared to up to 115 μmg% for cirrhotic ascites. Malignant and nonmalignant ascites have had equally low levels of prothrombin, Factors V, VII, VIII, and X, urokinase inhibitors, and alpha$_2$ macroglobulins. DIC may ensue after the fluid enters the circulation. Ascitic fluid may also perform as an anticoagulant, but this depends on the levels of FDPs in the solution. The patient's tolerance of the reinfusion seems to be modified by multiple host factors such as the ability of the reticuloendothelial system to clear abnormal substances, the levels of circulating procoagulants, and the level of inhibitors of fibrinolysins. Ascites can act as a substitute for complete thromboplastin in the prothrombin time, in the activated and the nonactivated partial thromboplastin time, and as incomplete thromboplastin in the two-stage thromboplastin generation tests. The infranatant and occasionally the supernatant from the ascitic fluids can replace the phospholipids in the coagulation tests. Not all fluids have this activity; thus each fluid should be tested in vitro before the shunt is placed so that the relative risks involved can be determined.

Patient G, a 50-year-old woman with ovarian carcinoma, had rapidly recurring ascites after multiple attempts at therapy. Frequent peritoneal taps were required to control the burdensome ascites. At this

advanced stage of disease, a Leveen shunt was placed. Within 24 hours, the patient developed pulmonary insufficiency, and peripheral blood manifestations of DIC. The shunt was ligated, and heparin was initiated. The patient died in two days. Postmortem examination demonstrated microthrombi throughout the pulmonary arterial circulation (Fig. 11.2).

Fibrinogenolysis and fibrinolysis in cancer patients. Fibrinogenolysis and fibrinolysis cause the dissolution of circulating or precipitated fibrinogen and fibrin. Plasminogen is converted to plasmin, which is then able by hydrolysis to cleave portions of Factors V and VIII, fibrinogen, and fibrin. When in excess, this process creates hypocoagulable states. Besides

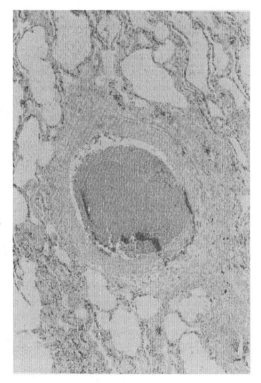

Fig. 11.2 Microthrombus within the pulmonary vasculature and adherent to the endothelial surface (Patient G).

causing depletion of these substances, the process produces potent anticoagulant by-products. Fibrinogen and fibrin give up their respective degradation products, FDPs and fdps. These substances interfere with coagulation and platelet thrombosis, and thus further potentiate an anticoagulated situation. The FDPs/fdps can be detected by several techniques. The commonly used, commercially available technique uses latex beads coated with antifibrinogen antibody. The latex beads agglutinate in the presence of FDP/fdp. Also available is the tanned red cell hemagglutination inhibition immunoassay. In vitro studies of the effect of the FDPs/fdps on the thrombin time assay, and less commonly on other clotting assays, reveal the anticoagulant effect of these substances. The platelet aggregometry will also show the effect of the FDP and fdp substances. The overall rate of fibrinolysis can be determined by the serial thrombin time and euglobulin lysis. The former measures active plasmin, whereas the latter is a measure chiefly of circulating activators of plasminogen. The actual substrate levels of plasminogen and plasmin also can be measured in the clinical laboratory. Plasminogen and plasmin levels may be depleted when fibrinolysis is flagrant.

When in physiologic balance, fibrinolysis helps to keep blood in a fluid form, but when excessively activated, excessive bleeding may ensue. Fibrinolysis may be secondary to DIC or may be primarily and initiated by tumor products released into the circulation. This may be dramatic when circulating tumor cells are released during surgery. Some tumors may actually have their own capacity to activate lysis.

Fibrinolysis may be primary with the fibrolytic stimulus released by the tumor directly, or it may be secondary to disseminated coagulation.

Several carcinomas have been described in association with an increased incidence of lysis. These include carcinomas of the lung, pancreas, breast, stomach, colon, ovary, kidney, lip, esophagus, thyroid, and liver, as well as melanoma and mesothelioma. Reports of these cases have not adequately distinguished between primary and secondary fibrinolysis. Plasminogen activator has been found to be elevated in carcinomas of the cervix, lung, prostate, and kidney, but was missing from invasive endometrial adenocarcinoma. Patients with advanced liver disease secondary to metastasis or to comorbid cirrhosis are more likely to develop fibrinolysis than DIC. The latter group of patients has a decreased capacity to generate plasminogen activator inhibitor, and often has a reduced capacity to clear the FDPs/fdps by the reticuloendothelial system.

Patient H, a 52-year-old man with known advanced cirrhosis of the liver, developed a hemorrhagic diathesis one hour after completion of a pneumonectomy for lung carcinoma. Bleeding occurred in the surgical wound, at venipuncture sites, and into the urine. The platelet count was 270,000 preoperatively and 240,000 postoperatively. The prothrombin time and the partial thromboplastin time were prolonged. Factor VIII level was 85%. Clot lysis was complete at 30 min by the euglobulin lysis test. The serial thrombin time was 18 sec at 0 time (control 15 sec), 29 sec after 30 min of incubation, and 62 sec after 45 min of incubation. Epsilon amino caproic acid five grams was initiated intravenously. This was continued at 1 gram IV every hour until the bleeding stopped six hours later. Laboratory values returned to normal

---

Liver disease promotes the likelihood of fibrinolysis in cancer patients.

The measurement of FDPs is a simple and generally available method for discovering whether fibrinolysis is present. In one study, 9 of 17 patients with prostatic carcinoma had FDP levels of 8 to 128 μgm%. Patients with benign prostatic disease had very much lower or absent titers of FDPs. Patients with renal cell carcinoma may have FDPs in the plasma and urine. Their FDPs are important only in the absence of glomerular lesions and in the absence of hematuria from any source. The persistence of elevated FDPs after surgery may be the first indication that residual metastatic cells are present.

Epsilon amino caproic acid (EACA, Amicar) is an effective therapeutic agent for neutralizing plasmin, but EACA will not prevent the release of activators from the tumor. Effective antitumor therapy therefore is necessary to arrest release of the substance. The doses of EACA necessary are unpredictable. As little as 500 mgm orally every six hours can occasionally correct abnormal laboratory findings. As much as 15 g in 12 hours may be required to control flagrant hemorrhagic fibrinolysis. Subsequent doses must then be determined by the clinical and laboratory findings.

Estrogen therapy and fibrinolysis. The fibrinolytic system is also important in relation to the estrogens used to treat metastatic prostate carcinoma. Patients who received high doses of diethylstilbestrol (DES) developed a higher than expected incidence of myocardial infarction, congestive heart failure, and central nervous system thrombosis. Estrogens cause a reduction in the fibrinolytic activity present in vein walls and a compensatory tendency for urokinase inhibitors to fall and for the plasminogen and alpha$_2$ macroglobulin levels to rise. Thus, only low doses of estrogens can be prescribed in an attempt to control metastatic prostatic carcinoma without encountering risks of these major sequelae. Patients may occasionally appear very sensitive, even to low doses of estrogen, and may develop thrombi. Such patients can be protected by giving oral anticoagulants in addition to the estrogens.

Patient I, a 68-year-old man with metastatic prostatic carcinoma for whom orchiectomy failed, was given 3 g of DES per day. His bone pain was rapidly controlled, and his bone lesions subsequently healed. After two months on DES, the patient developed angina pectoris. Before initiating DES, the prothrombin time was 12.0 sec (control 11.5 sec), and the partial thromboplastin time was 34 sec (control 33 sec). When examined again after two months of DES therapy, the prothrombin time was 9 sec, and partial thromboplastin time was 28 sec. Plasminogen levels were elevated. Warafin was given so as to extend the prothrombin time and partial thromboplastin. The DES dose was not changed. The patient had no further anginal attacks.

3.0 Platelets

Thrombocytosis occasionally presents in malignancy in the absence of metastasis to the bone marrow. In one series of 82 patients with thrombocytosis, 31 were found to have neoplasm. Thrombocytosis is sometimes mistakenly attributed to such myeloproliferative syndromes as polycythemia vera or primary thrombocytosis, and only later diagnosed as being secondary to carcinoma of the pancreas or lung. The platelets may function normally, or they may function poorly. Patients with hypofunctional platelets may have decreased platelet Factor III release, poor aggregation, poor clot retraction, and have prolonged bleeding times. Such findings are for the most part unexplained for patients with carcinoma. It may be postu-

lated that such platelets are partially activated and have partial release or that
they are inhibited by plasma FDPs. Bleeding, especially from the tumor-bearing
organ, may be associated with these
changes. Platelet function testing is required in each case to determine the risk
factors associated with each patient's
thrombocytosis. Rarely, in patients with
thrombocytosis, platelet transfusions may
be needed to temporarily control bleeding. The effectiveness of these "micro
Band Aids" is brief.

Thrombocytopenia and cancer. Patients
with cancer may develop thrombocytopenia because of coexistent but independent diseases, bone marrow displacement,
myelophthisic changes, splenic sequestration, consumptive coagulopathy, radiotherapy, or chemotherapy. The categories
are summarized in three levels: peripheral
(systemic) destruction, peripheral use,
and under production. (Table 11.1). Marrow suppression caused by chemotherapy
is the most common cause of thrombocytopenia in patients with carcinoma. Spurious thrombocytopenia or pseudothrom-
bocytopenia occurs in patients who usually do not develop bleeding. Dilutional
thrombocytopenia occurs when massive
blood transfusions are necessary, if the
transfusions employ banked blood that is
over three days old. Such blood has no
functionally normal platelets present. Immunologic thrombocytopenia in cancer
patients is caused by the production of a
globulin that causes platelet aggregation.
   Hemorrhage rarely occurs at platelet
counts greater than 20,000/mm^3, but occurs often if there is an associated thrombocytopathy due to myelophthisic
changes, circulating FDPs, partial release
of platelet granules, or pharmaco-inhibi-
tion from agents such as aspirin. The
potential for hemorrhage is increased also
if the thrombocytopenia is acquired rapidly or if it is associated with sepsis. The
risk of hemorrhage also seems increased if

Table 11.1 Causes of Acquired
Thrombocytopenia

I. Decreased Production
   A. Toxic marrow suppression
      1. Ionizing radiation
      2. Drug suppression
         a. Chemotherapeutic agents
         b. Alcohol
         c. Thiazides
         d. Chloramphenicol
   B. Maturation failure
      1. Aplastic anemia
      2. Megaloblastic arrest (Vitamin
         B$_{12}$ or folate deficiency)
   C. Infectious suppression
      1. Bacterial
      2. Viral
II. Marrow Replacement
   A. Epithelial carcinoma with
      myelophthisis
   B. Lymphoma including leukemia,
      myeloma
   C. Mesenchymal fibrosis
      (myelofibrosis)
III. Peripheral Extramedullary Use
   A. Platelet loss ex vivo
      1. Hemorrhage with insufficient
         replacement and dilution
      2. Extracorporeal circulation
   B. Sequestration
      1. Hypersplenism
      2. Hemangioma or angiosarcoma
      3. Hypothermia
   C. Enhanced destruction
      1. Immune destruction
         a. Drug sensitivity
         b. Ideopathic thrombocytopenia
      2. Nonimmune
         a. DIC
         b. Thrombotic
            thrombocytopenic purpura
         c. Hemolytic uremic syndrome
         d. Bacteremia

thrombocytopenia is induced by chemotherapy, possibly because of concomitant
damage to the endothelium.

Patient J, a 58-year-old-woman with disseminated leiomyosarcoma, was treated with cyclophosphamide and Adriamycin. At day 21 following chemotherapy, she had persistant thrombocytopenia (80,000) without clinical evidence of bleeding. The thrombocytopenia persisted at day 35, and bone marrow studies revealed adequate megakaryocytes. The blood smear showed clumping of the platelets in all fields. The patient was again treated with chemotherapy without incident although the spurious thrombocytopenia did not recede. A cold platelet agglutinin was subsequently identified in the patient's serum by special techniques.

Table 11.2 Factors that Accentuate the Hemorrhagic Tendency in Patients with Thrombocytopenia

I. Drugs Interfering with Platelet Function
  A. Aspirin
  B. Phenylbutazone
  C. Indomethacin
  D. Carbinicillin in high doses
II. Platelet Surface Inhibitors
  A. Fibrin(ogen) degradation products
  B. Macroglobulins
  C. Monoclonol protein spikes
III. Valsalva Maneuver
  A. Cough
  B. Straining to pass stool
  C. Lifting heavy objects
  D. Sexual intercourse
IV. Fever and Sepsis
V. Coincidental Protein Coagulopathy
  A. Primary
  B. Acquired
    1. Dysfibrinogeneia associated with liver disease
    2. Factor II, VII, IX, X deficiency
      a. Liver disease
      b. Vitamin K deficiency
    3. Others
VI. Systemic Pathologic Conditions
  A. Uremia
  B. Hyperbilirubinemia
  C. Primary thrombocytopathy

Thrombocytopenia associated with hypersplenism may be accentuated by chemotherapy.

The treatment of thrombocytopenic hemorrhage extends beyond transfusion. Sepsis and fever should be controlled. Low doses of steroids may improve capillary integrity. Prophlaxis against CNS bleeding involves instructions to avoid the Valsalva maneuver, with its pursuant increase of intrathoracic and intracranial pressure. This is accomplished by avoiding constipation, by suppressing coughs, by abstaining from sexual intercourse, and by not lifting or pushing heavy objects. By avoiding the precipitating factors listed in Table 11.2 the need for transfusion may be minimized.

A low platelet count alone is not an indication for giving platelet transfusions. If the patient is bleeding, or if clinical problems exist that make bleeding likely, platelet transfusions are appropriate. The physician can be aided in these judgments by measuring the bleeding time, capillary fragility, prothrombin consumption, and clot retraction. By using these assays, the physician can determine whether there is better hemostasis than implied by the platelet count alone. Some rules of platelet transfusion are outlined in Table 11.3. The single important feature is the concomitant reversal of factors contributing to thrombocytopenic bleeding, such as sepsis, an active ulcer, or a bleeding wound or artery.

Severe thrombocytopenia is associated with cerebral, gastrointestinal, and genitourinary tract bleeding.

Siblings, parents, and offspring are the most appropriate donors of platelets.

Table 11.3 Guides for Platelet Transfusion

Correct ancillary contributing factors such as sepsis, associated coagulopathy, or surgical bleeding.

Administer platelets if bleeding is active and occurs with prolonged bleeding time or poor prothrombin consumption.

Administer platelets prophylactically if maneuvers are required that may induce trauma or Valsalva reaction. These include laryngoscopy, bronchoscopy, intubation, sigmoidoscopy, and colonoscopy.

Administer platelets to form temporary "micro Band Aids" for patients who have bleeding coincidentally with processes such as uremia or aspirin ingestion.

Administer 6 to 10 units of platelets and repeat daily until bleeding stops; if given prophylactically, administer about twice weekly.

They can help to preserve the blood bank reservoirs, and generally offer the freshest cells. The HL-A match is rarely an issue for these patients with thrombocytopenia, as they usually do not require long-term exogenous platelet support. Transfusions across ABO barriers, though not ideal, are acceptable. Minor hemolytic reactions can occur. Platelet counts are usually about 50,000 or higher 24 hours after transfusion. If sepsis, hyperslenism, or antiplatelet antibodies are present, the counts will be much lower 24 hours after transfusion. If the patient has had a splenectomy, the platelet counts will stay elevated for four or five days. Thus, the clinical situation dictates the frequency with which the patient is to be transfused.

4.0 Red blood cells

Anemia is a common complication for patients with carcinoma and can cause significant morbidity. The etiology of anemia frequently involves many factors and thus may require multiple, but selective, therapies. Anemia may be due to deficiencies of iron, folic acid, vitamin B_{12}, protein, and trace materials; myelophthisis or leukoerythroblastosis; hemolysis associated with malignancy; unresponsiveness to erythropoietin; endocrine deficiencies; "anemia of chronic disease"; tumor-produced toxins that suppress red blood cell metabolism; chemotoxins that suppress red blood cell metabolism; and chemotherapy and radiation. The anemia associated with cancer is too often considered as an obligatory consequence of malignancy, and patients are encouraged to live within the limitations imposed upon their activity by reduced hemoglobin. These limitations, however, can be significant burden to an already burdensome disease. The physician can often improve the quality of the patient's life by diagnosing and selectively treating the anemia.

The most common malignancy associated with reversible anemia is iron deficiency.

Anemias due to deficiency states. A discussion of the details of iron, folate, or vitamin B_{12} deficiencies is beyond the scope of this chapter, except to point out the difficulties relevant to cancer patients. Chronic blood loss may result from any cancerous or benign lesion in the oropharyngeal, gastrointestinal, and genitourinary systems. The blood loss may be too small to cause obvious hematuria or melena. The stool guaiac for occult blood will be misleadingly negative if less than 10 cc of blood are lost to the aliquot of feces tested. Use of benzidine, a more sensitive reagent, or radioactive labeling of the red blood cells may be needed to detect very small quantities of blood lost to the stool. Barium contrast studies may then be indicated. Patients who have had resections of the stomach, jejunum, or ileum may develop iron, folate, or vitamin B_{12} deficiency, respectively, because they cannot mix and dissolve their food, have inadequate intrinsic factors, have blind loops, or have inadequate absorptive surfaces. Because chronically ill patients are often anorexic and therefore often refuse meats and leafy green vegetables, they lose their normal sources of iron and folate. In these cases, replacement of the missing nutrients is simple and will give gratifying results. Bile salt and pancreatic enzyme deficiencies due to obstruction or displacement of the biliary of pancreatic organ systems by the cancer can cause malabsorption, which in turn causes anemia. Treatment of malabsorption with bile salts or pancreatic enzymes administered orally will both correct the anemia and improve the patient's overall nutritional status. Severe malnutrition that mimics kwashiorkor may develop from the anorexia or malabsorption but this is rare. Such patients have hypocellular marrows, hypotransferrinemia, and deficiencies of trace materials. The serum transferrin level, which falls in malnutrition, is an excellent marker for the status of the patient's protein nutrition. It remains to be clarified what exact affect hypotransferrinemia has on normal iron metabolism in humans. Proteins and carbohydrates can be replaced with oral or intravenous supplements. These supplements should include the vitamins needed for erythropoiesis and normal red blood cell survival. These include riboflavin or vitamin B_2 (a cofactor for glutathione reductase and an enzyme that prevents oxidative denaturization of hemoglobin), pyridoxine, or vitamin B_6 (a cofactor for folic acid reductase and an enzyme needed for normal folic acid metabolism). Vitamin K is necessary to prevent bleeding, which may develop from hypoprothrombinemia. Even severe vitamin E deficiency has been associated with anemia. Appropriately selected multivitamins, given orally or parenterally each day, will guard against these deficiencies.

Myelophthisic anemia. The bone marrow is a fenestrated, spongelike network of "extravascular" channels juxtaposed to the intravascular space. The microenvironment of the bone marrow must conform to highly refined specifications to support normal red cell, white cell, and platelet production. Disruption of the physiologic "barriers" between the marrow channels and the efferent blood vessels is manifested as myelophthisic anemia. If the disruption is very severe, leukoerythroblastic anemia will occur. The peripheral cytologic changes may include anisocytosis, poikilocytosis, polychromasia, "tear drops," microspherocytes, and nucleated red blood cells. Leukocytosis with myelocytes and metamyelocytes, and thrombocytosis or thrombocytopenia often with metathrombocytes are usually present in the peripheral blood. Promyelocytes and myeloblasts are not normally part of this picture. Circulating megakaryocytes will occasionally be found. The reticulocyte count is slightly elevated but is not commensurate with the severity of the anemia. The tumor burden in the bone marrow is rarely commensurate with the peripheral blood's manifestations. The marrow's reaction to metastatic cells is variable: the peripheral blood smear may be nearly normal even though there is extensive marrow replacement with tumor, or the smear may show several alterations and pancytopenia with minimal metastatic cancer in the marrow. Absence of metastatic cells on a single random needle aspirate and biopsy of the marrow should not dissuade the physician from the diagnosis of metastatic disease to the marrow. In this situation a microscopic examination of a wedge biopsy of the marrow is appropriate. On the other hand, the presence of myelophthisic anemia should not be construed as proof of metastatic disease. Several diseases are associated with leukoerythroblastic blood picture; these include myelofibrosis, polycythemia vera, leukemia, hemolysis, sepsis, lipid storage disease, tuberculosis, and fungemia. Therapy for myelophthisic anemia is the appropriately selected antitumor therapy. Resolution of the myelophthisic picture may be the earliest sign of successful tumor suppression; the peripheral blood smear may improve before the anemia resolves. Unfortunately, successful control of tumor does not always mean that the bone marrow will fully recover. Such carcinomas as those of the breast or lung stimulate intense fibrotic reaction in the marrow, which remains after the tumor has left the marrow. There may also be transient or permanent marrow damage from chemotherapy or radiation therapy.

The treatment of malignancy-associated myelophthisic anemia is systemic chemotherapy of the tumor.

Distant effects of carcinoma on red blood cells. Carcinomas can adversely affect erythropoiesis and red blood cell survival unrelated to marrow invasion. These distant or remote effects can occasionally be corrected by simply removing the tumor mass. Several mechanisms exist that explain these distant effects: suppression of erythropoiesis by chronic inflammation, hemolysis, plasma volume expansion, defective iron metabolism, and increased reticuloendothelial activity.

Some tumors stimulate local inflammatory reactions, often with necrosis or superinfection. The tumor may be completely localized. When this occurs, there tends to be depression of erythropoiesis and decreased sensitivity to erythropoietin. Removal of the necrotic tumor mass may end the anemia.

Patient K, a 78-year-old woman, presented with carcinoma of the breast. The lesion, which had been present for eight months, was very large with necrotic and inflamed surfaces. Candida albicans and multiple bacteria were cultured from the wound. The contiguous axillary lymph nodes were palpable. The hematocrit was 28%; hemoglobin was 9.0 gm%; reticulocyte count was 0.5%. There was no evidence of metastases to the bones or other organs, and deficiency state could account for the anemia. The mass was surgically excised. Four months postoperatively, the hematocrit was 38% and the hemoglobin was 12 gm%. Local metastasis in the skin and distant metastasis to the lungs developed 10 months postoperatively. Anemia did not recur.

Hemolysis is another cause for anemia in patients with carcinoma. As many as 50 percent of patients with carcinoma may have some hemolysis. The anemia is characterized by red blood cell fragmentation (schistocytes), shortened red cell survival, hemoglobinemia, hemosiderinuria, elevated lactate dehydrogenase and mild reticulocytosis. Several mechanisms cause hemolysis. As already discussed, intravascular thrombosis and red cell fragmentation may occur with mucin-producing carcinomas of the breast, colon, prostate, pancreas, stomach, lung, and gallbladder. In these patients, the red cell survival may be only 12.5 days. Hemolysis may also be caused by toxins released from the tumor. Cell-free extracts from some breast carcinomas cause red cell lysis in vitro. Another cause for hemolysis is the acquired immune, warm-reacting antibody, hemolytic reaction rarely found with ovarian carcinoma. In all of these situations, removal of the tumor will help control the anemia. On the other hand, splenectomy and steroids usually fail to control the anemia.

The effect of the reticuloendothelial system (RES) on red blood cell survival is related to hypertrophy of the RES and is associated with shortened red cell survival. Heightened RES activity is found in patients with carcinoma, and fever from the cancer or from comorbid infections will accentuate RES activity. Portal hypertension, due to malignant diseases in the liver, will further accentuate the RES functions by causing congestive splenomegaly. Therapy should not be directed toward the role of RES in causing the anemia. Agents that suppress RES function may complicate cytotoxic therapy. The latter must have priority. Steroids, cyclophosphamide, azathioprine, and splenic radiation, while useful therapy for the tumor, may simultaneously suppress RES activity and improve the hematocrit.

Anemia of chronic disease. "Anemia of chronic disease" is a term used to classify anemias found in chronically ill patients, including those with carcinoma. The syndrome is characterized by a normocytic or microcytic anemia with low serum irons, low total iron binding capacity, increased serum ferritin, slow ferrokinetics, and increased deposition of iron in the bone marrow, liver, and spleen. The amount of iron stored in the tissues can be crudely estimated by evaluating the Prussian blue-stained hemosiderin and ferritin in tissue samples, the most available of which is bone marrow. The syndrome may occur without evident metastasis. This anemia is due to a metabolic shift in the handling of iron, such that iron is unavailable for incorporation into heme. The metabolic defect causing this shift is unknown. Response to erythropoietin is poor. Effective therapy is unavailable other than the successful treatment of the carcinoma and any associated inflammatory diseases.

Therapy-associated anemia. Therapy for cancer will frequently cause or worsen anemias. Many of the therapeutic modalities are toxic to the bone marrow and contribute to anemia, or more commonly to pancytopenia. By cataloging the chemotherapeutic agents whenever possible, one can predict those agents likely to be marrow toxic. The catalog includes purine analogs (thiopurines, 6-mercaptopurine, thioguanine, azathioprine), pyrimidine analogs (5-fluorouracil, 5-fluoro-2-dioxyuridine), nucleotide synthesis inhibitors (cytosine arabinoside, hydroxyurea, daunomycin, Adriamycin), alkylating agents (cyclophosphamide, nitrogen mustard, melphalan, Thiotepa, busulfan), and folate inhibitors (methotrexate). The duration and depth of the depression of the white blood cell, red blood cell, and platelet counts are determined by the drug used, the dose delivered, the duration of therapy, and the amount of marrow suppression already caused by prior chemotherapy or radiation therapy. The erythroblasts are the most sensitive cells to the effects of drug therapy. During the marrow-suppressive phases of therapy, adverse symptoms may be relieved by administering packed red blood cell transfusions. Care must be directed simultaneously to the problems of malnutrition, and deficiencies of iron, folate, and the vitamins discussed earlier. The indications for transfusions are dictated by the patient's symptoms. In practice, patients receiving chemotherapy generally tolerate as little as 9.0 gm% of hemoglobin without undue stress. Hemoglobin levels in this range rarely require transfusion support. Patients with atherosclerosis of the coronary arteries, the mesenteric arteries, or other major vessels may become symptomatic at this level of hemoglobin and thus may need earlier transfusion support. Patients with 8.0 gm% of hemoglobin or less are generally symptomatic from anemia. When and how frequently they are transfused is a clinical decision made by the physician and the patient. Normally only 1/120th of the circulating red cell mass is lost each day, but patients with cancer may have more rapid loss of red cells. Nevertheless, sudden hemoglobin decreases cannot be ascribed to marrow suppression, and such other causes of blood loss as bleeding and hemolysis must be sought. Any non-essential drug capable of causing hemolysis should be discontinued. Many patients receiving drug therapy have gastritis and esophagitis, both of which may cause bleeding.

Radiation therapy and anemia. Radiation therapy is toxic for any marrow in the path of the radiation beam. The degree of anemia or pancytopenia caused by radiation therapy is determined by the amount of bone marrow covered by the radiation ports and the dose of radiation given. Although all cellular elements of the marrow are affected by radiation, erythroid cells are the most sensitive. Because of the longer life span of the circulating erythrocytes, effects of radiation therapy may be missed for many days unless reticulocyte counts are performed. Stem cells are similarly sensitive to radiation. After significant doses, the portion of marrow irradiated will remain hypoplastic for many years. After 4500 rad, patients are known to maintain hypoplastic marrows in the area of therapy for up to 16 years. Productive bone marrow in the adult is confined to the skull, vertebrae, ribs, sternum, pelvic bones (iliac, ischium, and pubis), and upper ends of the femur and humerus. The more areas to receive radiation, the worse will be the anemia (or pancytopenia), and therefore, the pelvic bones and the vertebrae are the most important. The abscopal effect of radiation on bone marrow is a poorly defined suppression from small, sublethal doses of radiation. This suppression is commonly observed following splenic radiation for chronic myelogenous leukemia and is reversible.

Bone marrow biopsies should not be taken from areas that were previously irradiated, as the morphology may not represent the overall marrow status or capacity (Fig. 11.3). The marrow may re-

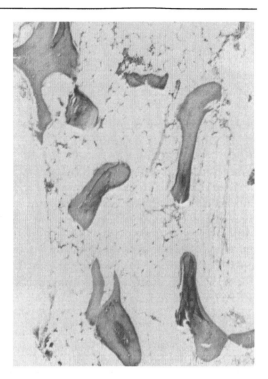

Fig. 11.3 *Bone marrow biopsy specimen of the iliac crest demonstrating interspicule space occupied by fat and occasional mononuclear cells in isolated foci.*

cover partially, but the radiation-induced alteration of the marrow milieu is not conducive to maturation of the stem cells. Transfusion support is the only effective therapy now available for patients with extensive radiation-induced marrow damage. Bone marrow transplantation, now available on an investigational basis for some forms of marrow aplasia, may be available in the future.

Endocrine deficiencies and anemia. In special circumstances patients may develop anemia due to endocrine deficiencies. Patients who receive radiation therapy to the oropharynx, neck, or superior mediastinum may develop hypothyroidism. Patients who require orchiectomy for testicular or prostatic carcinoma will develop androgen deficiencies. Patients now treated on investigational protocols for lymphoblastic leukemia may receive radiation therapy to the testicles to treat sanctuaries of lymphoblasts missed by chemotherapy. Patients may have adrenalectomy to control breast carcinoma. Selective hormone replacement therapy can be used for all of these patients, provided the replacement has no adverse effect on the cancer control.

Acquired Hemoglobinopathies. Very rarely patients with new malignancies may develop acquired hemoglobinopathy or pseudohemoglobinopathy. A patient with thymoma has been reported to have had an acquired Bart's hemoglobin (alpha thalassemia), and other rare cases have been reported. Any anemia, if severe, can result in the reappearance of expanded hemoglobin F production in the red blood cells.

Erythrocytosis. Hypernephromas, hepatocellular carcinomas, hemangioblastomas, and bronchogenic carcinomas, as well as benign tumors of the uterus, adrenal glands, and ovaries are capable of stimulating the marrow to cause erythrocytosis. The tumors excrete an $alpha_2$ macroprotein that acts like or is identical to erythropoietin. A peripheral blood picture of polycythemia, with or without thrombocytosis or leukocytosis, may be the first indication of malignancy or the first indication of recurrence of a malignancy. These patients lack signs and symptoms for other causes for erythrocytosis, such as hypoxemia due to lung disease, high-oxygen-affinity hemoglobinopathies, right-to-left shunts, renal cysts, and polycythemia vera. The erythropoietin level is elevated. Primary therapy for tumor-associated erythrocytosis is removal of the tumor. Because this is not always successful, phlebotomy to the point of iron deficiency becomes a useful adjunct whenever the patient is bothered by polycythemia. Erythrocytosis may

be used as a marker for recurrence of the tumor.

Patient L, a 65-year-old man, was found to have a hemoglobin level of 18.5 gm%. The cardiac and lung examinations were normal. No organomegaly was evident. The pO_2 was 89 mm Hg with 94% saturation; the vitamin B_{12} level was normal; the erythropoietin level was elevated. The bone marrow had erythroid hyperplasia. An intravenous pyelogram demonstrated a mass in the left kidney. The hypernephroma was removed surgically, and the hemoglobin levels returned to normal. The patient was followed frequently with IVPs, urinary cytologies, and hemoglobin levels. Four years after the first presentation, the erythrocytosis reappeared. Simultaneously, a mass was discovered in the remaining kidney. The erythropoietin level was again elevated.

5.0 White blood cells

The white blood cell mass, including neutrophils and lymphocytes, is crucial for the patient's defenses and is affected in a variety of ways by cancer and its therapy. In addition to quantitative changes in the circulating white blood cell pool, qualitative functional changes of the white blood cells are frequent, as are changes in the relative proportions of the types of white cells including the eosinophils, basophils, and monocytes.

The recent development of cell separation techniques for white blood cells has stimulated interest in the white blood cells of the cancer patient. In the past, platelet transfusion reversed hemorrhagic deaths secondary to thrombocytopenia; currently, the availability of granulocyte transfustions may cause a diminution in the infectious mortality that develops as a consequence of leukopenia, particularly in leukemic patients.

Leukemoid reactions and cancer. Leukemoid reactions secondary to carcinoma develop with localized or metastatic disease that almost invariably involves the bone marrow. The peripheral blood and bone marrow show a conspicuous increase of myelocytes and metamyelocytes but no significant increase of promyelocytes or myeloblasts. The term leukoerythroblastic anemia is applied when nucleated red blood cells appear on the peripheral smear. A concomitant shift to early erythrocyte forms generally appears in the bone marrow, and a moderate anemia is often present. Monocytosis is often evident but with no increase of eosinophils and basophils. Many cancers, including carcinomas of the lung, stomach, kidney, breast, pancreas, bladder, prostate, and rectum, can cause leukemoid reactions. Various and unproven explanations have been suggested to explain the reaction; these include marrow "irritation," marrow displacement, disruption of the barrier between the marrow and the intravascular circulation, and humoral products released by the tumor. These humoral factors have not yet been characterized. Two mechanisms appear to be involved: the tumor may secrete a colony-stimulating substance, or clearance of neutrophils from the circulating pool may be delayed. The humoral factors may create a leukocytosis, even when the tumor is still localized. This can be corrected after local therapy.

Patient M, a 58-year-old man with local pelvic extension of bladder carcinoma, had a white blood cell count of 19,500 with increased myelocytes and metamyelocytes. Few nucleated red blood cells appeared on the peripheral smear. There was no evidence of infection. The leukocyte alkaline phosphatase was 210 (normal $\leq$ 150). A needle biopsy of the bone marrow failed to demonstrate metastatic cells. Wide field radiation therapy caused

disappearance of the tumor and disappearance of the leukemoid reaction.

The leukemoid reaction associated with tumors must be distinguished from other causes of leukocytosis, as the therapies are so divergent. The list of causes includes bacterial and fungal infection, primary or secondary Cushing's syndrome, tumor necrosis, idiosyncratic drug reactions, physiologic drug reactions (e.g., to steriods or lithium), hyperthyroidisn, hemolysis, recovery after replacement therapy for folic acid or vitamin B_{12} deficiency, recovery from recent marrow suppression by chemotherapy, functional or anatomic asplenia, rheumatic diseases, hyperosmolality, and chronic myelogenous leukemia (CML). Whereas almost all causes of leukocytosis show a normal or elevated leukocyte alkaline phosphatase (LAP), patients with chronic leukemia have low LAPs. The distinction between CML and leukemoid reaction may be subtle, however, and karyotyping may be essential.

Patient N, a 68-year-old woman, had been treated 15 years earlier for breast carcinoma metastatic to the bones. Radiation therapy had been used to control symptomatic bone pain. The patient presented 15 years later with a leukemoid reaction. Estrogen therapy successfully reduced the leukemoid shift from 50,000 to 20,000 white blood cells/mm³. Bone marrow biopsy confirmed the presence of marrow metastases. Three months later the white blood cell count rose to 150,000 cells/mm³, and acute myeloblastic phase of CML was documented on the basis of a Philadelphia-positive chromosome and a bone marrow biopsy showing tumor and leukemia (Fig. 11.4).

Cytologic evaluation of the neutrophils can occasionally distinguish between the leukocytosis associated with inflam-

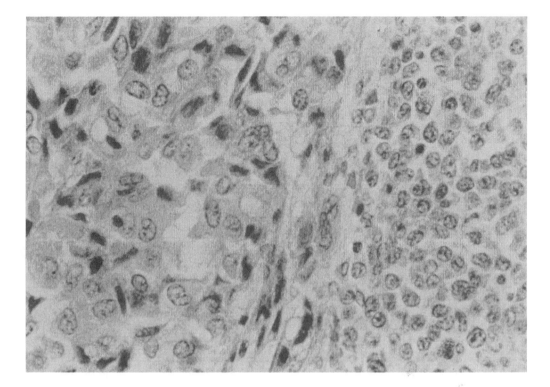

Fig. 11.4 Bone marrow biopsy demonstrating a colision tumor with metastatic breast cancer to the marrow space (left) and a myeloproliferative expansion of the marrow cavity (right), most probably representing chronic myelogenous leukemia.

matory responses and that associated with tumors. With malignancy-associated changes, the polymorphonuclear cells have nuclear projections containing chromosomal subunits when viewed by electron microscopy. Light microscopy shows that the cells have increased nuclear size, discontinuity of the nuclear membranes, translucent nuclear inclusion, and increased spacing between nuclear bands.

Little is known about abnormalities of neutrophilic function in patients with carcinoma. It has been demonstrated that the sera of patients with prostatic carcinoma inhibit the migration of leukocytes and that this inhibition is related to the level of alpha$_2$ globulins. Malnutrition, which develops with advanced cancers, may cause depression of neutrophilic response to infectious agents.

Eosinophils, basophils, and cancer. Eosinophilia often accompanies the myeloproliferative disorders and Hodgkin's disease. It may occasionally be seen in patients with carcinomas of the lung, bronchus, thyroid, or cervix. More than 10 percent of patients with carcinoma of the lung have eosinophils greater than 500/mm^3 with no concomitant evidence of allergy or parasitic infestation. The presence of eosinophils in the peripheral blood or pleural effusions makes an underlying occult carcinoma suspect. These are nonspecific findings, however, and their significance has not been established. Some tumors have been shown to contain eosinophil chemotactic factors, which may explain the accumulation of the eosinophils. The eosinophils, as sites of plasminogen synthesis, may promote tumor invasiveness.

Basophilia is an uncommon finding in leukemoid reactions associated with solid tissue malignancy. The presence of basophilia should therefore raise the possibility of such other disease processes as tuberculosis, hypersensitivity reactions, and myeloproliferative disease, including chronic myelogenous leukemia.

Monocytes and macrophages. Monocytosis, which can occur in patients with solid tissue neoplasms, may represent an immunologic attempt to control the neoplasm, or it may be a consequence of such a coexistent infection as tuberculosis, cryptococcosis, or pneumocystis pneumonia. The monocyte and the monocyte-derived macrophage are found in higher than expected concentrations in the environment of the tumor; this observation may have immunologic implications. Activated macrophages are known to be able to destroy tumor in vitro. The macrophages attach with Fc receptors to cytophilic antibodies, which are bound to those tumors. The macrophages then phagocytose small particles from the tumor, which is then used as an antigenic template for the afferent limb of the immune process. Some therapeutic agents, such as bacillus Calmette-Guerin (BCG), are known to stimulate these macrophage functions. Tumor products, however, are capable of inhibiting some macrophage functions, including chemotaxis. Future studies of macrophages may offer an improved understanding of the immune suppression of malignant cells and a means of obtaining more specific immune stimuli that can be used therapeutically.

Lymphocytes and cancer. Lymphocytosis occasionally appears in patients with primary carcinomas of the breast, gastrointestinal tract, and bronchus. Patients with malignant lymphocyte disorders, such as lymphomas and lymphocytic leukemias, have an increased likelihood of developing a second malignancy, one that usually involves the colon, rectum, breast, bladder, skin, endometrium, or prostate. Although a discussion of the many possible roles lymphocytes play in protecting against the development of malignancy is beyond the scope of this chapter, a few clinical observations should be noted. Patients with carcinoma often have decreased lymphocytic reactivity to phytohemagglutination, and with disease progression the PHA reactivity decreases further. Likewise, patients with advanced carcinoma often develop cutaneous anergy as an indication of failure of the T-lymphocytes.

Patients with such functional defects generally have a poor prognosis, usually based upon the lymphocyte function. Asymptomatic coin lesions of the lung, for example, may prove to be malignant when quantitative and qualitative depressions of the lymphocytes exist in the patient's peripheral blood. After the tumor is removed from such patients, the concentration of T cells in the circulation rises. This suggests that the tumor has suppressive effects on lymphocyte differentiation. While these many similar concepts have not been proven to be clinically reliable, they do hold great promise. Therapies may ultimately be derived from these studies. Levamisole, a drug capable of recruiting T cells, is currently undergoing clinical trials.

Leukopenia and cancer. Leukopenia may appear in patients with carcinoma as a consequence of another independent process such as immune neutropenia or folate deficiency. More commonly the tumor or therapy leads to leukopenia and granulocytopenia (Table 11.4).

Table 11.4 Differential Diagnosis of
Neutropenia in Cancer Patients

I. Decreased Granulopoiesis
   A. Marrow hypoplasia secondary to
      cytotoxic drugs or radiation
   B. Metabolic deficiency
      (megaloblastic)
   C. Idiosyncratic drug reaction
II. Increased Peripheral Consumption
   A. Sepsis
   B. Hypersplenism
   C. Immune destruction
      1. Antibody—antigen specific
      2. Hapten mediated
   D. Connective Tissue Disorders
   E. Leukophagocytosis of Histiocytic
      Medullary Reticulosis

Chemotherapy is inherently associated
with myelosuppression and subsequently
with secondary leukopenia because of
a narrow therapeutic index for the majority
of the agents. Because of a dose-response
relation for most agents and combinations
of agents, the effect of cytotoxic drugs
may be minimized with dose and schedule
adjustments. Therapeutic goals differ
between those tumors that occupy the
marrow space and those solid tumors that
do not involve the marrow. In patients
whose marrow is not invaded by tumor,
marrow suppression and secondary leukopenia are dose related. In patients whose
marrow is invaded, as for patients with
leukemia or breast cancer metastatic to the
marrow, the stem cell population tends
to be already diminished. Functional
depression or reduced population of stem
cells may occur when the bone marrow
is occupied by the tumor. Therefore, major
marrow suppression occurring at the
lesser doses of therapy makes close monitoring for leukopenia essential.

The antitumor drugs employed as single
agents are relatively specific in the chronologic evolution of leukopenia. The five
commonly used drugs which are generally

associated with marrow suppression are
listed in Table 11.5. In patients with compromised bone marrow prior to therapy
or in patients receiving drug combinations, the likelihood of marrow suppression is increased. For the five classes of
drugs the nadir of leukopenia is variable.
For some drugs such as mitomycin C
and the nitrosoureas, leukopenia may be
delayed and have a cumulative effect
on the marrow as therapy continues.

In monitoring patients on chemotherapeutic programs, the blood counts must
be evaluated on the day of the anticipated
nadir to insure a "safe" level of leukopenia and to provide closer monitoring if
excessive leukopenia develops (Table
11.6). With radiation therapy to marrow-
bearing areas, particularly to the pelvis
and vertebral column, secondary leukopenia commonly develops above doses of
2000 R. Interruption of therapy may be
essential to prevent major secondary complications as infection.

Neutropenic patients are exposed to
fewer infections with resistant organisms
if they are left in their homes rather than
returned to the hospital to await marrow
recovery. If fever develops, hospital observation and treatment are essential. White
blood cell counts of less than 1000 cells/
mm³ can be sustained without infectious
consequence if the patient's immune
mechanisms are otherwise intact. Counts
of 400 to 500 white blood cells/mm³ almost uniformly lead to infection, commonly from self-colonization from the
gastrointestinal tract.

No evidence currently indicates that
antibiotics given prophylactically protect
neutropenic patients against developing
infection unless the effort is coupled with
complex efforts to sterilize the skin, and
gastrointestinal and genitourinary tracts,
while maintaining the patient in a life-
island environment. Studies designed to
test the effectiveness of prophylaxis with
antibiotics have generally been inconclusive because of inadequate stratification

Table 11.5 Chronologic Patterns of Marrow Suppression Secondary to Chemotherapy Following Single Course Exposure from day 0 of Therapy

Non−Marrow-Suppressive Drugs *
    Bleomycin
    Vincristine
    Streptozotocin
    Corticosteroids
    Dacarbazine (DTIC)

Marrow-Suppressive Drugs	*Nadir†* Day	*Duration†*
Alkylating Drugs		
Cyclophosphamide		
Nitrogen mustard	5−8	Variable
Mitomycin C	10−21	Cumulative
Antibiotics		
Adriamycin	12−14	5 days
Actinomycin		
Antimetabolites		
5-fluorouricil	5−10	< 5 days
Ara C (cytosine arabinoside)		
Methotrexate		
Natural Products		
Vinblastine	8−12	3 days
Other		
Nitrosoureas	14−28	Cumulative
Hydroxurea	Variable	
Procarbazine	Variable	

*This group of drugs may be myelosuppressive if used in combination with other drugs or if the host marrow reserve is limited.
†The nadir day may be earlier and the duration longer in patients with limited marrow reserve.

of patient and control groups. Patients who develop sepsis in spite of prophylactic antibiotics run the risk of infection with microbes resistant to the agents used in the prophylactic regimen.

The mortality rates for neutropenic patients with bacteremia approach 75 percent. Extensive cultures for fungi and for aerobic and anaerobic bacteria as well as microscopic examinations of fluid smears should be obtained from skin, mouth, nose, pharynx, sputum, blood, stool, and urine. While it is always best to treat bacteria with appropriately selected antibiotics, aggressive efforts to obtain internal fluids, such as cerebrospinal and pleural fluids, may introduce bacteria into an otherwise sterile location. Areas of cellulitis should be cultured judiciously to insure minimal skin damage. Prostatic, rectal, and pelvic examinations should be deferred unless truly justified. Patients with neutropenia have an obviously limited capacity to generate pus. Thus, the classic signs of pneumonia, cellulitis, meningitis, and peritonitis are often missing, and more subtle signs must be accepted as indications of correct diagnosis and therapy. Minimally localized erythema may be the only indication of ex-

Table 11.6 Clinical Monitoring of Leukopenia

Observed White Blood Count	Follow-up	Adjusted Chemotherapy Dose
1000–2000	Repeat in one week.	Allow recovery to > 3000; treat with 100% of dose.
500–1000	Observe daily until same on consecutive days.	Allow recovery to > 3000; treat with 50% of dose.
100–500	Hospitalize for observation.	Allow recovery to > 4000; treat with 25% of dose.

tensive bacterial infection. Organisms cannot often be isolated, even after extensive sampling. In this situation it is assumed that the pyrogenic agents enter through the gastrointestinal or genitourinary tracts. Consideration should be given to unusual organisms including *Mycobacterium tuberculosis, Pneumocystis carinii*, herpes, and the agent of Legionaire's disease (see Chapter 16).

The failure of antibiotics to control the infection may be heralded by changes in systemic signs. The patient will have significant worseing of malaise and fatigue, and hyperthermia will increase. Hypotension may develop in the absence of hypovolemia. Thrombocytopenia may be present due to chemotherapy-induced bone marrow suppression, but may also develop because of septic platelet consumption. DIC or resistance to platelet transfusion may develop as well. Patients with absolute neutropenia and who remain febrile after 48 hours of antibiotic therapy, those in whom bacteremia is proven, and those who develop any of the above-mentioned systemic signs of clinical deterioration are possible candidates for leukocyte transfusions.

Patients who receive chemotherapy for solid tumors and who develop neutropenia can be expected to have a relatively brief leukopenic nadir, as compared to that experienced by patients treated for acute leukemia. Leukocyte transfusions have been shown experimentally to be useful in preventing death from sepsis in neutropenic patients, but controversy remains regarding the role of leukocyte transfusion in patients with short duration nadirs of three or four days. The transfused cells sequester in the areas of infection for patients with occult infection and neutropenia. Bacteremia in neutropenic patients carries a dire prognosis; up to 75 percent of all patients can die within the first 48 hours of onset of septicemia. Thus, leukocyte transfusion therapy can be extremely valuable.

Technical elements of this therapy still to be resolved include collection technique, frequency of transfusions, duration of transfusions, and optimal dose of cells relative to the recipient's body size. Once-a-day transfusions of 1×10^{10} cells/m^2 body surface area for at least four or more consecutive days is considered appropriate. Cells gathered by centrifugation techniques are well received by the patient, while those gathered by fiber filtration are associated with hyperthermia. Using only HLA- and ABO-compatible cells may increase the percentage of granulocytes recovered in the recipient's circulation 1 hour after transfusion, but this has little effect on the clinical response to the transfusion. For practical reasons, transfusion with only HLA-compatible cells is difficult to arrange, so that to maximize compatiblity, siblings and close blood relatives are preferable cell donors. The transfusion is clinically beneficial if the fever subsides, the preexisting sites of infection clear, or the secondary signs of septicemia recede. Once the white blood cell count rises over 500/mm³, leukophoresis is generally not needed. If sepsis persists in spite of leukocyte transfusions, the transfusions should be continued and possibly increased to every 12 hours.

Patient O, a 38-year-old woman with carcinoma of the stomach, developed neutropenia to 600 white blood cells/mm³ after receiving Adriamycin and methyl-CCNU(lomustine). She remained afebrile at home for seven days. Thereafter, her oral temperature rose to 102°F. Upon hospitalization the white blood cell count was 200 cells/mm³. Cultures failed to isolate a pathogen, and empric triple-drug antibiotic therapy was begun. On the third hospital day the white blood cell count was 350/mm³. She developed a severe shaking rigor and the oral temperature spiked to 104°F. Leukocyte transfusions were given at 24-hour intervals for four days. She became afebrile on the fourth day, when the white blood cell count was 600/mm³ with 15% PMNs and 40% monocytes. Antibiotics were discontinued four days later, and the patient was discharged with a white cell count of 2200/mm³ and rising.

Plasma proteins. Changes in the plasma proteins can have diagnostic or clinical implications in patients with malignancies. The most common of these changes is reflected in the erthrocyte sedimentation rate (ESR). This nonspecific, inexpensive, easy-to-perform assay is often the first indication of an inflammatory, infectious, or neoplastic disease, and the last should be high on the list of differential diagnoses. The ESR also functions, although poorly, as a marker for patient improvement after therapy. A sudden decrease in the ESR may reflect diminution of fibrinogen in patients developing a consumptive coagulopathy. Patients with cancer also have alterations of serum protein concentrations with a decrease in albumin and an increase in alpha$_1$ and alpha$_2$ globulins, the beta$_2$ macroglobulins, transferrin, and the haptoglobulins. Albumin decrease may or may not reflect malnutrition. The globulins are a heterogeneous mixture of glycoproteins, coagulation factors, and enzymes. The glycoproteins contain alpha fetoprotein (AFP) and carcinoembryonic antigen (CEA) fractions, which serve as plasma markers for several carcinomas. Hepatocellular and embryonic carcinomas are gauged by AFP; CEA is used to measure adenocarcinomas of the gastrointestinal organs and breast.

Monoclonal gammopathies are frequently seen in the plasma cell dyscrasias (multiple myeloma), the lymphocyte dyscrasias (lymphomas and chronic lymphocytic leukemia), and the plasma-lymphocyte disorders (Waldenström's macroglobulinemia). Monoclonal (M) spikes can also occur in patients with chronic infections and collagen vascular diseases and in patients with no apparent disease but who later acquire these diseases. Monoclonal gammopathies have also been described with various carcinomas. Spikes of IgG have been found in carcinomas of the lung, stomach, jejunum, liver, bile ducts, pancreas, colon, urinary bladder, prostate, oropharynx, tongue, and thyroid. Spikes of IgA have been found with carcinomas of the breast, uterus, and ampulla of Vater. "Myeloma kidney" in the absence of Bence-Jones (light chain) proteinuria has been described in patients with acinar carcinomas of the pancreas and thyroid carcinoma. Thus, the finding of an M spike is not diagnostic of myeloma, lymphoma, or Waldenström's macroglobulinemia unless supported by other appropriate studies. It is not clear why patients with carcinoma develop M spikes when they have no demonstrable myeloma. To demonstrate the classic morphologic findings of myeloma, the malignant clone must have adequate bulk. The bulk may not be adequate for diagnosis at the time the work-up is conducted. Alternatively, the M spike may be a selective immunologic reaction to the tumor. This may be reflected histologically in the increase of plasma cells in the immediate vicinity of the tumor. As yet, such M spikes have not been shown to have immunologic specificity for the tumors.

Hormones made by cancers. Many tumors are capable of producing or stimulating the production of hormonally active substances found in the patient's plasma. These include ACTH, ADH, melanocyte-stimulating hormone, parathormone, serotonin, erythropoietin, thyrocalcitonin, gastrin, masculine and feminine hormones, and insulin. Management of the patient often requires simultaneous management of the tumor and manifestations of the tumor's excretory product (see Chapter 19).

Cryoprecipitable proteins and cancer. Cryofibrinogen and cryoglobulins may be found in the plasma and the serum of patients with various neoplasms. These proteins occasionally exist in high titers and can contribute to thrombosis and hemorrhagia in cool extremities and appendages. Heparin-dependent cryofibrinogen, normally up to 20 mgm%, but occasionally even as high as 80 mgm%, may be found in normal plasma and thus has little importance in the absence of clinical signs. Cryofibrinogens found in plasma anticoagulated with EDTA is less likely to be demonstrable in normal donors. When present, it should be investigated. Cryofibrinogens also appear in the presence of coincidental acute and chronic infections, inflammation, and fibrinolysis. In these instances, the fibrin and fibrinogen degradation products are cryoprecipitates.

Therapy to reduce the amount of cryofibrinogen should be initiated if high titers of cryofibrinogens are found with temperature-dependent vascular occulusive syndromes in the extremities or appendages. Even retinal vein thrombosis can occur. A simple viscometer can be used to monitor the effect of cold, and therapy on the propensity for sludging due to hyperviscosity. Therapy should be directed at both the underlying neoplasm or infection and the protein simultaneously. Keeping the patient warm is the first priority. This can be easily accomplished with blankets or gentle heat. Great care must be used for patients on cooling blankets for hyperthermia, as they may have major skin problems. If allowed to remain on the blanket too long, they may develop necrosis of the cooled skin. Plasmaphoresis can be used to reduce the concentration of the cryoprotein to levels below those causing intravascular sludging. Anticoagulation with heparin can be attempted, with the reservation that the process may be worsened instead of improved if the in vitro observations apply.

Cryoglobulins are another class of cryoprecipitants seen in patients with neoplasm, coexistent infections such as syphilis or mononucleosis, or coexistent collagen-vascular diseases. The most common neoplasms causing this syndrome are multiple myeloma and Waldenström's macroglobulinemia. Plasma samples for cryoglobulin analysis are collected into a prewarmed syringe without added anticoagulant. They are then allowed to clot for 60 minutes and are centrifuged at 37°C to remove the fibrin clot. Samples for cryofibrinogen are likewise handled at 37°C, but calcium chelators are added for anticoagulation. Thereafter, the sample is incubated at appropriately selected temperatures for 24 to 72 hours. The appearance of a cold-sensitive gel or glocculus is a positive finding. Quantitation of the cryoprecipitate can be made by measuring whole plasma for fibrinogen or the serum for globulins before and after cold incubation.

Patient P, a 48-year-old woman, was referred for evaluation of multiple and recurrent thrombosis in the fingers and feet. The attacks were painful, caused cyanosis of the affected digit, and resolved spontaneously within two or three days. Thrombi had begun two months earlier and had increased in frequency. They occurred when she was home and walking barefooted. The cryoglobulins were highly concentrated, and metastatic breast cancer was found. No light chains were evident in the urine, and no increase of plasma cells appeared in the bone marrow sample. Keeping her extremities warm provided temporary relief from the thrombi and plasmaphoresis successfully controlled the thrombotic attacks for many weeks. Chemotherapy was initiated for the breast cancer.

Cryoglobulins are often monoclonal IgG, IgM, mixtures of IgG with IgM, or IgG with IgA with attached kappa chains. Although cryoglobulins appear commonly with lymphoproliferative and plasma cell dyscrasias and rarely in apparently healthy people, they may add a significant morbidity to patients with cancer. Their presence does not indicate the status of the neoplasm, but may lead to hemorrhage or thrombotic complications. Abnormalities may appear in platelet aggregation and adhesion, bleeding time, and clot retraction. There may be circulating anti-

coagulants, interference with Factor VIII and Factor X, abnormal fibrin polymerization, and diminished fibrinolysis. Thrombi are due to the hyperviscosity and sludging that develops in such cool areas as the extremities. The Ostwald viscometer can be used to monitor the cold-dependent changes of viscosity as well as therapeutic response. Therapy, as with the cryofibrinogen, should be simultaneously directed to the underlying process and the cryoglobulins. Hydration and increased warmth to the extremeties are the first line of therapy, for hydration is especially effective if the IgG is subclass three. Plasmaphoresis can be clinically useful for both hemorrhage and thrombotic complications, especially for cryo-IgM, which is 80 percent intravascular, as opposed to IgG, which is only 50 percent intravascular. Dextran, which reduces viscosity and may help diminish the recurrent thrombotic process, involves a small risk of immune complex diseases. The dosage is 500 ml of low–molecular-weight dextran given as an eight-hour infusion on three consecutive days. Dextran will transiently increase the intravascular fluid by its osmotic effects and will alter the viscous properties of the microcirculation

7.0 Summary

The hematologic complications of cancer are diverse and common manifestations of malignancy. The hematologic system may be a marker of tumor activity in such instances as erythrocytosis or leukemoid reactions to the tumor. These secondary manifestations are probably induced by a humoral tumor secretion. Systemic alterations of the coagulation mechanism, particularly disseminated intravascular coagulation, are similar reflections of tumor activity and probably result from the release of thromboplastic material.

Anemia, leukopenia, and thrombocytopenia are also common secondary hematologic manifestations of tumors, but are more commonly manifestations of tumor therapy. Support with transfusion has helped enormously to provide blood elements and inhibit the secondary complications of asthenia, infection, and hemorrhage.

In the management of hematologic complications specific replacement therapy is necessarily supplemented by therapy directed at the tumor. Intramedullary tumors, particularly the hematologic neoplasms, are managed differently from solid or extramedullary tumors with secondary hematologic effects, but in all instances, the therapeutic management depends on a tumor-specific sensitivity to therapy.

References

Ablin, R. J.; Guinan, P. D.; Bush, I. M.; and Bruns, G. R. Inhibition of leukocyte migration by serum from patients with prostatic cancer. *Allerogal. Immunopathol.* 379–384, 1975.

Astedt, B.; Svanberg. L.; and Nilsson, I. M. Fibrin degradation products and ovarian tumors. *Br. Med. J.* 4:459, 1971.

Astedt, B.; Svanberg, L.; and Nilsson, I. M. F. D. P. *Lancet* 11:1312, 1972.

Brugarolas, A.; Mink, I. B.; Elias, E. G.; and Mittleman, A. Correlation of hyperfibrinogenemia with major thromboembolism in patients with cancer. *Surg. Gynecol. Obstet.* 136:75–77, 1973.

Clauson, K. P., and von Haum, E. Fine structure of malignancy-associated change (MAC) in peripheral human leukocytes. *Acta. Cytol.* 13:435–442, 1969.

Levin, J., and Conley, C. L. Thrombocytosis associated with malignant disease. *Arch. Intern. Med.* 114:497, 1964.

McCfedie, K. B., and Hester, J. P. White blood cell transfusion in the management of infections in neutropenic patients. *Clin. Haematol.* 5:379–394, 1976.

Mertins, B. F.; Greene, L. F.; Bowie, E. J.; Elveback, L. R.; and Owne, C. A. Fibrinolytic split products (FSP) and ethanol gelatin test in preoperative evaluation of patients with prostatic disease. *Mayo Clin. Proc.* 49:642–645, 1974.

Pengelly, C. D. P., and Zureski, Z. A. Hemolytic anemia associated with carcinoma of the pancreas. *Br. J. Cancer Pract.* 27:141–144, 1973.

Rieche, K., and Wand, H. Comparative studies on the behavior of the plasmatic clotting system and platelet function in surgically treated cancer patients. *Arch. Geschwulstforsch.* 45:153–162, 1975.

Sproul, E. E. Carcinoma and venous thrombosis: the frequency of association of carcinoma in the body and tail of the pancreas with multiple venous thrombosis. *Am. J. Cancer* 34:566–585. 1938.

Veterans Administration Cooperative Urologic Research Group. *Surg. Gynecol. Obstet.* 124:1011, 1967.

Weiss, G., and Beller, F. K. Localization of fibrinolytic activity in uterine cancer. *Am. J. Obstet. Gynecol.* 103:1023–1027, 1969

Chapter 12

Cutaneous Complications of Malignancy

B. Wintroub
A. Hood

1.0 Background

The cutaneous complications of cancer can be clasified as: (1) cutaneous (dermal, subcutaneous, or both) infiltration by malignant cells; (2) dermatologic syndromes associated with internal malignancy; and (3) cutaneous changes associated with cancer therapy, including radiation and cytotoxic drugs. Some cutaneous alterations are characteristic and occasionally pathognomonic of a specific syndrome such as necrolytic migratory erythema associated with alpha cell tumors of the pancreas, but more often the cutaneous manifestation of malignancy is a commonplace lesion that changes with the activity of the tumor. Such lesions include seborrheic and other forms of keratoses, psoriasiform lesions, and sympathetic nonspecific xanthems. Although these lesions are associated with an internal malignancy, their significance and

mechanism of production have not been established.

The skin, a common site for primary and secondary tumors and their complications, is readily accessible to observation by inspection and biopsy. This chapter will focus on the cutaneous complications and manifestations of malignancy exclusive of primary tumors of the integument such as squamous cell carcinoma, basal cell epithelioma, and malignant melanoma.

2.0 Cutaneous infiltration by malignant cells

Infiltration of the dermis by cancer cells may arise as a consequence of direct extension from subcutaneous tumor, of hematogenous dissemination, or secondary to such local trauma as surgery, paracentesis, or direct blunt injury. External trauma with secondary cutaneous hemorrhage can lead to secondary implantation of tumor.

Tumor invasion of the skin occurs in direct proportion to the relative frequency of the primary tumor. In decreasing order of frequency, skin invasion can occur with carcinoma, hematologic neoplasm (lymphomas and leukemias), and sarcoma. Cutaneous manifestations of sarcoma generally derive from subcutaneous mesenchymal tissues, but the tumor may disseminate hematogenously to implant in the skin from a distant site.

Cutaneous metastases can affect any area of the body from the scalp to the toes, including the gingiva, buttocks, phalanges, and even mucosal surfaces such as the anogenital area. The skin in proximity to the underlying carcinoma is commonly affected. Breast and lung carcinomas often metastasize to the chest wall by contiguous growth, and lesions from gastrointestinal carcinomas often involve the abdominal wall in continuity with the viscera. Nodules sometimes implant along the unbilicus. These "Sister Marie Joseph's nodules" generally result from pancreatic carcinoma but can be observed in association with any intra-abdominal visceral malignancy. Umbilical nodules can also develop as a consequence of laparoscopy, which is commonly employed for the staging of intra-abdominal tumors, particularly ovarian cancer. Ovarian carcinoma is the one malignancy prone to implant nodules subcutaneously as a consequence of surgical interruption of the cutaneous integument. It is extremely rare for nonovarian tumors to implant in surgical scars or at sites of paracentesis or thoracentesis.

Skin metastases from carcinoma. The frequency of cutaneous metastasis ranges from one to five percent. Although carcinomas arising in any organ can metastasize to the skin, the tumors most often producing cutaneous metastases are lesions of the breast, lung, gastrointestinal tract, kidney, uterus, and ovary (Table 12.1). In general, cutaneous metastases are observed after recognition of the primary tumor, but tumors that invade veins, such

TABLE 12.1 Frequency and Relative Incidence of Cutaneous Metastases

	Estimated Frequency	Relative Incidence
Lung	5%	15%
Breast	10–15%	25%
Colon	<5%	15%
Melanoma	20%	10%
Kidney	<5%	6%
Other gastrointestinal tract	<5%	11%
Sarcoma	5–10%	5%
Other	–	13%

as carcinoma of the kidney and lung, may initially present with distant cutaneous metastases. In contrast, cancers that invade the lymphatic ducts, such as tumors of the breast and oral cavity, may appear in the skin overlying the primary tumor later in the course of the disease. Occasionally, cutaneous lesions can be the singular manifestation of a malignancy and can represent an accessible source of biopsy tissue for an unknown primary tumor.

Patient A, a 64-year-old man, presented with a five-week history of progressive weight loss and was discovered to have hypercalcemia. Routine radiographic studies failed to demonstrate any significant abnormality. Careful examination of the skin by palpation revealed multiple subdermal lesions of the anterior thorax, and biopsy of the lesion demonstrated undifferentiated small cell carcinoma.

Innocuous dermal or subdermal tissue lesions may represent cutaneous metastases.

Irrespective of the primary tumor site, clinical manifestations of cutaneous lesions are generally similar. A skin metastasis may appear to be an innocent, nonspecific papule and may have been perceived by the patient prior to discovery of the primary malignancy. In general, cutaneous metastases are firm, dermal or subcutaneous nodules. The lesions can be single or multiple, although they are generally discrete and rarely ulcerated. Tumor appearance varies from flesh color to mildly erythematous to violaceous. Histologic examination of the cutaneous lesion may classify the tumor as epithelial (adenocarcinoma or squamous carcinoma), mesenchymal, or lymphomatous; clinically, however, cutaneous manifestations are similar.

Two special forms of cutaneous metastases are carcinoma en cuirasse and in-

flammatory carcinoma. Carcinoma en cuirasse, derived from the French and meaning leatherlike shield, refers to extensive tumor infiltration of the chest wall and has been associated almost exclusively with carcinomas of the breast. Lymphatic permeation by cancer cells causes extensive thickening and fibrosis of the dermis and subcutaneous tissue.

Patient B, a 57-year-old woman with a previous history of breast carcinoma, developed a small nodule at the lateral margin of the scar and subsequently developed extensive inflammation over the anterior and posterior chest wall. Secondary edema of the arm developed. Successful systemic chemotherapy resulted in resolution of the lesions for eight months (Fig. 12.1).

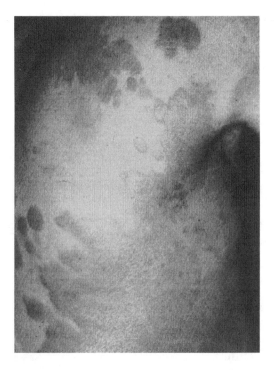

Fig. 12.1 Lateral thorax and back demonstrating extensive nodular lesions of the skin that have coalesced to form a pattern referred to as en cuirasse.

En cuirasse metastases are flat or nodular and represent dermal cutaneous and lymphatic tumor implants.

Tumors other than breast cancer rarely cause an en cuirasse tumor because hematogenous metastases do not characteristically permeate lymphatic ducts.

Inflammatory carcinoma is a characteristic form of breast cancer, but an inflammatory component can develop in primary mesenchymal tumors and in metastases to the subcutaneous tissue. Clinical observation shows that breast lesions are sharply demarcated, erythematous, warm, and tender. The lack of a definitive tumor mass underlying the dermal inflammation often suggests a clinical diagnosis of cellulitis or erysipelas, but the lack of response to systemic antibiotics is a clue to the potential presence of underlying tumor. Increased sedimentation rate and leukocytosis are similarly common.

Patient C, a 49-year-old man, had a malignant fibrous histiocytoma removed from the left supraclavicular area, and postoperatively received radiation and systemic chemotherapy. He was well for three years, but at follow-up he had developed increasing pain and limitation of motion in the left shoulder. These symptoms were followed in rapid succession by increasing erythema and warmth over the left shoulder, in addition to a daily temperature of 101° and leukocytosis to 25,000 cells/mm³ with a sedimentation rate of 62 mm per hour. The patient was treated for two months with different antibiotic regimens but without success. He subsequently underwent a surgical biopsy, at which time extensive tumor necrosis underlying the shoulder muscles and, with characteristic pathologic changes of malignant fibrous histiocytoma, was observed (Fig. 12.2).

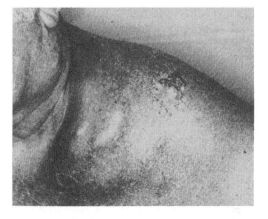

Fig. 12.2 *Inflammatory mass of lymph nodes involving the left supraclavicular fossa and cervical area characteristic for recurrence (Patient C) with soft tissue sarcoma.*

Inflammatory reactions to cutaneous or subcutaneous tumors may be confused with cellulitis, especially in recurrent sarcomas or in primary breast cancer.

In addition to the unique cutaneous manifestations of malignancy, such common cutaneous lesions as wens, acneiform lesions, or even alopecia may be secondary to metastatic lesions. In unexplained circumstances in which these lesions do not respond to appropriate therapy, biopsy of the lesion is worthwhile.

Cutaneous infiltration by lymphoma. The lymphomas include Hodgkin's disease, lymphosarcoma, and reticulum cell sarcoma. Various pathologic subclassifications (Rappaport or Lukes and Butler) are based on lymph node morphology rather than on organ infiltration and are not considered in the context of skin infiltration. All subtypes of Hodgkin's disease and non-Hodgkin's lymphoma are associated with cutaneous infiltration, although skin lesions are more common with the latter. In all types of lymphoma, the cutaneous lesions are clinically similar; they are papules, nodules, and tumor plaques. The lesions can involve any part of the integument and are generally violaceous without secondary inflammation or ulceration. Histologic examination is helpful although Reed-Sternberg cells in the skin are rarely identified in Hodgkin's disease.

Patient D, a 32-year-old woman who presented with mixed-cell Hodgkin's disease involving cervical nodes and mediastinum, was treated with mantle radiation therapy. The patient was well for two years after therapy when she developed unilateral swelling of the face with intermittent swelling of the upper or lower lip (Fig. 12.3). Biopsy revealed a pleo-

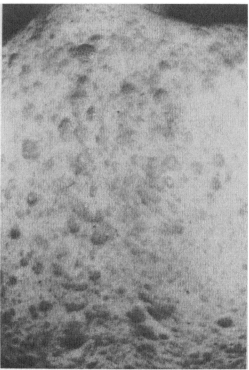

Fig. 12.4 Multiple cutaneous lesions of the skin forming discrete nodules consistent with lymphoma or leukemia.

morphic infiltrate of inflammatory cells, including mononuclear cells, but no evidence of Reed-Sternberg cells. The patient was treated with MOPP chemotherapy (mechlorethamine + Oncovin (vincristine) + procarbazine + prednisone). Her facial lesions rapidly resolved and abated for two years.

Cutaneous infiltation in lymphoma (Fig. 12.4) generally occurs late in the course of the disease, although skin lesions have been identified in patients with histiocytic and lymphocytic lymphoma months and even years before visceral involvement is identified. So-called lymphoma cutis often recurs intermittently. Although it has been reported to be contained within the skin (primary cutaneous lymphoma),

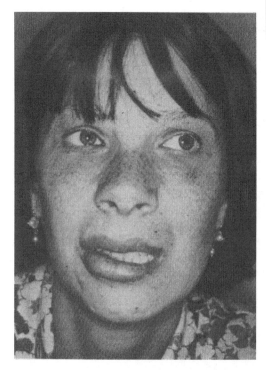

Fig. 12.3 Subcutaneous infiltration of the lips and perioral area without skin involvment (Patient D) in a woman with Hodgkin's disease.

most cases of lymphoma cutis eventually disseminate.

Patient E, a 59-year-old woman, presented with recurrent unilateral erythema of the malar eminence that waxed and waned for 18 months. The lesion was intermittently responsive to systemic steriods, and biopsy revealed typical features of lymphosarcoma, with cleaved lymphocytes invading the dermis and subcutaneous tissues. With combination chemotherapy, the lesion partially regressed (Fig. 12.5) but promptly returned, with rapid dissemination of disease to visceral sites, including the lungs and liver.

Cutaneous lymphoma (lymphoma cutis) is most commonly associated with lymphosarcoma and is rarely a primary lesion.

Mycosis fungoides and the related Sézary syndrome are also lymphomatous skin diseases that subsequently disseminate. Mycosis fungoides generally evolves

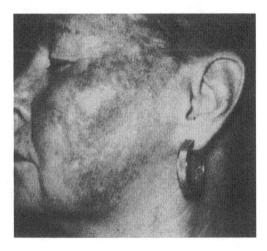

Fig. 12.5 Coalescent erythema of the malar eminence (Patient E) secondary to cutaneous and subcutaneous infiltration with lymphoma.

through three clinical stages. In the earliest stage the lesions may resemble psoriasis or eczema or may be clinically diagnosed as parapsoriasis en plaques or poikiloderma. After a variable but usually long course, infiltrative plaques appear. These become progressively indurated and may be arcuate with central clearings. This second or plaque stage may regress spontaneously, or the lesions may wax and wane. As the cell infiltrate increases, the lesions elevate and are thereafter designated as tumors. These tumors may evolve progressively from previously existing plaques or may develop spontaneously in previously unaffected skin. During this third stage, dissemination to visceral sites in the lungs or liver often develops terminally or preterminally.

The diagnosis of mycosis fungiodes is made by histologic examination of skin biopsy specimens that are generally not diagnostic early in the disease. With the appearance of the plaque or tumor stage, the pathognomonic Pautrier's microabscesses develop in the epidermis; a dermal infiltrate composed of polymorphic cells and atypical T cells confirms the diagnosis. The prognosis of mycosis fungoides is based partially on the stage of the disease and on the patient's response to therapy. At the time of histologic diagnosis, median survival is approximately five years, but with the development of the tumor stage, the median survival is two and one half years. When the viscera become involved, median survival is less than one year.

Patient F, a 45-year-old man, developed circumscribed eczematous and psoriasiform lesions on the chest, abdomen, and back, which responded to topical steriods. Skin biopsy revealed only psoriasiform dermatitis with a perivascular inflammatory infiltrate and occasional atypical cells. The lesions occurred intermittently for 10 years, after which infiltrative

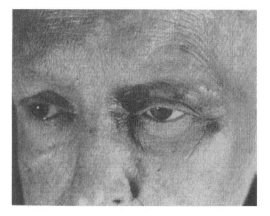

Fig. 12.6 Nodular stage of mycosis fungoides with periorbital lesions involving the canthus and lateral margin of the line of the eyebrow.

plaques developed (Fig. 12.6). Skin biopsy confirmed the diagnosis of mycosis fungoides. The patient was treated with electron beam therapy, photo-chemotherapy, and systemic chemotherapy. He died 15 years after the appearance of the first skin lesions.

Therapy for mycosis fungoides depends on the stage or biologic expression of the disease. In the absence of visceral involvment, treatment is directed to the cutaneous disease and includes topical steroids, immunochemical therapy with nitrogen mustard sensitization, photochemotherapy with psoralen and ultraviolet light, electron beam x-ray therapy, and topical chemotherapy including the nitrosoureas. Systemic chemotherapy is sometimes effective in mycosis fungoides, although response rates and duration of response are lower than for the noncutaneous lymphomas.

Skin infiltration by leukemia. The cutaneous complications of leukemia often occur secondary to thrombocytopenia and leukopenia. These include cutaneous hemorrhage, petechiae, purpura, and in-

fection. Candidiasis is a characteristic infection in leukemia patients. Cutaneous infiltration by leukemic cells is uncommon, but sometimes occurs in monocytic and myelomonocytic leukemias (Fig. 12.7). The cutaneous lesions are generally violaceous and appear as macules, papules, nodules, or plaques. As in lymphomatous infiltration of the integument, the type of leukemia can be diagnosed only after histologic study. The lesions often respond rapidly to antileukemic therapy.

Patient G, a 56-year-old woman, presented with a white blood cell count of 150,000 cells/mm^3, severe thrombocytopenia, and fever. Physical examination revealed hepatosplenomegaly and cervical lymphadenopathy. A violaceous to purpuric cutaneous eruption was also evident. The nodular exophytic lesions were discrete (Fig. 12.8). Cytosine arabinoside and daunomycin were administered and the patient's lesions regressed within three days.

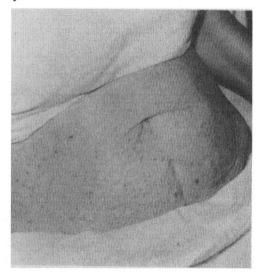

Fig. 12.7 Multiple small maculopapullar and punctate lesions of the anterior abdominal wall in a patient with acute myelomonocytic leukemia.

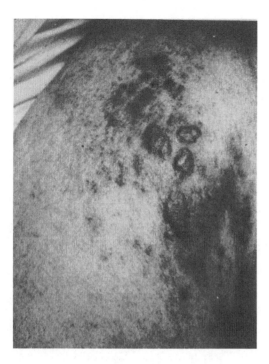

Fig. 12.8 Large, nodular, nontender lesions of the right posterior thorax with a typical violaceous coloration.

The chloroma is pathognomonic of leukemia and occurs primarily in association with acute myelocytic leukemia. Chloromas are generally found on the face and are primarily observed in children and young adults. They affect the periorbital and retro-orbital areas and can lead to proptosis. Chloromas can also present as discrete mass lesions in continuity with bone or in the ovaries or testicles. Chloromas are named for the green color that is caused by the presence of myeloperoxidase in the leukemic cell.

Rare and unusual cutaneous malignancy. One group of cutaneous malignancies represents neither primary, metastatic, nor infiltrating lesions of the integument (Table 12.2). These tumors are rare and frequently involve the skin appendages or supporting stromal struc-

Table 12.2 Rare and Unusual Cutaneous Malignancies

Stewart-Treves syndrome
Kaposi's sarcoma
Paget's disease
Adnexal tumors
Leiomyosarcoma

tures. The tumors are resistant to systemic and radiation therapy, although the natural history of these lesions is generally protracted.

The Stewart-Treves syndrome is a lymphangiosarcoma that develops in chronically edematous extremities. More than one-half of the reported cases have occurred in patients who had prior mastectomy and local radiation therapy with secondary lymphedema of the arm, but the syndrome has also been reported in patients with filariasis-associated leg edema. The lesion is often superficially purpuric or hemorrhagic, and progresses to a discrete cutaneous nodule followed by pulmonary metastases. Edema is presumably a consequence of lymphatic obstruction with tumor.

Patient H, a 62-year-old woman, had a carcinoma of the left breast removed five years previously. She presented for evaluation of lymphedema and was observed to have a purpuric lesion of the inner aspect of the arm (Fig. 12.9). A biopsy was performed, the characteristic features of lymphangiosarcoma were demonstrated. Systemic therapy was unsuccessful, and the patient succumbed three years later.

The rare skin tumors are derived from mesenchymal tissues and are often sarcomas.

Another rare cutaneous lesion is Kaposi's sarcoma. The lesion is embryologi-

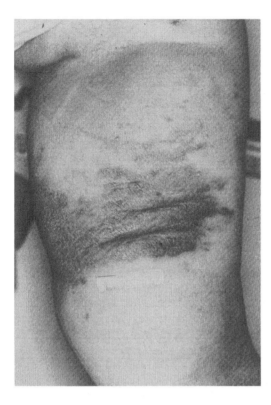

Fig. 12.9 Massive lymphedema of the proximal arm with purpuric discoloration in an irregular area proximal to the antecubital fossa. The lesion was raised and infiltrated the subcutaneous tissue.

cally derived from vascular structures. The tumor commonly has a protracted history and, like lymphangiosarcoma, is associated with edema of the extremities. The lesions are violaceous and often appear on the soles of the feet or anywhere along the extremity. Kaposi's sarcoma is exquisitely responsive to irradiation and to vinblastine chemotherapy. The disease occurs most frequently in Africa.

Patient I, a 69-year-old man, complained of edema of the left leg for approximately 10 years. During this time he had carried on his activities and then noted the development of a lesion on the sole of his foot. Because of the edema he was unable to

observe the lesion and contacted the physician only after his podiatrist noticed multiple violaceous lesions (Fig. 12.10). Initial treatment with local radiation therapy induced regression of the lesions on the skin surface, but subsequent recurrence necessitated cryosurgery. No evidence of metastases developed during the observation period.

Kaposi's sarcoma can metastasize to lymph nodes and the viscera, and is a rare cause of gastrointestinal blood loss.
Another unusual sarcomatous lesion of the integument is leiomyoma or low-

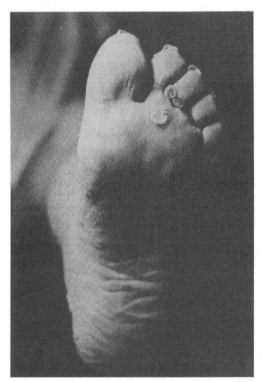

Fig. 12.10 Typical distribution of Kaposi's sarcoma lesions involving skin and subcutaneous tissues of the sole of the foot. Central umbilication and desiccation of the lesions evolves with time and psoriasislike scaling appears over the surface of the sole and dorsum of the foot.

grade leiomyosarcoma of the skin. Like Kaposi's sarcoma, these lesions are often indolent and generally unresponsive to local therapy, including radiation and perfusion chemotherapy. The protracted clinical course that is characteristic of these low-grade malignancies dictates caution and suggests intervention only in the presence of major symptomatology (Fig. 12.11).

Tumors of the adnexal structures including the apocrine and eccrine (sweat) glands are uncommon. They can develop as cutaneous lesions and can appear at any site, including the subungual area. The clinical appearance of the lesions is typically papular with infiltrating features and an erythematous or violaceous hue.

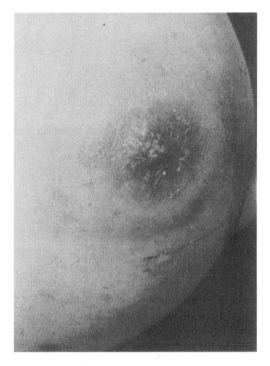

Fig. 12.12 Scaling erosion of the nipple of the left breast characteristic for Paget's disease.

Wide local excision, including amputation for subungual lesions occasionally in association with lymph node dissection, is indicated.

Paget's disease of the breast primarily affects the nipple and areola, and results from intra-epidermal invasion by underlying intraductal carcinoma. The primary tumor extends within mammary duct epithelium into the epidermis of the areola and causes an eczematoid lesion resembling contact dermatitis (Fig. 12.12). Paget's disease does not respond to topical steriods and is thus distinguished from eczema. Biopsy is diagnostic and demonstrates clear cells containing mucopolysaccharide within the epidermis. Extramammary Paget's disease is clinically and histologically similar and can occur on the pubis, perineum, genitalia, or axilla (Fig. 12.13). Such lesions are often associ-

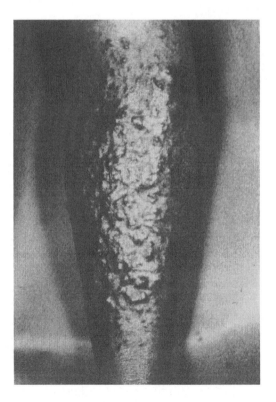

Fig. 12.11 Irregular confluent and generally tender lesions involving the dermis and subcutaneous tissues of the leg and not associated with edema.

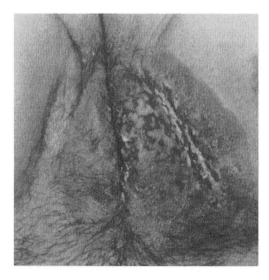

Fig. 12.13 Characteristic appearance of Paget's disease of the vulva involving the left labia majora.

Table 12.3 Therapeutic Modalities for Management of Cutaneous Neoplastic Lesions

Surgery, including cryo- and electrocautery
Radiation
Topical cytotoxic drugs
    1. 5-Fluorouracil
    2. Nitrosourea compounds
    3. Bleomycin
Systemic or perfusion chemotherapy
Immunotherapy
    1. DNCB or HN_2 sensitization
    2. Intralesional or epilesional immune potentiators

ated with underlying apocrine or eccrine gland carcinoma.

Therapies for cutaneous malignancy. A summary of the therapies for dermal lesions is found in Table 12.3. Primary cutaneous tumors, such as basal cell and squamous cell carcinomas, can be treated by simple surgical excision, curettage and electrode desiccation, cryosurgery, or local radiation therapy. The choice is based on the size and site of the lesion. Malignant melanoma, another primary skin tumor, is generally treated by surgical excision with a wide margin and, in appropriate instances, the use of a split-thickness graft. In the case of metastatic skin lesions, cryosurgery or electrocautery are applicable, particularly in circumstances for which palliation is the primary consideration. For example, in large cutaneous or even subcutaneous lesions of the extremities where local infection or significant local morbidity exist, limited surgical excision by cryosurgery or electrocautery may provide adequate pallia-

tion and preclude the necessity for amputation.

Therapies for secondary skin malignancy are palliative, and may require local or regional application of cryo- or electrocautery surgery.

Irradiation can be administered either by electron beam therapy, which penetrates the superficial layers of the skin and precludes secondary radiation effects on tendons, muscles, or underlying structures; or it can be given as implantation (contact radiation). Tumor implantation with radon seeds or other radiation sources has been used in the local management of primary breast cancer and sarcomas. The radiation source is implanted in the tumor for a finite period. This technique permits administration of a large local dose of radiation.

Cytotoxic drug therapy can be administered systemically, topically, or by arterial infusion in extremity lesions. Topical therapy using 5-fluorouracil, nitrosoureas, or bleomycin mixed in an orabase would appear to be ideal. Although topical therapy is effective, particularly for ulcerative lesions, the morbidity of the treatment is substantial. The drugs induce a local inflammatory reaction and must be applied daily over a protracted period. Arterial perfusion for cutaneous lesions of the extremities has been used for melanoma and other skin lesions. In the presence of extensive or diffuse lesions in one extremity, arterial perfusion or isolated infusion of the chemotherapeutic agent is theoretically ideal.

Immunotherapy for cutaneous lesions involves a potentially innocuous substance that promotes host resistance. Although the use of nonspecific immune potentiators or stimulants on uninvolved areas of the skin has not been effective, intralesional or epilesional injection of the nonspecific immune stimulants, such as bacillus Calmette-Guerin (BCG), the methanol-extracted residue (MER) of BCG, purified protein derivative (PPD) of tuberculin, or vaccinia preparations, has been successful. These immunologic agents may cause cutaneous tumor involution in more than 80 percent of lesions, depending on the size and depth of the lesion as well as on the dose of the immune stimulant. In general, the regression of tumors by intralesional application of immune stimulants is most probably mediated as a result of a general inflammatory reaction (Fig. 12.14). Little data support the concept that intralesional therapy promotes regression by an immunologic mechanism.

3.0 Cutaneous syndromes associated with internal malignancy

Three categories of cutaneous lesions can be associated with malignancy at internal sites: (1) lesions resulting from tumor secretion of a humoral substance or a metabolic alteration, (2) specific skin manifestations of an internal malignancy, and (3) nonspecific cutaneous lesions associated with malignancy (Table 12.4). The

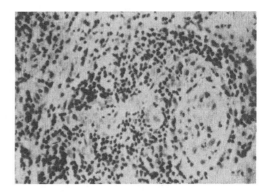

Fig. 12.14 *Multiple noncaseating granuloma appearing in conjunction with mononuclear inflammatory cells in a patient receiving intralesional MER-BCG. No evidence of viable melanoma cells was observed.*

cutaneous lesions associated with an increased incidence of internal malignancy may be a result of a genetically linked abnormality affecting the skin and the affected organ; alternatively, the pairing may reflect a concomitant carcinogenic stimulus to the skin and the primary tumor site. In some cutaneous manifestations associated with internal malignancy, the actual incidence of malignancy has varied and therefore the associations may be controversial.

Cutaneous alterations due to secondary metabolic effects. Many endocrine and nonendocrine tumors secrete humoral substances that can be manifested in the skin or subcutaneous tissues. Tumors that secrete ACTH, particularly oat cell carcinomas of the lung, can produce hyperpigmentation. The effect results from secretion of ACTH and β-MSH-like peptides; oat cell carcinoma, however, is uncommon, and pigmentation requires an extended time to develop. More often, patients with Cushing's syndrome secondary to oat cell carcinoma succumb to the disease before hyperpigmentation develops.

Table 12.4 Cutaneous Syndromes
Associated with Malignancy

I. Cutaneous Changes Due to
   Secondary Metabolic Effects
   A. Hyperpigmentation
      1. ACTH-secreting tumors
      2. Postadrenalectomy ablation for
         breast cancer
      3. Melanosis secondary to
         malignant melanoma
   B. Carcinoid syndrome
   C. Nodular fat necrosis
   D. Necrolytic migratory erythema
   E. Pachydermoperiostosis
II. Specific Cutaneous Syndromes
    Associated with Internal Malignancy
    A. Dermatomyositis
    B. Acanthosis nigricans
    C. Acquired ichthyosis
    D. Alopecia mucinosa
    E. Bowen's disease
III. Nonspecific Cutaneous Conditions
     Associated with Malignancy
     A. Infections
     B. Pruritus
     C. Urticaria and angioedema
     D. Xanthomatosis
     E. Vesiculobullous
     F. Erythroderma
     G. Keratosis

Patients who undergo adrenalectomy
as an ablative procedure for metastatic
breast cancer have increased ACTH levels
and diffuse hyperpigmentation in these
patients is common. Dermal melanosis
has also been associated with disseminated malignant melanoma; here the pigmentation develops as a consequence
of melanin deposits in the dermal tissues.
Patients with dermal melanosis excrete
detectable melanin in their urine, but
metastases develop rapidly, and death
may ensue before pigmentation is
apparent.

Intermittent flushing is characteristic of
the carcinoid syndrome, which develops

in less than five percent of patients with
carcinoid tumors of a variety of sites. The
total syndrome includes abdominal
cramps, diarrhea, and hypotension, and a
flushing episode lasts approximately 10
to 30 minutes. Both serotonin and kallikrein mediate the syndrome; kallikrein
cleaves bradykinin from kininogen, which
is the predominant mediator of the cutaneous flush.

Nodular fat necrosis comprises a syndrome of tender subcutaneous nodules,
fever, eosinophilia, and polyarthritis; the
condition has been associated predominantly with tumors of the pancreatic duc-
tal system. Glucagonoma, a pancreatic
tumor localized to the alpha cell component of the islet cells, causes necrolytic
migratory erythema. This syndrome is
composed of a specific dermatitis, weight
loss, stomatitis, diabetes mellitus, and
anemia. The lesions are typically erythematous with erosions and crusts on the
lower abdomen, groin, buttocks, thighs,
perineum, distal extremities, or central
third of the face (Fig. 12.15). The lesions
begin as erythematous macules and subsequently form blisters and erosions that
generally heal but leave areas of hyperpigmentation. The early lesions are histologically typical for glucagonoma; subcorneal
and mid-epidermal separation of keratin-
izing cells in the absence of acantholysis
is characteristic. These cells evidence
pyknotic nuclei and cytoplasm varying
from pink to blue when stained with he-
matoxylin and eosin. In addition, a psoriasiform epidermal hyperplasia and a
perivenous inflammatory infiltrate can be
observed. The specific role of alpha cell
glucagon secretion in producing cutaneous lesions is not known. Patients with
increased levels of glucagon, however,
may have a depletion of amino acids that
are essential to epidermal replication.
Early recognition of the syndrome is important, as most glucagonomas are malignant. In at least 1 of the 27 reported cases,

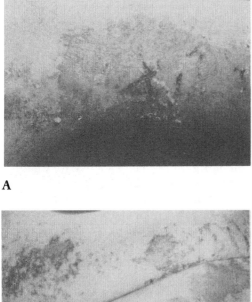

A

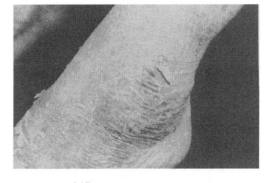

B

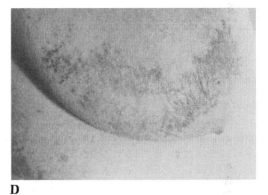

C

D

Fig. 12.15 Necrosis (A), scaling (B), and irregular circumscribed flat lesions of the epidermis of the buttocks as well as the breasts. This is typical for erythema that is necrolytic and migratory and is associated with glucagonoma.

a familial inheritance was established (autosomal dominant); in 2 cases, multiple endocrine neoplasia was identified with endocrine adenomas in the parathyroid or adrenal glands.

Patient J, a 40-year-old man, presented with a four and one-half-year history of psoriasiform lesions of the face and perineum. The lesions were typical of migratory necrolytic erythema and did not respond to topical therapy. The postprandial blood sugar was elevated, and plasma and glucagon levels were seven times normal. At exploratory laparotomy, a glucagon-secreting islet cell tumor was found in the tail of the pancreas. The patient's rash resolved completely after tumor resection. He is alive now, three years after surgical excision.

A common cutaneous manifestation of malignancy is hypertrophic osteo-arthropathy, which may be associated with acromegalic features. When thickening of the skin of the hands, the forearms, and the legs occurs, the syndrome is then designated as pachydermoperiostosis. This disorder is commonly familial and unrelated to malignancy, but in the acquired form and particularly in patients over age 40, the relationship to malignancy must be investigated (see Chapter 19).

Characteristic cutaneous syndromes. Cutaneous manifestations of internal malignancy having specific diagnostic features are restricted to five distinct entities (Table 12.4). The relationship between the cutaneous manifestation and the malignancy has not, however, been clearly established. A group of four familial syndromes is also associated with internal neoplasia (Table 12.5). Although the dermatologic manifestations of the familial syndromes are not pathognomonic, the constellation of cutaneous soft tissue and visceral lesions with a family history of cancer necessitates evaluation for neoplastic disease.

Dermatomyositis is an inflammatory disorder of the skin and muscle and is associated with malignancy in approximately 50 percent of affected patients. Dermatomyositis develops in the fifth and sixth decades of life, and the relative incidence of cancer for these patients is seven times that of the normal population. In general, the cancer arises after the dermatomyositis has been diagnosed. Tumors of the breast, lung, and genitourinary and gastrointestinal tracts are most commonly associated with dermatomyositis. Clinical manifestations of dermatomyositis include a heliotrope suffusion and edema of eyelid margins and periorbital tissue, and periungual erythema with linear telangiectasis and papules of the dorsum of the interphalangeal joints. Psoriasiform lesions, macular scaling in a butterfly distribution, and calcinosis cutis may also be observed. The cutaneous and myopathic manifestations of dermatomyositis and malignancy may resolve with treatment of the tumor, but improvement is the exception rather than the rule. Thus, the etiologic interaction between the two processes is unclear.

A clinically spectacular and rare syndrome related to dermatomyositis is erythema gyratum repens. Patients with this syndrome have concentric arcuate lesions resembling wood grain, and the few reported cases have all been associated with malignancy. With removal of the tumor, the lesions may regress. Acanthosis nigricans is a dermatosis that can occur in association with endocrine disorders or obesity, is often congenital, and is frequently inherited. When the lesions develop in a lean adult, the association with internal malignancy is significant: ap-

Table 12.5 Familial Syndromes Associated with Neoplasia

Syndrome	Dermatologic Manifestations	Neoplastic Lesion
Gardner's	Sebaceous cysts of face and trunk; fibromas, especially in scars	Colon
Cowden's	Lichen and papillomata of pinna, dorsum of hands and feet	Breast, thyroid
Torre's	Sebaceous adenoma of trunk, head, and neck	Gastrointestinal
Peutz-Jeghers	Freckling lips, fingertips, and buccal mucosa	Gastrointestinal polyps, rarely malignant

proximately 65 percent of those patients who get cancer develop gastric carcinomas. Approximately 25 percent develop other intra-abdominal tumors, and less than 10 percent develop extra-abdominal malignancies. In general, the dermatosis develops simultaneously with the tumor, although in approximately 20 percent of patients the tumor precedes diagnosis of the skin reaction. Generally, patients with concomitant cancer and acanthosis nigricans survive less than 12 months. The typical skin lesions appear in flexural areas, including the neck, axilla, groin, and antecubital space. The lesions are verrucose and have a velvety appearance, suggesting hyperpigmentation. The cutaneous lesions may occasionally progress and regress in relationship to the status of the primary tumor (Fig. 12.16).

Acquired ichthyosis is frequently associated with Hodgkin's disease, although tumors of the lung, breast, and cervix have also been reported. The ichthyotic lesions are scaly and involve large areas of skin; they have characteristic lambdoid shapes and free edges.

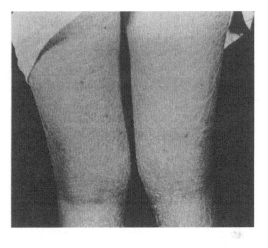

Fig. 12.17 Icthyosis developing (Patient K) with metastatic breast cancer and resolution with tumor-specific therapy.

Patient K, a 67-year-old woman, had a primary adenocarcinoma of the breast removed six months before she developed a nonpurpuric scaling rash of the skin. There had been no previous history of familial or individual dermatologic problems. Examination revealed generalized lambdoid scales with free edges, and the lesions were most prominent on the arms and legs. Because metastatic disease was evident, the patient was treated with Adriamycin and cyclophosphamide, and her ichthyosis appeared to improve (Fig. 12.17). In spite of six courses of chemotherapy, the metastatic lesions in the liver and bone, as well as the ichthyosis, were exacerbated.

Alopecia mucinosa is an uncommon disorder in which dermal papules develop with follicular accentuation and secondary hair loss. Histologically, acid mucopolysaccharide develops in the outer root sheath of the hair follicles, and an inflammatory infiltrate ensues. The acquired variant, particularly in patients over 40, is often associated with lymphoma or mycosis fungoides.

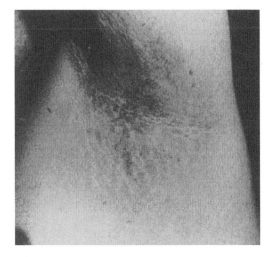

Fig. 12.16 Typical axillary pigmentation in acanthosis nigricans.

Uncommon, acquired skin lesions include Bowen's disease and ichythyosis, among others. These syndromes are associated with internal malignancy in 20 to 50 percent of patients.

Bowen's disease of the skin, an epidermoid carcinoma-in-situ, has similarly been associated with internal cancer. In approximately five percent of patients, the squamous cell carcinoma itself becomes invasive, and 30 percent of such patients develop visceral metastases. More important is the observation that 30 to 40 percent of patients with Bowen's disease have an independent primary malignancy arising in almost any site and derived from epidermal, mesenchymal, or lymphatic tissue. The likelihood of carcinoma increases if the skin lesions occur in a covered area as opposed to a sun-exposed, uncovered area. Typical Bowen's lesions are circumscribed areas of scaling, erythematous plaques that resemble eczema or psoriasis and which expand gradually over a protracted period. The latent period before carcinoma develops varies from 1 to 10 years.

Nonspecific cutaneous lesions associated with malignancy. A variety of cutaneous lesions without specific characteristics may be associated with malignancy although they are not necessarily diagnostic of an internal process (Table 12.4). In general, these nonspecific lesions are more commonly associated with nonmalignant processes, but patients with malignancy are prone to develop these lesions.

The infectious complications of many malignant processes result in cutaneous manifestations. Specific skin lesions, characterized by central necrosis and a black eschar, are seen in patients with pseudomonas infection. Disseminated fungal infection occurs in patients with candidiasis, sporotrichosis, or aspergil-

losis. These skin infections are observed particularly in patients with hematologic malignancies, especially leukemia and lymphoma, for whom immunosuppressive therapy is employed. For the most part, the cutaneous manifestation is secondary to deterioration of health and is not a clue to the detection of an occult malignancy. Pyoderma gangrenosum is a noninfectious lesion associated with leukemia (and ulcerative colitis) and represents a sterile inflammatory reaction in the skin. Herpes zoster, a cutaneous infection along a nerve, is commonly observed in patients with hematologic malignancy, particularly Hodgkin's disease. Disseminated zoster infection occurs infrequently and predominantly in patients with profound immunosuppression or disseminated disease (Fig. 12.18).

Pruritis is the most common dermatologic symptom although most causes of pruritis are not related to malignancy. Nonetheless, pruritis can be one of the "B" symptoms associated with Hodgkin's disease and has been observed in more than 10 percent of patients. It is currently not considered a single "B" symptom in this disease, but rather only in association with the other typical "B" symptoms:

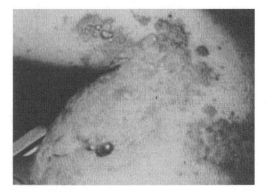

Fig. 12.18 Disseminated vesicular lesions originating in a dermatome with sudden dissemination throughout the body representing herpes zoster infection.

fever, weight loss, and night sweats. The most common cause of pruritis in patients with malignancy is bile salt deposition in the integument as a result of obstruction of the biliary tree. The patient usually has associated jaundice, but occasionally anicteric pruritis is observed. Pruritis is also a manifestation of the early erythroderma syndrome that may progress to mycosis fungoides or one of the other variants of lymphoma cutis.

Urticarial skin lesions result from the accumulation of fluid in the superficial dermis and present clinically as circumscribed, raised, erythematous lesions lasting 12 to 24 hours. When the fluid accumulation involves the deep dermis or subcutaneous tissue, the lesions are designated as angioedema. Such lesions are rarely related to malignancy although lymphoma patients with recurrent angioedema have recently been shown to have a deficiency of the inhibitor of the first component of complement.

Common, nonspecific, acquired skin lesions, such as keratosis, pruritis, and urticaria may be associated with visceral malignancy.

Xanthomatosis is common in patient populations at risk for cancer. In patients who have normal circulating lipid levels, the potential for underlying malignant disease approaches 50 percent. Multiple myeloma is most frequently associated with xanthomatosis, but patients with lymphoma and histiocytosis have also been reported. Vesicobullous disease has been reported in association with internal malignancy, but no evidence indicates that cancer incidence is increased in patients with bullous pemphigoid. Nonetheless, for patients with bullous pemphigoid and a primary malignancy, surgical removal of the cancer may result in regression of the bullous lesions.

Erythroderma, an extremely common cutaneous process, is rarely associated with underlying malignancy; only eight percent of such patients develop cancer. The most common cancers occurring with erythroderma are mycosis fungoides, the lymphomas, and the leukemias. The lesions are often present for a protracted period, and skin biopsy may identify only nonspecific changes. Therapy for the often pruritic erythroderma is generally topical ointments.

Palmar and plantar hyperkeratoses also have been associated with an increased likelihood of malignancy; the relationship, however, remains controversial. Punctate keratoses have been related to internal malignancies as well.

4.0 Cutaneous complications of cancer chemotherapeutic agents

Cutaneous complications from cancer chemotherapeutic agents occur commonly but rarely limit use of the drug. Table 12.6 contains the categories of cutaneous reactions and the medications that cause them; the range of cutaneous reactions to the individual drugs is collated in Table 12.7. Because many cutaneous alterations can be induced by chemotherapy, only the most common reactions will be reviewed here.

Cutaneous complications of cancer drugs are generally idiosyncratic, immunologic, or dose related.

Replication rates of tissues such as the bone marrow, gastrointestinal mucosa, and hair follicles approximate tumor growth rates and are susceptible to the toxic effects of anticancer drugs. Therefore, two common cutaneous complications associated with chemotherapy are stomatitis and alopecia. Stomatitis or

Table 12.6 Cutaneous Complications Associated with Selected Chemotherapeutic Agents

Antiobiotics	Antimetabolites
Bleomycin	5-Fluorouracil
Edema and erythema of extremities	Stomatitis
Infiltrated plaques, violaceous	Alopecia
nodules on hands	Hyperpigmentation
Raynaud's phenomenon	Photosensitivity
Morbilliform eruption	Onycholysis
Hyperpigmentation	Hydroxyurea
Nail changes	Stomatitis
Desquamation, particularly of hands	Nail dystrophy
Dactinomycin	Lichen planus
Stomatitis	6-Mercaptopurine
Alopecia	Stomatitis
Acne	Annular lichenoid papular eruption
Adriamycin (doxorubicin)	Methotrexate
Alopecia	Stomatitis
Subungual vesicles	Alopecia
Onycholysis	Hyperpigmentation
Hyperpigmentation	Vesiculation and ulceration of skin
Transverse banding of fingernails,	overlying pressure areas
palms, soles, mucous	Generalized pruritic, macular
membranes, and diffuse or	erythematous eruption with
generalized hyperpigmentation	desquamation
of skin	Exfoliative erythroderma
	Urticaria
Alkylating agents	Photosensitivity
	Acne
Busulfan	
Cheilosis	Natural products
Glossitis	
Anhidrosis	Vinblastine
Diffuse hyperpigmentation of skin	Alopecia
and mucous membranes	Photosensitivity
Exfoliative erythroderma	Vesiculation
Chlorambucil	Vincristine
Urticaria	Alopecia
Periorbital edema	
Exfoliative erythroderma	
Cyclophosphamide	
Alopecia	
Transverse ridging of nails	

Table 12.7 Cutaneous Complications of Cytotoxic Drug Therapy

Stomatitis	*Radiation recall*
Methotrexate	Adriamycin (doxorubicin)
5-Fluorouracil	Actinomycin D
Adriamycin (doxorubicin)	
Actinomycin D	*Photosensitivity*
	Adriamycin (doxorubicin)
Alopecia	Methotrexate
Adriamycin (doxorubicin)	5-Fluorouracil
Cyclophosphamide	
Vincristine	*Hyperpigmentation**
Actinomycin D	Adriamycin (doxorubicin)
	5-Fluorouracil
Chemical cellulitis	Bleomycin
Adriamycin (doxorubicin)	Cyclophosphamide (rare)
Actinomycin D	Busulfan
Vincristine	
Nitrogen mustard	*Onychodystrophy or onycholysis*
Mitomycin C	Bleomycin
	Cyclophosphamide
	5-Fluorouracil
	Exfoliative dermatitis
	Methotrexate
	Bleomycin
	Chlorambucil

*Includes mucous membrane and nail beds.

mucositis affects the mucosa of the oral cavity and anogenital area, and the extent and severity of the reaction depends on the characteristics of the drug and the dose administered. Lesions can occur on the vermilion border of the lip, the buccal mucosa, the tongue, or the oropharynx. Lesions begin with a prodrome of oral (or anogenital) pain and erythema or arise as white or yellow plaques that soon ulcerate. The ulcerations are usually less than one centimeter in diameter and are often surrounded by a zone or erythema. They are always painful and may interfere with the patient's ability to ingest food, fluids, or medications, or to urinate or defecate.

In evaluating mucosal ulcerations in a patient receiving cytotoxic and immunosuppressive medication, other causes of stomatitis must be considered. Infectious agents such as candida, gram-negative bacteria, and herpes simplex can produce painful oral ulcerations, and cultures for these organisms should be obtained when possible. The treatment of ulcerations includes maintenance of oral hygiene and adequate analgesia. Frequent tooth brushing or other mechanical debridement will help prevent buildup of necrotic tissue, and a broad-spectrum antibiotic can be a useful prophylactic measure to reduce the incidence of bacterial super-infection. Topical analgesia can be provided with viscous Xylocaine® or liquid diphenhydramine hydrochloride (Benadryl®). The diet should comprise soft, bland, nonirritating foods.

Chemotherapeutic agents transiently inhibit cell metabolism and mitosis in actively growing hair follicles; this inhibition results in focal narrowing of the hair shaft. The structurally weakened hair is susceptible to fracture with even the mildest trauma. At any one time, 80 percent of the scalp hairs are in anagen (growth) phase; therefore, a transient growth inhibition produced by antimitotic drugs causes diffuse alopecia. This process is called anagen effluvium. As cytotoxic medications affect only anagen hair follicles, major hair loss occurs on the scalp where the anagen count is highest, but alopecia also affects the axillary, pubic, and facial areas. The eyebrows and lashes remain in a resting or catagen phase for long periods and are rarely affected. The most potent inducer of alopecia is Adriamycin, which at therapeutic dose and schedule always produces total hair loss. Other drugs produce only prominent thinning of the hair, which evolves over 6 to 12 weeks. Anagen effluvium is a reversible process, and regrowth always occurs when the offending medication is discontinued. In some instances limited regrowth will begin while drug therapy proceeds. Drug-induced anagen effluvium is often dose dependent. Scalp alopecia can be reduced by the use of a scalp tourniquet at the time of drug administration, but the effectiveness of this approach is limited and hazardous.

Actinomycin D is associated with a particular folliculitis or acneiform lesion that is often confined to the trunk and dose related (Fig. 12.19). In addition, actinomycin D is a radiation-sensitizing drug and may "recall" a skin reaction to previous radiation outlining the treatment portals (Fig. 12.20). The radiation-sensitizing effect is not dose related but may be due to the inhibition of radiation-damage repair systems within the cell. Almost all chemotherapeutic drugs can sensitize and "recall," but actinomycin D and Adriamycin are most commonly implicated. Rarely, sunlight may "recall" previous

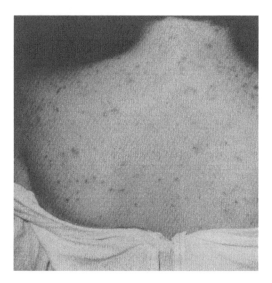

Fig. 12.19 Typical acniform or folliculitis lesions in a patient treated with Actinomycin D.

radiation portals in the presence of actinomycin D.

Photosensitivity after the administration of 5-fluorouracil, methotrexate, and Adriamycin has been observed. In at least one instance, an injection of vinblastine has caused immediate sensitivity to the sunburn range (280–320 nm) of ultraviolet light. Skin eruption may be prevented by the use of sunscreen agents. If exposure to bright sunlight is expected after administration of the drugs mentioned above, a sunscreen containing five percent para-aminobenzoic acid should be applied to the exposed skin.

Cancer chemotherapy commonly causes hyperpigmentation. The pattern of hyperpigmentation is variable, and the discoloration can affect the mucosal surfaces. In addition, a wide variety of drugs produces the reaction. Busulfan causes diffuse hyperpigmentation of sun-exposed and unexposed skin. Occasionally, the pigmentary changes are accompanied by an Addisonian-like syndrome. Diffuse hy-

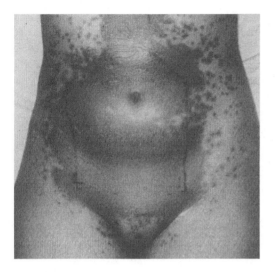

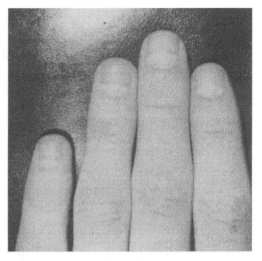

Fig. 12.20 Confluent erythema over the anterior abdominal wall appeared approximately five days following exposure to Actinomycin D and conformed to the previous area of radiation delivered for treatment of para-aortic and iliac nodes.

Fig. 12.21 Pigmented bands across the nails in patients treated with Adriamycin representing growth-arrest lines.

perpigmentation can also be seen with cyclophosphamide, Adriamycin, and 5-fluorouracil (Fig. 12.21). Parallel horizontal and vertical bands, single or multiple, as well as diffuse hyperpigmentation have been reported. Drugs producing mucous membrane hyperpigmentation and other localized changes are listed in Table 12.7. Bleomycin produces linear or "flagellate" hyperpigmentation on the trunk as well as hyperpigmentation over the small joints of the hands and occasionally over the elbows and knees (Fig. 12.22). The phenomenon may be a postinflammatory change associated with scratching, but it is not reproducible. The pigmentation usually fades after discontinuance of the chemotherapeutic agent.

Drug-induced changes are generally transient, with the exception of hyperpigmentation.

Cutaneous reactions associated with chemotherapy are generally not dose related and are rarely dose limiting. The exceptions are the skin reactions to actinomycin D and methotrexate. Most skin reactions to chemotherapeutic agents, including 5-fluorouracil, bleomycin, and chlorambucil, are idiosyncratic or immunologically mediated and necessitate discontinuance of the therapy. The paradoxical occurrence of an allergic reaction to an immunosuppressing agent is an intriguing enigma.

5.0 Summary

The cutaneous complications of cancer are of diagnostic as well as therapeutic importance. The cutaneous syndromes, specific and nonspecific, sporadic and familial, can imply the presence of an internal malignancy and lead to early detection. Furthermore, they represent a monitor of the malignancy. Occasionally, the skin manifestation can be the major symp-

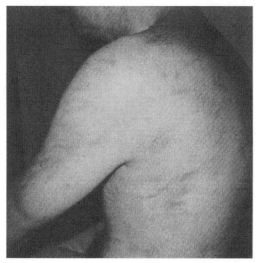

Fig. 12.22 Linear hyperpigmentation across the thorax and upper torso related to bleomycin therapy.

tomatic complication of the malignancy, particularly for patients with disfiguring cosmetic lesions or lesions resulting in chronic pruritis, such as the erythroderma syndromes.

Because the skin comprises an enormous surface area, it is a frequent site of complications from malignancy and its treatment. Furthermore, the availability of the skin to inspection and biopsy offers the opportunity to evaluate pathologically the dynamics of malignancy in terms of growth rate and the impact of therapy on the tumor.

References

Barnes, B. E. Dermatomyositis and malignancy. Ann. Intern. Med. 84:68–76, 1976.

Braverman, I. M. Skin signs of systemic disease. Philadelphia: W. B. Saunders Co., 1970.

Brownstein, M. H., and Helwig, E. B. Metastatic tumors of skin. Cancer 29:1298–1307, 1972.

Dreizen, S.; Bodey, G. P.; Rodriguez, F.; and McCredie, K. B. Cutaneous complications of cancer chemotherapy. Postgrad. Med. 48:150–158, 1975.

Flint, G. L.; Flam, M.; and Soter, N. A. Acquired ichthyosis: a sign of non-lymphoproliferative malignant disorders. Arch. Dermatol. 111:1446–1447, 1975.

Greenwald, E. S. Cancer chemotherapy. Medical Outline Series. 2nd ed. Flushing, N.Y.: Medical Exam. Pub. Co., Inc., 1973.

Kahan, R. S.; Perez-Figaredo, R. A.; and Niemanis, A. Necrolytic migratory erythema: distinctive dermatosis of the glucagonoma syndrome. Arch. Dermatol. 113:793–797, 1977.

Koranda, F. C.; Dehmel, E. M.; Kahn, G,; and Penn, I. Cutaneous complications in immunosuppressed renal homograft recipients. JAMA 229:419–424, 1974.

Lutzner, M,; Edelson, R.; Schein, P.; Green, I.; Kirkpatrick, C.; and Ahmed, P. The Sezary syndrome, mycosis fungoides, and related disorders. Ann. Intern. Med. 83:534–552, 1975.

Marshall, V. Premalignant and malignant skin tumours in immunosuppressed patients. Transplantation 17:272–275, 1974.

Part IV

Special Problems in Cancer Management

Chapter 13

Management of Serous Effusions

J. McCaffrey

1.0 Background

Effusions of the serous surfaces are common complications of advanced cancer. Major and somtimes life-threatening symptoms can develop as a consequence of pleural, peritoneal, or pericardial effusions. As many as 50 percent of patients with breast and lung cancers develop pleural effusions, and this complication is common for patients with lymphoma and carcinoma of the ovary as well. Peritoneal effusion, or ascites, occurs most frequently in patients with ovarian cancer; it also appears often in patients with gastrointestinal neoplasms, particularly gastric and pancreatic cancer. Pericardial effusions develop most commonly in association with lung and breast cancer, and its progression to cardiac tamponade is a critical, life-threatening syndrome (see Chapter 3).

A serous effusion may be the first clinical evidence of malignancy, but the presence of an effusion invariably represents incurable metastases or heralds widespread extrathoracic disease. The prognosis in patients with effusions is determined in part by the type of tumor, the source of the primary lesion, the responsiveness of the tumor to systemic therapy, and the mechanism of fluid accumulation. Pleural effusions are associated with a median survival of six to eight months, peritoneal effusions with a median survival of less than six months, and pericardial effusions with a median survival of less than three months. Median survival times differ, however, depending on the type of primary tumor and the extent of visceral disease.

Fluid accumulates in the potential space between the visceral and parietal envelopes of the pleural, peritoneal, or pericardial surfaces when the normal fluid volume within the closed space increases either by virtue of increased production or by decreased absorption. Increased production is determined by alterations in the hydrostatic or oncotic pressure intravascularly or by an alteration in capillary permeability. The nonmalignant effsions, such as those associated with congestive heart failure or hepatic cirrhosis, develop as a consequence of increased hydrostatic pressure accentuated by salt and water retention. A similar decrease in plasma oncotic pressure as a consequence of protein loss or impaired albunin synthesis leads to secondary fluid accumulation within the serosal surface and results in interstitial peripheral edema.

Cancer-related effusions commonly result from an alteration in capillary permeability. Pleural or peritoneal surface implantation by metastatic tumors can lead to secondary inflammatory responses and local hemorrhage. Because of permeability, these metastases can cause exudates. The second most common mechanism involved in the development of malignant effusions is decreased clearance of normal fluid secondary to obstruction of the normal lymphatic ducts. Obstruction of lymphatic drainage of the pleural surface through the pulmonary parenchyma may develop with lymphangitic tumor that plugs the local parenchymal lymphatic channels or can occur from second level obstruction, as in tumor replacement of the mediastinal and hilar nodes.

The pathophysiologic mechanism for malignant effusion is either tumor obstruction of lymphatic drainage or direct exudation from tumor implants on the serosal surface.

The intra-abdominal drainage pathway is the cisterna chyli, which passes through the thoracic duct into the jugular venous system. A second drainage pathway of the abdomen is the diaphragmatic lymphatic ducts to the internal mammary lymph node chain. Obstruction of lymphatic ducts along the diaphragmatic surface is a common mechanism of ascitic fluid accumulation in ovarian cancer.

2.0 Diagnostic evaluation and differential diagnosis

Pleural effusion. Pleural effusions may develop acutely and generally lead to clinical symptoms of dyspnea only when the fluid volume compromises a major proportion of functioning lung units. In patients with chronic lung disease, relatively small amounts of fluid result in disproportionate symptoms (less than 500-cc accumulation). Effusions that compromise an entire lung ("white out") may be unassociated with clinical symptoms if the opposite lung is normal, but in the presence of a secondary problem, such as pulmonary embolus or pneumonia, clinical symptoms may develop. The typical radiographic finding that distinguishes pleural effusion from lobar collapse is the position of the mediastinum. In the presence of an effusion without collapse, the mediastinum remains mid-line or shifts to the contralateral side; in the presence of lobar collapse, the mediastinum shifts to the ipsilateral side of the collapse. The lateral decubitus film is helpful in identifying small amounts of fluid but is less useful in distinguishing between radiopacity secondary to pleural effusion and that secondary to collapse or tumor mass if the fluid is loculated.

In addition to dyspnea, cough and pain with pleuritic characteristics may develop as fluid accumulation prevents contact irritation by separating the parietal and visceral surfaces. Pain is unusual, and the pain syndrome generally implies the presence of a local tumor with secondary inflammation or neural invasion of the intercostal nerves. Characteristically, patients with pleural effusion assume a supine position in which the fluid-laden side is down, thus allowing for adequate respiratory excursion on the normal side.

Peritoneal effusion. Ascites is more insidious than pleural effusion and results in many more complications and secondary symptoms. In addition to the cosmetic embarrassment of abdominal distention, the patient may develop pain as a consequence of the distention. With extremely large intra-abdominal volumes, the elevation of the diaphragm may cause secondary dyspnea. As a consequence of increased abdominal pressure, the fluid may compress the abdominal contents, particularly the gastrointestinal tract and the venous system, and may result in peripheral edema as well as nonspecific gastrointestinal symptomotology including anorexia, nausea, vomiting, early satiety, and diarrhea. Finally, ascites with the sequestration of protein-rich fluid leads to depletion of normal nutrients and consequent malabsorption with secondary marasmus.

Differential diagnosis. Pleural effusions are encountered clinically in many diseases (Table 13.1). Cardiovascular disease is a common cause of pleural effusion in the cancer patient, as both diseases frequently occur in the older age group. In addition, cancer therapy may involve modalities that affect cardiac function.

Patient A, a 49-year-old woman with

chronic diabetes, developed ovarian carcinoma and was treated for a Stage III tumor with cyclophosphamide and Adriamycin. After completing eight months of chemotherapy, she was in complete remission and was monitored thereafter at monthly intervals. At four months (12 months after the original diagnosis), the patient presented with progressive dyspnea and was found to have bilateral pleural effusions. Diagnostic thoracentesis and cytologic evaluation failed to demonstrate malignant tumor cells, and the patient was treated with diuretics and digitalis with complete resolution of the effusions.

Pleural effusions are not necessarily malignant, and congestive heart failure as well as other benign causes must be ruled out.

Adriamycin, an anthracycline anti-

Table 13.1 Differential Diagnosis of Pleural Effusions

Etiology	Mechanism
Neoplasm	Pleural implants Mediastinal lymphatic obstruction
Infection	Bacterial pneumonia Opportunistic infections: viral, protozoal, fungal
Congestive heart failure	Unrelated disease (Coronary artery disease) Pericardial disease Treatment related
Pulmonary embolism	
Collagen vascular disease	
Other fluid overload states	Iatrogenic Renal disease Hepatic disease Secondary to ascites

biotic, is known to have a cumulative effect on cardiac function and is one of the most effective anticancer drugs. At dosages beyond 450 mg/m², however, Adriamycin progressively compromises cardiac function. Radiation therapy to the heart in patients treated by mantle port for Hodgkin's disease or for lung cancer may induce a cardiomyopathy and accelerate coronary artery disease. Other benign causes of pleural effusion, particularly infection and pulmonary embolus, generally occur acutely and are associated with fever and pleuritic pain.

The causes of neoplastic peritoneal effusions include: (1) diaphragmatic lymphatic blockage, (2) diffuse peritoneal implants, and (3) obstruction of the cisternal chyli (Table 13.2). The third cause generally results in a characteristically milky appearance of chylous ascites. Chylous ascites invariably implies not only obstruction of lymphatic pathways but also a presumed interruption or rupture of the lymphatic pool in the cisterna chyli, which permits the introduction of chyle (fat globules) into the abdominal cavity. Chylous fluid must be distinguished from so-called "chyliform" fluid; the latter is an opaque liquid containing lipids (predominantly esterified triglycerides) secondary to the breakdown of large numbers of cells, thus creating debris within the fluid. Chylous ascites occurs most frequently in patients with lymphoma and can be associated with a long clinical course.

Patient B, a 72-year-old woman, had had abdominal distention for one year prior to seeking medical attention. Abdominal paracentesis yielded chylous ascites, and a lymphangiogram demonstrated extensive retroperitoneal lymphadenopathy. Combined radiation and chemotherapy resulted in control of the ascites for an additional two years without the development of extra-abdominal disease (Fig. 13.1).

Table 13.2 Differential Diagnosis of Peritoneal Effusions

Etiology	Mechanism
Neoplasm	Diaphragmatic lymphatic block Peritoneal implants Mass obstruction of cisterna chyli
Infection	Bacterial Mycobacterial
Special forms	Chylous ascites Pseudomyxoma peritonei Budd-Chiari
Other diseases	Iatrogenic Renal disease Hepatic disease

Pseudomyxoma peritonei is another unusual form of malignant ascites characterized by the development of gelatinous fluid within the abdominal cavity. The gelatinous fluid may or may not be associated with tumor cells, but the most frequent tumors associated with pseudomyxoma are mucoceles of the appendix, ovary, and bile duct. Pseudomyxoma peritonei should be distinguished from mucinous tumors derived from the stomach or colon, as these may produce a similar viscid material. Although the natural history for pseudomyxoma peritonei is protracted over many years, the disease is often difficult to manage.

Patient C, a 55-year-old man, had a mucocele of the appendix removed; one year later he developed progressive abdominal distention. Reexploration failed to identify a tumor; abdominal contents were displaced by large gelatinous mass lesions, which were easily freed from the bowel. Over the next three years, the pa-

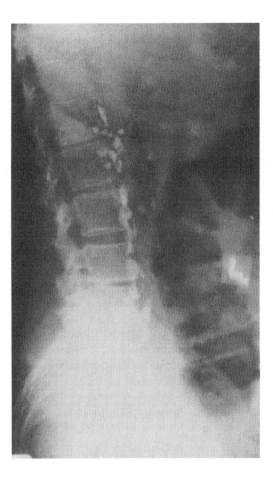 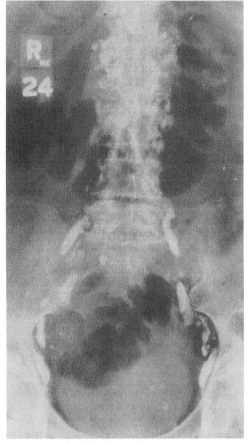

Fig. 13.1 Lymphangiogram in a patient with chylous ascites (Patient B) demonstrating displacement of the normal flow of contrast and filling defects in many of the retroperitoneal lymph nodes. No evidence of dye extravasation into the free peritoneal space.

tient required two additional laparotomies for removal of fluid. The ascites eventually became less viscid and was removable by periodic paracentesis.

Nonneoplastic ascitic fluid generally develops as a consequence of such hepatic disease as cirrhosis, but vascular insults and particularly the Budd-Chiari syndrome may result in acute ascites. The latter may develop with malignancy as a consequence of the hypercoagulable state or may result from direct venous invasion by the tumor (particularly with hepatoma or renal cell carcinoma) and obstruction of the inferior vena cava.

The development of pleural or peritoneal fluid does not necessarily imply the development of progressive tumor. An unusual but important clinical circumstance is the development of pleural or peritoneal effusions as a consequence of effective therapy.

Patient D, a 50-year-old woman, had a primary breast cancer in 1974 and developed multiple pulmonary nodules in 1976. She was treated by ablative surgery

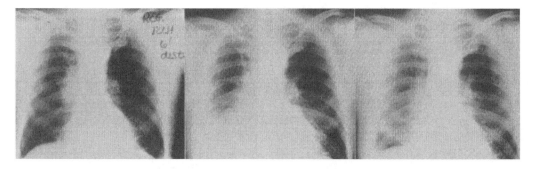

Fig. 13.2 An example of pleural effusion developing as a consequence of cytotoxic effect of chemotherapy. Oat cell cancer with parahilar and mediastinal adenopathy (A), treated with chemotherapy re-sulted in massive right pleural effusion at two weeks (B), and which following thoracentesis did not recur and the paratracheal lesions regressed (C).

and two weeks later developed a left pleural effusion (Fig. 13.2). Diagnostic thoracentesis failed to reveal evidence of malignant cells, and the pulmonary nodules in the right-lung field had disappeared. The effusion did not recur, and the patient did not develop pulmonary lesions during the remainder of her life.

Patient E, a 52-year-old woman, developed multiple pulmonary and liver metastases two years after having been treated for primary breast cancer. A combined chemotherapy and hormonal therapy program was administered, causing complete regression of the pulmonary abnormalities and progressive improvement in the liver scan. At the same time, cytologically normal ascites developed, which eventually required a peritoneal-venous shunt.

Reactive effusion (pleural and peritoneal) may develop as a consequence of tumor necrosis from the inflammatory reaction to drug-tumor interaction.

The mechanism for the development of serous effusions in the presence of an antitumor response is unknown but may be a consequence of sclerosis and healing of tumor sites or a secondary inflammatory response to tumor necrosis. This phenomenon has been observed most commonly in patients with breast tumors, but has also been seen in other cancers.

The diagnostic evaluation of serous effusions is reviewed in Table 13.3. The most crucial examination is of the fluid itself. Cytologic evaluation with the Papanicolaou smear and a preparation of a cell block for fixed tissue cytologic examination may identify the neoplastic cells

Table13.3 Diagnostic Evaluation of Serous Effusions

Fluid Evaluation
  Cytology and cell block
  Chemical characteristics
    Lactic dehydrogenase
    Protein quantity and electrophoresis
    Glucose
    Quantitative lipid/cholesterol content
  Chromosomal evaluation
Pleural Biopsy
Sonogram (ultrasonic evaluation)
Lymphoscintigraphy

as well as their architecture. Malignant effusions will have a postive diagnosis made from the fluid in 50 percent of patients, and both a cytologic and cell block pathologic analysis are important. Because of sampling or technical error, either may be positive for malignancy when the other is negative. Both should therefore be employed. The importance of critical cytologic evaluation cannot be overstated. Normal mesothelial cells may have all the pathologic features of malignant cells including phagocytosis, active mitosis, and cytoplasmic and nuclear anaplasia (Fig. 13.3). The cell block, however, permits evelution of architectural relations among malignant cells; for example, the identification of glandular formation may be appreciated. Histochemical staining can also be important in distinguishing leukemic infiltrates from lymphoma and in identifying unknown primary tumor sources.

Chemical characteristics of the fluid may distinguish an exudate from a transudate. Traditionally, the presence of any of the following characteristics indicates that pleural fluid is an exudate: elevated lactose-dehydrogenase (LDH) level greater than 200 IU; pleural fluid/serum LDH ratio greater than 0.6; or pleural fluid/serum protein ratio greater than 0.5. The absolute protein level is diagnostic of an exudate if it exceeds 3.0 gm%, and occasionally an electrophoresis of the protein may identify a monoclonal pattern. Glucose determination is useful in that decreased levels are generally found in highly proliferating tumors, infection, and effusions from collagen vascular disease. The identification of fats, specifically triglycerides and cholesterol, and the determination of esterified and nonesterified fats are useful in evaluating chylous and chyliform effusions. Recent studies on the measurement of carcinoembryonic antigen (CEA) activity in pleural and peritoneal fluid indicates that CEA may be a useful adjunct in evaluating malignant effusions. Pleural effusions with CEA levels greater than 12 ng/ml are usually associated with malignancy, although some neoplastic effusions may contain less CEA activity. Fluid from nonmalignant effusions rarely exceeds CEA levels greater than 12 ng/ml.

Chromosomal evaluation of the effusion cells may increase the diagnostic yield of fluid analysis by the identification of tumor marker chromosomes or aneuploidy. Techniques involving the evaluation of protein receptors and immunologic markers on the cell wall are also available in special centers, but their usefulness has not been definitively established.

Clarification of the etiology of an effusion can sometimes be achieved by pleural biopsy, and ascitic fluid evaluation may be supplemented by laparoscopy and biopsy of the peritoneal surface. The biopsy allows more definitive evaluation of the pleural surface. Random samples may not identify tumor because the effusion may be secondary to obstruction rather than to a metastatic implant on the serosal surface. Such biopsy procedures may successfully yield the diagnosis in somewhat less than 30 percent of patients.

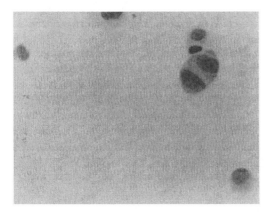

Fig. 13.3 Normal mesothelial cells demonstrating the cytologic features of anaplastic tumor cells.

The use of ultrasonic evaluation to quantify fluid, particularly in the abdominal and pelvic areas, is quite useful especially in identifying small amounts of fluid. Extensive ascitic fluid generally displaces the bowel anteriorly, however, and precludes an adequate evaluation of mass lesions in the retroperitoneal space or pelvis. Generally, the specific etiology of ascitic effusions may be usefully evaluated by ultrasonography only after adequate fluid removal.

Lymphoscintography is a method of evaluating the pleural, pericardial, or abdominal space employing radionuclides. Generally technetium sulphate is injected into the cavity following removal of the fluid, and the gamma camera image is obtained at one and six hours. The radionuclide coats the cavity and outlines the lung, heart, and abdominal viscera (Fig. 13.4). Lymphoscintography has been particularly useful in the study of the mechanism of ascitic fluid production and may be a dynamic method of evaluating ascitic fluid production. The radionuclide is introduced into the abdominal cavity and is absorbed by the nodal and peritoneal lymphatic channels. Subsequently, the radioisotope is transmitted to the diaphragmatic lymphatic ducts and then to the internal mammary or parasternal lymph nodes. The absence of identifiable radioisotope in the parasternal lymph nodes at four to six hours following intraabdominal injection suggests the presence of obstruction in the diaphragmatic lymphatic ducts. In such patients, radiation therapy to the diaphragm may result in relief of ascites. In this instance, specifically identifying the cause of the ascitic fluid can permit introduction of appropriate therapy.

Malignant effusion (pleural and peritoneal) without an identifiable primary tumor. Occasionally, a pleural effusion that reveals Class V malignant cytology develops when no primary tumor has been

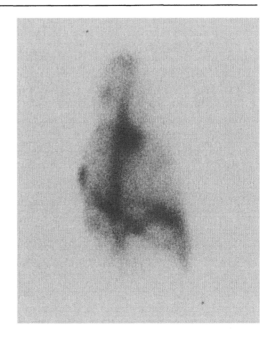

Fig. 13.4 Technetium (^{99m}Tc) radioisotope was introduced into the pleural space following thoracentesis. The radionuclide is distributed throughout the pleural cavity with increased activity in the areas of loculated fluid or fissure drainage areas such as the hilum and supradiaphragmatic areas.

identified. The cytologic diagnosis is generally adenocarcinoma, and the patient undergoes an evaluation for the potential sources of adenocarcinoma. The source of such tumors is usually shown at postmortem examination to be primary adenocarcinoma of the lung. Primary mesotheliomas of the pleura, however, are commonly confused with adenocarcinoma, especially on cytologic evaluation. Such tumors may appear as anaplastic glandular tumors on cytologic examination.

Patient F, a 58-year-old chronic smoker, presented with cough and pleuritic chest pain. Chest x-ray revealed a pleural implant with effusion, and pathologic anal-

ysis of a pleural biopsy was consistent with adenocarcinoma (Fig. 13.5).

Ascitic fluid can be malignant even when a primary source is not identifiable. While peritoneal mesothelioma may be considered, cancer of the ovary is more often the source of the ascites, as ovarian cancer is the most common cause of malignant ascites. Germinal tumors may arise in the retroperitoneal space along the urogenital ridge; these cancers represent ovarian tissue that has been deposited during embryonic life and has undergone malignant degeneration. Malignant ascites in the absence of an identifiable tumor in the ovary, pancreas, or stomach should be presumed to indicate an ovarian malignancy, particularly as ovarian tumors are quite responsive to chemotherapy. Malignant ascites can also be caused by occult carcinoma of the breast, another responsive tumor.

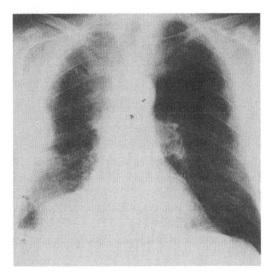

Fig. 13.5 Chest radiograph demonstrating right mid-lung field pleural-based mass that was associated with pain and on biopsy was consistent with adenocarcinoma (Patient F).

3.0 Treatment principles

In general, the therapy of malignant effusions has been remarkably effective, with control of the effusion in approximately 50 percent of cases. Of course, management depends upon the specific tumor class, mechanism of effusion production, and responsiveness to systemic or local radiation therapy. The major therapies have involved surgical drainage, intracavitary therapy, and local or regional radiation therapy. Prior to the application of one of these modalities, however, a general sequence of diagnostic and therapeutic trials should be undertaken (Table 13.4).

Thoracentesis or paracentesis is not only a diagnostic procedure but may also be therapeutic. In a small proportion of patients, fluid may not reaccumulate, because of the sealing contact of the serosal surfaces following fluid removal. In this context, it is important that removal of the entire fluid volume be achieved. The concern that secondary hypotension or intravascular fluid depletion may develop is less important in malignant effusions than in effusions developing as a consequence of cirrhosis. In cirrhotic effusion, fluid is continuously produced, whereas in malignant ascites, fluid accumulation may be intermittent. Intravascular volume and pressure are therefore not compromised with malignant ascites. Nonetheless, the removal of excessive amounts of fluid may be attended by some

Table 13.4 General Principles of Treatment for Malignant Effusions

Thoracentesis or paracentesis of all sequestered fluid

Trial of diuretics

Systemic treatment of the specific cancer

Local treatment (radiation) of the effusion if obstruction is the mechanism orthostatic effects in the elderly patient with extensive ascites. Following removal of the fluid, a period of observation is recommended before a secondary form of treatment is introduced. The second step may be a trial of diuretics, which are occasionally useful in diminishing the rate of fluid reaccumulation.

The major method for controlling an effusion should be systemic treatment of the malignancy, particularly for those effusions developing as a consequence of such responsive tumors as lymphoma, breast cancer, or ovarian cancer. Successful treatment of these tumors is achieved in more than 50 percent of patients; therefore, the use of the more morbid surgical, intracavitary, or radiation therapies may be avoided.

Patient G, a 42-year-old woman, developed progressive dyspnea and was found to have a pleural pericardial effusion with adenopathy. A lymph node biopsy revealed histiocytic lymphoma. The patient was initiated on a program of combination chemotherapy, which led to rapid resolution of the pleural effusion within three weeks (Fig. 13.6.)

Patient H, a 72-year-old woman, presented with progressive dyspnea. Cytologic examination of the pleural fluid revealed a small cell carcinoma. Bronchoscopy identified extrinsic compression, and the patient was initiated on combination chemotherapy. She also had a therapeutic thoracentesis. The pleural fluid did not return during the course of her subsequent therapy (Fig. 13.7).

The primary treatment of effusions is tumor-specific drug therapy.

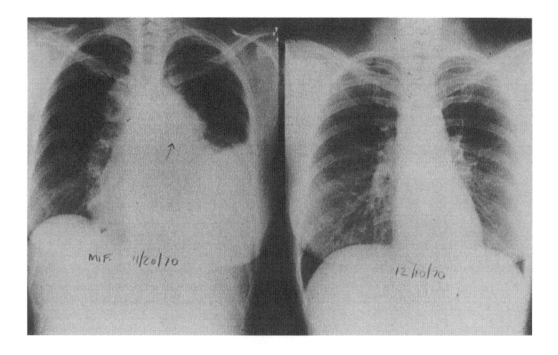

Fig. 13.6 Sequential chest radiographs in a patient with histiocytic lymphoma (Patient G) with rapid regression over a period of less than three weeks of both effusion and mediastinal and hilar adenopathy.

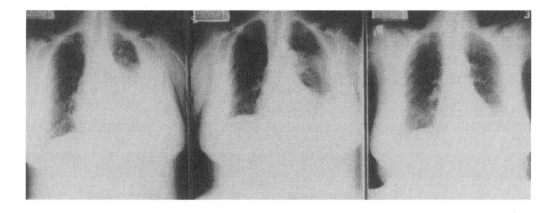

Fig. 13.7 Sequential radiographs in a patient with oat cell carcinoma (Patient H) with rapid resolution of pulmonary nodules and left pleural effusion.

4.0 Intracavitary therapy

All agents intended for instillation in the thoracic and abdominal cavities, whether cytotoxic antitumor drugs, inert substances, or radioactive isotopes, act functionally by sclerosing the visceral and parietal surfaces, thereby obliterating the potential space in which fluid can accumulate. Generally, these treatments are most successful when the pleural cavity is entirely drained of fluid by a tube thoracostomy, the chosen therapeutic substance is introduced, and the cavity is redrained after a short time. Following instillation of the agent, the tube is clamped, and the patient is rotated to assure adequate distribution of the intracavitary substance over the entire serosal surface. Depending upon the character of the instilled agent, a transient reactive pleuritis and effusion may develop in association with fever and may require a secondary drainage procedure before adequate control of the effusion is achieved.

The therapies and side effects for intracavitary treatment are listed in Table 13.5. Many cytotoxic drugs have been used for intracavitary therapy of malignant effusion. Originally the antineoplastic drugs, particularly nitrogen mustard, 5-fluorouracil, and triethylene thiophosphoramide (Thiotepa), were presumed to affect malignant effusions by tumor cell destruction, as the treatment was most effective in the presence of cellular effusions. It is probable, however, that the major effect of such drugs is independent of the cell composition of the fluid and is related more specifically to the induction of an irritative serositis.

Nitrogen mustard was the first agent to be used extensively, but it is systemically absorbed and may result in secondary marrow suppression and adverse gastrointestinal effects. The antimetabolite 5-fluorouracil is less irritating to the serosa and therefore causes less pain and fever, but it appears also to be somewhat less effective. More recently the antitumor antibiotic bleomycin was evaluated for intracavitary treatment and was effective in controlling more than 60 percent of pleural effusions and more than 36 percent of peritoneal effusions.

Quinacrine (Atabrine), an antimalarial drug, has also been popular as an instillation agent because of its lack of hematopoietic suppression. Nonetheless, the agent has several serious disadvantages in that it is quite painful and requires prolonged hospitalization for administration daily or

Table 13.5 Intracavitary Agents for the Management of Serous Effusions

Agent	Dose	Side Effects	Comments
Nitrogen mustard	0.4 mg/kg	Marrow depression, nausea, vomiting, severe serositis	Reduce dose if marrow already compromised.
5-Fluorouracil	2–3 g	Marrow depression	Possibly less effective agent.
Bleomycin	60–120 mg in 100 cc saline	Minimal marrow depression, fever, hypotension	
Quinacrine	Pleural effusion: 100–200 mg q.d. or q.o.d.	Pain, fever, hypotension, ileus, seizures	Requires longer hospitalization as dosage is escalated to induce serositis.
	Ascites: 200–400 mg q.d. or q.o.d.		
Tetracycline	500 mg in 30 cc saline	Fever, pain	Probably least toxic sclerosing agent.
Talc	Sterile packet in 200 cc saline	Fever, pain, reactive effusion	
Radioactive phosphorus (^{32}P)	Pleural effusion: 5–10 mc	Mild if any radiation sickness	Should not be used with open wound or draining fistula. Half life 14 days, beta radiation.
	Ascites: 10–15 mc		
Radioactive gold (^{198}Au)	Pleural effusion: 75–100 mc	Same as ^{32}P	Short half life (2.7 days) with gamma radiation requiring isolation.
	Ascites: 150–225 mc		

every other day to a total of two to five doses. It has been associated with fever, hypotension, hallucinations, and even sudden death.

More recently the antimicrobial agent tetracycline has become increasingly popular for intracavitary treatment. The method of instillation generally involves the use of 0.5 gm of tetracycline dissolved in 50 cc of saline and introduced into the pleural space following fluid removal.

A successful control of the effusion is achieved in more than 70 percent of patients. A randomized trial of intrapleural quinacrine versus tetracycline in malignant effusions demonstrated less toxicity from tetracycline, although the therapeutic effect was comparable for both drugs.

Talc, an inert silicate related chemically to asbestos, is another sclerosing agent that has significant activity when instilled intrapleurally. Talc poudrage controls

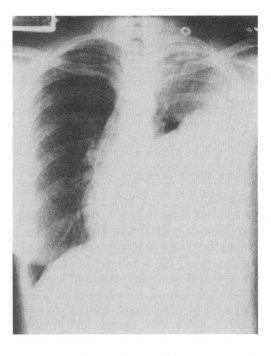 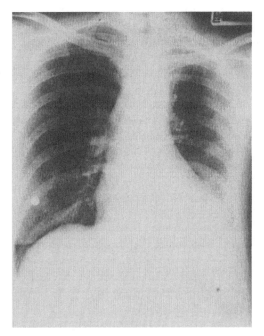

Fig. 13.8 Chest radiograph (Patient I) of massive left pleural effusion with medias-tinum displaced to the right (A) treated by thoracentesis and talc instillation demonstrating complete and persistent improvement over a nine-month period (B).

up to 90 percent of pleural effusions, but the method must be performed during thoracotomy. Insufflation of talc at the bedside following tube thoracostomy is somewhat less effective, but its effect is comparable to those of the other agents.

Patient I, a 47-year-old woman, devel-oped recurrent inflammatory breast can-cer of the left chest wall six years following left mastectomy. Soft tissue and nodal metastases were initially controlled for 18 months with combination chemotherapy, but she then developed a disabling left pleural effusion and progressive meta-static disease. Four liters of cytologically positive fluid were removed by tubal thor-acostomy. Sterile talc suspended in 200 cc of saline was instilled through the chest tube. No pleural effusion has reaccumu-lated nine months following this proce-dure despite continued progression of metastatic disease (Fig. 13.8).

The level of effectiveness for intracavi-tary therapy is different for pleural and abdominal effusions. The pleural effusions can be controlled in 60 to 70 percent of patients with intracavitary therapy, whereas abdominal effusions can only be controlled in less than 40 percent. Ab-dominal effusions are more difficult to control because of the danger of introduc-ing sclerosing substances such as nitro-gen mustard into the abdominal cavity: the secondary effects on the bowel may result in perforation or necrosis of intra-abdomi-nal viscera.

Intracavitary therapy with radioisotopes or cytotoxic drugs is effective in 60 to

70 percent of pleural effusions and 20 to 30 percent of peritoneal effusions.

5.0 Radiation therapy

External radiation therapy to the thorax or abdomen has been employed for peritoneal as well as for pleural effusions, but the technique is associated with major morbidity from radiation sickness because of the large treatment area. In addition, secondary effects on the viscera may ensue with radiation fibrosis of the lung, liver, bowel, or kidneys. Thus, the chronic morbidity or progressive fibrosis and the acute toxicity of the technique generally preclude the use of large-volume radiation therapy to treat effusion.

Nonetheless, several clinical problems may respond well to external radiation therapy. In such radiation-sensitive tumors as lymphoma or breast cancer, the use of tangential beam therapy to the chest wall may allow specific treatment of the pleural surface while sparing the underlying lung. In addition, radiation therapy directed at a tumor mass that is causing obstruction and increased lymphatic pressure may result in reduction of pleural fluid. Radiation of the diaphragmatic surface, particularly in patients with ovarian carcinoma, may inhibit the accumulation of malignant ascites by eliminating the obstruction to diaphragmatic lymph nodes.

External beam radiation therapy is of limited effectiveness in serous effusions.

More commonly, radiation therapy involves the use of radioactive isotopes administered as intracavitary agents. Colloidal suspensions of radioactive gold (^{198}Au) and radioactive phosphorus (^{32}P) are effective sclerosing agents that have only minimal side effects. The advantage of radioisotopes over external radiation therapy is that the radiation is confined to the serosal cavity and selectively affects the tumor while sparing the normal tissue. The suspended radioisotope particles are absorbed into the serous lining, thus creating an obliterative fibrosis that prevents reaccumulation of fluid. Radioactive gold emits gamma and beta rays and has a half life of 2.7 days with only one to three millimeters of tissue penetration. Phosphorus-32 is superior to radioactive gold in that it is a pure beta emitter; the radiation hazard is therefore minimal to hospital staff and the patient need not be isolated. The half life of ^{32}P is 14.3 days, and the tissue penetration is up to seven millimeters.

The shallow tissue penetration of both agents suggests that they would be ineffective in the treatment of large tumor masses. Certainly tumor accumulations beyond one centimeter are ineffectively managed by the colloidal suspensions.

6.0 Surgical methods of management

As indicated previously, thoracentesis and paracentesis have each been reported to effectively control effusions, but simple drainage generally yields only short-term palliation. Repeated thoracentesis or paracentesis may result in severe hypoproteinemia, development of secondary infection, and the potential complication of pneumothorax.

Tube thoracostomy alone may allow sealing of the visceral and parietal surfaces of the pleura. It has been demonstrated that with tube drainage a significant serositis and secondary fibrosis develop. Chest tubes must be maintained for 48 to 72 hours and are removed after optimal fluid evacuation. A major complication of tube drainage with or without talc instillation and the development of chronic fibrositis is the trapped-lung syndrome. Crippling respiratory insufficiency may develop as a consequence of the progressive fibrosis that restricts lung expansion and limits aeration of the alveolar spaces. In such patients, pleurectomy with decortication of the trapped lung is necessary and involves open thoracotomy and stripping of the entire parietal pleura. This procedure should be used judiciously, as the operative mortality approaches 10 percent. Thus pleurectomy with decortication should be attempted only for patients who have localized or controlled disease and for whom long-term survival is expected.

The surgical methods described thus far apply to patients with malignant pleural effusions and are not generally useful in the treatment of malignant peritoneal effusion or ascites. The peritoneal cavity can contain huge volumes of fluid and many loops of freely flowing bowel serosa studded with tumor implants, Realistically, the visceral surface cannot be fibrosed to the parietal peritoneum, as the visceral surface represents the serosa of the bowel. Instillation of intracavitary agents into ascitic fluid frequently causes only a localized serositis and loculated accumulation of the drug.

Ileo-entectropy is a surgical procedure for malignant ascites in which an isolated loop of ileum is exposed to ascitic fluid by everting the mucosa, thus promoting internal absorption of the fluid. Use of this approach to ascites is not widespread, however, in spite of success in a small group of patients.

The surgical management of ascites has recently become more effective with the development of peritoneal venous shunts. Many shunt mechanisms have been developed, but technical and mechanical problems involving clotting of the shunts have precluded a general application.

The development of a one-way valve shunt for patients with benign ascites secondary to chronic liver disease was developed by LeVeen and co-workers. It involves a simple surgical procedure using local anesthesia. A large tube with multiple drainage holes is placed, free-floating in the peritoneal cavity. An attached one-way valve is secured outside the peritoneum, and a silicone tube is tunneled beneath the skin along the anterior or lateral chest wall to the jugular vein. Flow proceeds only from the abdominal cavity to the thoracic cavity; fluid shift is a consequence of increased abdominal pressure as compared with negative intrathoracic pressure. The shunt thus promotes flow of the ascites from the abdominal cavity to the systemic venous system.

The major complications of the peritoneal venous shunt relate to acute fluid overload, which may be obviated by removal of most of the fluid at placement of an intra-abdominal catheter. Fluid removal is also important to obviate the direct infusion of a large quantity of thromboplastic material into the vascular space.

Patient J, a 64-year-old woman, developed progressive ascites secondary to ovarian cancer. Although initially responsive to therapy, her tumor was relentless after recurrence. Inanition, abdominal distention, and the need for recurrent paracentesis necessitated consideration of a peritoneal venous (PV) shunt. Analysis of the peritoneal fluid revealed high levels of thromboplastic activity, and surgical introduction of the shunt was deferred. At the patient's persistent request, a PV shunt was placed with the understanding that intravascular coagulation was a major risk. The patient died of intractable pulmonary insufficiency two days following placement of the shunt. Postmortem examination revealed disseminated pulmonary artery thrombosis (Fig. 13.9), which developed in spite of ligation of the shunt at 24 hours.

Complications of PV shunts include the potential for systemic dissemination of tumor in patients in whom malignant cells are free-floating in the fluid, and the

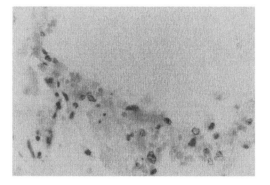

Fig. 13.9 Postmortem histologic section of
the lungs demonstrating a hyaline case
of thrombosis within the pulmonary
arterioles.

development of disseminated intravascular coagulation as a consequence of the
infusion of thromboplastic material. The
implantability of the free-floating tumor
cells in viscera has never been established,
and in the small series of cases thus far
reported in whom PV shunting has been
performed for cytologically positive malignant ascites, the development of disseminated tumor has not been observed

The following two cases illustrate the
success and the failure of PV shunts and
the specific role of these shunts in the
management of ascites.

Patient K, a 39-year-old woman, developed breast cancer metastatic to the liver
and with secondary ascites. She was
treated with combination chemotherapy
and had dramatic improvement of liver
function tests and regression of liver size,
but the ascites persisted and was consistently cytologically negative. Thromboplastic activity was not demonstrated in
the fluid, and the patient underwent a
PV shunt because of progressive marasmus and the need for a weekly eight-liter
paracentesis. At operation, the liver was
noted to be diffusely studded with tumor.
The shunt functioned immediately, caus-

ing a major diuresis. She has not required
paracentesis for two years.

Patient L, a 36-year-old man, presented
with ascites, weight loss, and jaundice
secondary to extensive intra-abdominal
anaplastic carcinoma of unknown primary origin. The tumor was controlled
initially by combination chemotherapy
and later by total abdominal irradiation
when jaundice and ascites recurred. Following three months of response, he developed intractable ascites and abdominal
pain requiring continuous hospitalization
for frequent paracenteses. Although the
ascitic fluid cytology was positive for
malignant cells, no significant thromboplastic activity was detected in the fluid,
and a LeVeen PV shunt was placed. A
radionuclide scan confirmed shunt function (Fig. 13.10). The patient returned
home three days following the surgery and
remained there until he died two months

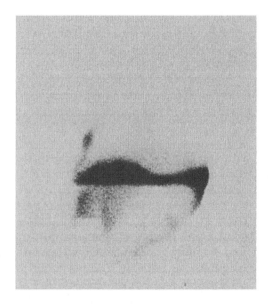

Fig. 13.10 A radioisotope is injected into
the ascitic fluid following placement of
the PV shunt with up-take demonstrated
throughout the course of the shunt.

later. Significant ascites did not recur, and autopsy revealed only 500 cc of fluid in the abdominal cavity.

These cases illustrate the successful use of a shunt in spite of malignant cells in the fluid. The use of a shunt for a patient whose ascites results from regression of tumor with presumably secondary fibrosis causing portal hypertension is unusual. This effect has been observed in at least two cases of breast cancer, which is generally a responsive tumor.

7.0 Summary

Pleural, peritoneal, and pericardial effusions cause significant debility because of pain, dyspnea, and marasmus; furthermore, they may be life threatening. Localized disease to the pleura or peritoneal surface is common with some tumors (particularly ovarian cancer), and the tumor may remain localized at the serous surface for some time. The management of ascitic effusions is much more problematic than that of pleural effusions, not only because of the degree of debility but also due to the therapeutic options available. The most important option, as for many other complications of malignant disease, depends on therapy directed at the primary tumor. Ancillary palliative procedures are for the most part only transiently effective.

References

Bayly, T. C. et al. Tetracycline and quinacrine in the control of malignant pleural effusions. *Cancer* 41:1188–1192, 1978.

Black, L. The pleural space and pleural fluid. *Mayo Clin. Proc.* 47:493–506, 1972.

Card, R. Y.; Cole, D. R.; and Henschke, U. K. Summary of 10 years of the use of radioactive colloids in intracavitary therapy. *J. Nucl. Med.* 1:195–198, 1960.

Coates, G.; Bush, R. S.; and Aspin, N. A study of ascites using lymphoscintigraphy with ^{99}Tc-sulfur colloid. *Radiology* 107:577–583, 1973.

Dollinger, M. Management of recurrent malignant effusions. *Cancer* 22:138–147, 1972.

Fracchia, A. A. et al. Intrapleural chemotherapy for effusion from metastatic breast carcinoma. *Cancer* 25:626–629, 1970.

Goldberg, B. B. Ultrasonic evaluation of intraperitoneal fluid. *JAMA* 235(22):2427–2430. 1976.

Lambert, C. J. et al. The treatment of malignant pleural effusions by closed trocar tube drainage. *Ann. Thorac. Surg.* 3:1–5, 1967.

LeVeen, H. H. et al. Peritoneo-venous shunting for ascites. *Ann Surg.* 180:580–591, 1974.

Leff, A.; Hopewell, P. C.; and Costello, J. Pleural effusion from malignancy. *Ann. Intern. Med.* 88:532–537, 1978.

Light, R. W. et al. Pleural effusions: The diagnostic separation of transudates and exudates. *Ann. Intern. Med.* 77:507–513, 1972.

Paladine, W. et al. Intracavitary bleomycin in the management of malignant effusions. *Cancer* 38:1903–1908, 1976.

Rittgers, R. A. et al. Carcinoembryonic antigen levels in benign and malignant pleural effusions. *Ann. Intern. Med.* 88:631–634, 1978.

Salyer, W. R.; Eggleston, J. C.; Erozan, Y. S. Efficacy of pleural needle biopsy and pleural fluid cytopathology in the diagnosis of malignant neoplasm involving the pleura. *Chest* 67:536–539, 1975.

Shedbalkar, A. R. et al. Evaluation of talc pleural symphysis in management of malignant pleural effusion. *J. Thorac. Cardiovasc. Surg.* 61:292–297, 1971.

Strober, J. S. et al. Malignant pleural disease: A radiotherapeutic approach to the problem. *JAMA* 226:297–299, 1973.

Suhrland, L. G., and Weisberger, A. S. Intracavitary 5-fluorouracil in malignant effusions. *Arch. Intern. Med.* 116:431–433, 1965.

Weisberger, A. S. Direct instillation of nitrogen mustard in the management of malignant effusions. *Ann. N.Y. Acad. Sci.* 68:1091–1096, 1958.

Chapter 14

Management of Nutrition: Hyperalimentation

B. Bistrian

A. Bothe

1.0 Background

The anorexia-cachexia syndrome occurs with distressing regularity in many cancer patients, and the devastating impact of the resultant protein-calorie malnutrition (PCM) has recently become evident. Tolerance of and response to specific therapy can be dramatically influenced by nutritional status. Recent developments in clinical nutrition have made nutritional support to reverse PCM possible for most cancer patients. Advances include new techniques such as total parenteral nutrition and infusion pumps, and new products such as commercial tube feeding formulas of varied composition, intravenous fat emulsions, and isotonic amino acid solutions. This chapter will briefly consider the etiology of PCM for cancer patients and its effects on their function, particularly immunocompetence, the assessment of nutritional status, recom-

mended needs for protein and energy, techniques for nutritional support, and methods of monitoring therapeutic effectiveness.

Etiology of PCM in cancer. One of the earliest recorded observations of the interrelation between cancer and nutrition is attributed to Hippocrates. He noted that if a patient with malignant disease was unable to gain weight, the prognosis was poor. Although many theories have attempted to account for the nearly universal occurrence of weight loss in cancer patients, no specific underlying mechanism has been found. Hypotheses have suggested that the increased Cori cycle activity of glucose recycling through lactate to glucose is an energy-inefficient process, but a finer appreciation of the stoichiometry of this process confirms the trivial nature of the resultant calorie loss. A widely espoused theory has been the so-called "nitrogen trap" hypothesis, whereby the tumor is able to grow while the host's nutritional stores are depleted. Tumors do exhibit some degree of autonomy, but subsequent research has shown that although tumor tissue has a higher priority for endogenous protein, tumor nitrogen does recycle through the host.

Certain rare tumors, particularly those with thyroidlike activity and some leukemias, cause an increased metabolic rate. In most instances, however, energy expenditures of cancer patients do not exceed resting metabolic expenditure by more than 10 to 20 percent. Thus, as in other forms of hospital PCM, four basic causes for PCM exist (Table 14.1). It appears that the major factor producing weight loss is inadequate intake due to cancer-related anorexia, particularly when gastrointestinal symptoms are present. Anorexia accompanies most disease and can be considered part of a short-term (7- to 10-day) metabolic response to injury. This response is effective in mobilizing body energy and protein during acute stress but becomes counterproductive

---

Cancer cachexia is primarily related to anorexia with insufficient protein and calorie intake.

---

when persistent, as in chronic illness. Some characteristics are unique to cancer anorexia, such as early development of

Table 14.1 Etiology of Hospital PCM

Reduced intake
  Anorexia
  Disorders of ingestion, digestion,
    absorption
  Iatrogenic semistarvation

Increased expenditure
  Catabolic effects of illness

---

distaste for meat proteins and relative preservation of taste for milk-based proteins. A second important characteristic of cancer anorexia is the rapid development of taste fatigue with generally good long-term acceptance of vanilla flavor. Occasionally, bland products such as Isocal® will be tolerated in preference to highly flavored products.

A second factor in the development of PCM is the numerous gastrointestinal tract disturbances that impair function; these include obstruction, ileus, and fistula formation. Malabsorption syndromes occur in patients with cancer of the pancreas (reduced enzymes), biliary tract obstruction (reduced bile), gastric hypersecretion (deconjugation of bile salts), infiltration of bowel mucosa (e.g., lymphomas), and a variety of more unusual syndromes such as blind loops and bypass of significant portions of the bowel as a result of fistula formation. Fat malabsorption secondary to PCM itself, however, is usually minor. Endocrine or paraendocrine tumors may secrete peptide hormones that stimulate secretions of the gastrointestinal tract (e.g., pancreatic cholera, Zollinger-Ellison syndrome, or carcinoid) leading to malabsorption diarrhea. These hormonal syndromes suggest the possibility that tumors can produce substances that also induce anorexia and weight loss, but no such substance has so far been identified. Finally, it must be recognized that certain characteristic weight loss patterns occur in particular cancers. For example, oat cell tumors of the lung can produce extreme wasting disproportionate to tumor bulk, whereas patients with breast cancer maintain their lean tissue reasonably well.

Third, iatrogenic malnutrition plays a major role for patients with the kwashiorkor-like illness characterized by hypoalbuminemia and anergy. This condition develops when stress is imposed on a malnourished, semistarved patient. The various modalities of therapy, particularly radiation therapy and surgery, place stress on the metabolism and reduce the efficiency with which protein and calories can be used. When this stress is compounded by common semistarvation regimens employed for the seriously ill, such as low-calorie and low-protein diets, hypoalbuminemia and anergy rapidly ensue. The PCM resulting from specific treatment further limits tolerance to the therapy, and ultimately, alters the prognosis.

The first three elements in the genesis of PCM pertain to limitation of nutrient intake. The fourth major etiologic factor relates to the other aspect of the equation, an increase in caloric and protein expense. The catabolic effects of illness are protective and supportive in the early phase of response to injury, but potentially harmful if persistent or occurring in a previously compromised patient.

Effect of PCM on patient function. The two primary variables in the production of hospital malnutrition are the severity of

the stress response and the amount of dietary protein restriction. When dietary energy supply is inadequate, deficit calories are provided from three body stores: skeletal muscle, viscera, and fat (Fig. 14.1). Fat tissue is the largest fuel deposit, containing more than 150,000 stored calories in most normal adults and is therefore considered dispensable. Though important for mobility, carcass skeletal protein can be expediently sacrificed during stress and semistarvation, as this process provides amino acids for protein synthesis and energy production by the liver. Although visceral organs represent only a small proportion of total available energy, they perform vital functions that can be impaired by even mild loss of substance.

In the absence of adequate dietary energy, the deficit is met principally by fat with a small contribution from muscle protein. If stress from injury or infection is superimposed on semistarvation, protein losses increase from both skeletal

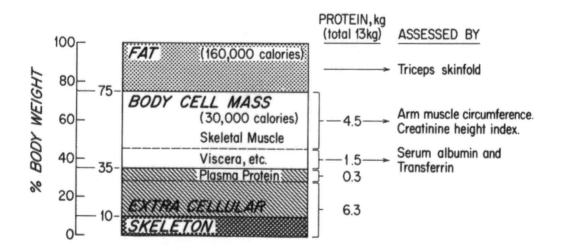

Fig. 14.1 *Body composition and energy expense in a 70-kg reference man. In malnourished patients, body compartments are altered, but the major energy stores (skeletal muscle protein, viscera, fat) can be simply estimated by anthropometrics or secretory protein levels. The sizes of the various body compartments are approximate values. (Source: Bistrian 1977. Reprinted by permission).*

muscle and viscera. When dietary protein alone is lacking but energy intake is adequate, muscle and viscera are more slowly depleted but similarly respond to stress by an increase in protein loss.

Skeletal and visceral protein loss is manifested by impaired organ function. In skeletal protein loss, symptoms and signs appear primarily as muscle weakness, including respiratory problems. In visceral protein attrition, dysfunction resulting from PCM has been described for most visceral organs including cardiac atrophy, pancreatic insufficiency, gastrointestinal mucosal atrophy, and the development of a fatty liver. Probably of more clinical importance is the significant impairment of the patient's immune function, particularly phagocytic activity and cellular immunity, which can be reduced by even mild degrees of PCM.

Cell immunity and hospital PCM. Both in vitro and in vivo correlates of cell-mediated immunity are impaired by PCM in direct relation to the degree of visceral depletion. This is true not only of the primary PCM prevalent in less developed countries, but also for the PCM secondary to disease in industrial nations. In hospitals caring for the acutely ill, 25 to 30 percent of all patients are significantly malnourished by standard anthropometric criteria for PCM, and at least the same percentage applies to cancer patients.

Cell immunity is important to the body's defense against infectious disease; its depression has been associated with increased morbidity and mortality from infection. PCM is the most common cause of acquired immunodeficiency. Two well recognized variants of PCM result from the dietary deficiency of calories (marasmus), protein (kwashiorkor), or both. In kwashiorkor, significant impairment of secretory protein synthesis is reflected in hypoalbuminemia and cellular immunocompetence. In marasmus, the response to semistarvation is more adaptive, with

fat and muscle providing most of the deficit calories while secretory protein levels and immune function are better preserved.

PCM can result in secondary compromise of metabolic and immunologic functions.

Similar syndromes occur in hospitalized adults with disease. Moderate-carbohydrate, low-protein diets in patients undergoing the stress of injury or infection may produce hypoalbuminemia and impaired immunocompetence in 7 to 10 days. This hypoalbuminemic malnutrition in adults resembles kwashiorkor. Adult marasmus, or cachexia, is characterized by depression of the weight/height index, the triceps skin fold, and the arm muscle circumference, but serum albumin levels are maintained and immune function is less severely impaired. This condition results from insufficient intake uncomplicated by a marked catabolic response to illness.

In both forms of PCM, nutritional repletion can restore cell immune function in several weeks. A major implication of this fact is the desirability of rapid nutritional repletion in any malnourished patient who is anergic. Because nutritional repletion is difficult in the presence of catabolic stress, the results of any elective procedure that produces such stress (surgery or radiation therapy) may be improved by prior nutritional repletion. When such nutritional therapy is undertaken concomitant with or prior to cancer therapy, tolerance to treatment may be improved.

Patient survival and tumor response to chemotherapy, surgery, or radiation therapy are related to maintenance of the patient's immunocompetence in a wide variety of tumor types. The relative proportion of cancer patients whose anergy is due to the primary disease or to PCM is not known, but a preliminary estimate would be that anergy in 35 to 40 percent of patients with solid tumors is secondary to PCM.

It has been shown over the short term that nutritional reversal of PCM-induced anergy can improve response to specific antitumor therapy. What is not known is whether improved survival is likely over the longer term for these patients or for other patients who have been maintained skin-test–positive by continued nutritional support, or even whether it would be possible to maintain long-term immunocompetence by nutritional support.

In Hodgkin's disease and other lymphomas, a defect in the thymus-derived lymphocyte function responsible for cell-mediated immunity has been consistently noted. This is characterized by an impaired in vitro response and by anergy to primary sensitizing and recall antigens. Delayed hypersensitivity usually remains intact with multiple myeloma, whereas severe deficiencies in cellular immunity are commonly seen in solid tumors. Immunologic responsiveness sometimes can be correlated with extent of tumor, whereas in other instances, immune depression is observed even in the earliest stage of malignancy.

2.0 Nutritional assessment

Static measures. Weight/height determinations are useful because of the ease of measurement and availability of generally accepted standards (Table 14.2). Weight/

Table 14.2 Recommended Weight in Relation to Height

| Height* | | Men | | Women | |
Feet	Inches	Average (lb)	Range (lb)	Average (lb)	Range (lb)
4	10	—	—	102	92–119
4	11	—	—	104	94–122
5	0	—	—	107	96–125
5	1	—	—	110	99–128
5	2	123	112–141	113	102–131
5	3	127	115–144	116	105–134
5	4	130	118–148	120	108–138
5	5	133	121–152	123	111–142
5	6	136	124–156	128	114–146
5	7	140	128–161	132	118–150
5	8	145	132–166	136	122–154
5	9	149	136–170	140	126–158
5	10	153	140–174	144	130–163
5	11	158	144–179	148	134–168
6	0	162	148–184	152	138–173
6	1	166	152–189	—	—
6	2	171	156–194	—	—
6	3	176	160–199	—	—
6	4	181	164–204	—	—

*Height without shoes, weight without clothes.
SOURCE: Adapted from the Tables of the Metropolitan Life Insurance Co.
(Courtesy of the Metropolitan Life Insurance Co.)

height is a composite measure of fat, protein-containing tissue, and water. It is particularly unfortunate that this simple parameter is so often neglected or disregarded in hospital patients. Weight/height can be used to help diagnose PCM and obesity. Generally, greater than 120 percent of ideal body weight (IBW) signifies obesity; less than 85 percent IBW signifies PCM. The usefulness of weight/height values is impaired by many pathologic conditions leading to water retention such as cardiac, renal, and hepatic disease which leads to weight increase not reflecting active metabolic tissue.

Each of the three energy-containing tissues described earlier (Fig. 14.1) can also be easily assessed individually and reflects the state of body energy and protein stores. Approximately 50 percent of the body fat is located subcutaneously. Physical anthropometry using skin fold calipers defines this compartment with acceptable accuracy. Standards and the percentiles signifying PCM for the U.S. population are given in Table 14.3.

An estimate of skeletal muscle reserves can also be derived from anthropometry [arm muscle circumference = arm circumference – (π × triceps skin fold)]. Again, standards and the percentile signifying PCM are in Table 14.3. The arm muscle circumference is a sensitive measure of protein nutrition and is correlated with other estimates of protein status such as serum albumin and transferrin.

The simplest parameters for PCM assessment are percentage of ideal body weight, anthropometry, serum albumin, and delayed hypersensitivity skin testing.

Serum albumin has been used as the primary index of significant PCM and, although less sensitive to nutritional repletion, it remains the benchmark for other measures of PCM. A serum albumin less than 3 g/dl represents significant PCM, as other changes characteristic of PCM occur at about this level. A serum transferrin less than 170 mg/dl also represents significant PCM but is more sensitive to early nutritional repletion.

Delayed hypersensitivity skin tests with three recall antigens (SK/SD, Candida, mumps) complete the static nutritional profile. Failure to manifest a reaction of greater than 5 mm at one or more sites is considered anergy and is believed to represent the most functionally important parameter of nutritional and clinical status.

Three of these parameters can be used to chart the course of nutritional therapy

Table 14.3 Standards* for Arm Muscle Circumference and Triceps Skin Fold†

Upper arm muscle circumference	*Standard (mm)*	*Lower 5th percentile (mm)*	*Percentage of standard represented by 5th percentile*
Male	270	220	81
Female	213	177	83
Triceps Skin fold			
Male	11	4	36
Female	19	9	47

*Standard is 50th percentile of 30-year-olds.
SOURCE: A. Frisancho, *Am. J. Clin. Nutr.* 27:1052, (1974).

because they respond rapidly; these include weight change, change in serum transferrin, and skin test responsiveness. A day-to-day measure of the effectiveness of nutritional therapy can be obtained by nitrogen balance measurements that reflect whether the body is adding or losing protein (nitrogen). A reliable estimate of nitrogen balance can be derived from the equation

$$\text{Nbal} = \frac{\text{protein intake}}{6.25}$$
$$- \text{(24-hour urine urea nitrogen} + 4).$$

Urine urea nitrogen can be easily measured in all hospital laboratories

Dynamic measures. Catabolic stress is a major variable in the development of PCM and also reflects the severity of illness. A simple procedure for estimating rates of lean tissue breakdown has been developed based on 24-hour urine urea nitrogen excretion:
Catabolic Index = 24-hour urine nitrogen − (0.5 dietary nitrogen intake + 3 g), where CI < 0 = no significant stress, 0−5 = moderate stress, and > 5 = severe stress. The integration of nutritional status and degree of stress is illustrated in Fig. 14.2. The recommended nutritional support under varying conditions of stress or nutritional status can be developed on a scientific basis using these variables.

Goal of nutritional support. Although more than 30 nutrients are necessary in human nutrition, only energy and protein needs are difficult to provide clinically because of the large volume required. Mineral and vitamin requirements can be easily met by daily oral supplements or as additions to intravenous feeding solutions. Commercial feeding formulas intended for enteral use contain on the average one calorie per centimeter, requiring an intake in excess of two liters for most patients. Parenterally, peripheral veins

only tolerate isotonic or mildly hypertonic solutions, which are hypocaloric. Each liter of five percent dextrose contains 170 calories, whereas near-isotonic amino acid solutions (3.0 to 3.5%) contain approximately 130 calories per liter. Isotonic fat emulsions (Intralipid® 10%) contain one calorie per centimeter, but are quite expensive, require refrigeration prior to administration, and are recommended only in limited amounts (1500 cc maximum daily). Hypertonic glucose and amino acids along with other essential nutrients can also be provided through a high-flow central vein; the method is called intravenous hyperalimentation. Each of these techniques has its own indications, risks, and risk/benefit ratios. Although minor differences may exist in the efficiency of nutrient use, the benefits of effective nutritional support generally derive from provision of an adequate diet, and not from any particular feeding route or technique.

Restoration of protein stores, particu-

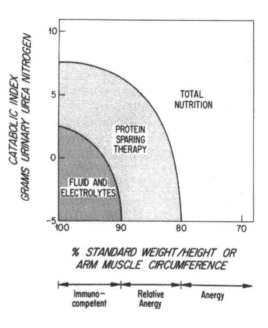

Fig. 14.2 *Nutritional status and degree of stress.*

larly in the viscera and occasionally in the respiratory musculature, is the major goal of nutritional therapy. Protein and energy needs are interrelated in that fulfillment of one reduces the other. Although both are essential, increased protein intake is more efficient at improving anabolism than is an equivalent amount of energy. The first priority in effecting protein anabolism, however, is meeting protein needs. The proportion of dietary protein that is used to replete lean tissue depends on the nitrogen intake, the nonprotein calorie intake, the metabolic rate, and the severity of catabolic stress. One can choose either the fed or semistarved state and either the enteral or the parenteral route (Table 14.4). Each of these combinations of nutrient intake and routes of administration can be viewed as a separate feeding module. Nutritional therapies are then designed using the most appropriate individual module or combination of modules. Use of the "modular concept" allows more flexibility in the planning of optimal nutritional support.

Similar amounts of protein and energy are recommended, 1.5 g protein per kilogram and 40 to 45 kilocalories per kilogram, respectively, to replete malnourished individuals and also to minimize the catabolic effects of severe stress. Except in the case of extensive body burns, energy and protein in excess of these amounts are inefficiently used and may occasionally be harmful.

An important area of nutritional support is the proper manipulation of the semi-starved state for maximal preservation of the visceral protein compartment. Whenever energy requirements are below 50 percent of estimated needs, provision of protein up to a level of one and one-half to two times the recommended daily allowance (i.e., 1.2 to 1.6 g/kg) either intravenously or enterally will maximize the sparing of body protein. Although nitrogen equilibrium may not be possible for patients with small fat reserves, nitrogen sparing is significantly better than can be anticipated with isocaloric amounts of other nutrients. Whenever nitrogen intake must be limited because of hepatic or renal disease, the addition of hypocaloric glucose (five percent) to lesser amounts of protein (<1 g/kg) is desirable. For example, a solution of two percent amino acids in five percent glucose will improve nitrogen sparing over isonitrogenous (two percent) amino acids only. Similar responses can be expected from oral feeding of whole protein with or without dietary carbohydrate.

3.0 Techniques for nutritional support

Oral feeding. By the time weight loss

Table 14.4 Modular Feeding

Type of feeding	Adequate diet	Semistarvation regimen
Enteral	House diet House diet and supplement Defined formula diet Meal replacement	Clear liquids Fruit juice and gelatin High protein

Parenteral	Intravenous
	  hyperalimentation
	Peripheral system with
	  Intralipid®
		5% dextrose and
		  water
		Crystalloid solutions
		Isotonic crystalline
		Amino acids

has occurred in patients with cancer, there is little or no likelihood that regular food can be made attractive enough to prevent further weight loss, particularly in the hospital. Patients' likes and dislikes should be considered, but a therapeutic maneuver will invariably be necessary to meet needs for proteins and calories. The first alternative for those with intact intestinal function is the use of liquid formula diets (Table 14.5 and 14.6). These can be defined-formula diets (DFD) such as Precision LR®, which is the one DFD that can be tolerated in reasonable amounts without a feeding tube due to its use of whole protein. The more usual alternative is a meal replacement that contains whole protein, and 25 to 30 percent fat along with carbohydrate. Ensure® and Nutri 1000® are two of this genre that are exceedingly well tolerated as either supplements to food or as the only items in the diet. For the occasional cancer patient for whom bland taste is desirable, Isocal®, a similar item containing medium chain triglycerides, is often well tolerated orally, although it is usually tube fed. Proposed reasons for the effectiveness of liquid formulas are their acceptable taste, their consistency that makes chewing unnecessary, and the patient's ability to quantify intake and to spread the task of eating over a prolonged period. Essentially this therapy involves no side effects other than the occasional production of osmotic diarrhea from the hyperosmolar formulas (i.e., DFD), or steatorrhea and diarrhea from the fat content of meal-replacement formulas for those patients with pancreatic or biliary dysfunction. Most of the formulas are low in sodium content but high in potassium. If the gastrointestinal tract is functional, enteral nutrition is adequate to maintain protein stores.

Patient A, a 53-year-old woman with pancreatic carcinoma, was referred for evaluation of a 20-lb weight loss during out-patient radiation therapy. She was provided with five 8-oz cans of Ensure® per day to supplement her spontaneous oral intake. Using several different flavors, she was able to consume enough meal replacement to arrest weight loss during her x-ray treatment although she was unable to regain to her previous weight level.

Tube feeding. For many patients receiving radiotherapy or chemotherapy, voluntary oral feeding with the above items is unsuccessful in meeting nutritional needs because of taste distortion with food rejection, difficulties with swallowing, or poor tolerance of large volumes by the stomach. For these individuals, the second major development in enteral nutrition has been the introduction of small (seven to nine French), well tolerated, silastic feeding tubes, which in some designs (Hedeco®) have a weighted mercury tip. This permits passage without the need for an accompanying larger tube. In cases of difficult passage, such as a constricted esophagus, these tubes can be made somewhat stiff by chilling or by placing a small, flexible guide wire inside the tube before passage. After placement and confirmation of the location of the tube by conventional means, it is usually best to feed continuously either with gravity drip from a reservoir or with infusion pump. Flow rates are usually begun at 40 cc per hour with slow increase over several days to full flow rates. Meal replacement formulas can usually be fed undiluted from initiation, but DFD should be begun at one-half dilution because of their higher osmolarity. Diluted feeding formulas can first be brought to anticipated full flow rates to meet fluid needs as soon as possible. The concentration can then be increased to full strength. Concern about aspiration can be essentially eliminated if the head of the bed is always elevated to 30° and the feeding is continuously infused.

Table 14.5 Composition and Indications for Use of Defined Formula Diets

Defined formula diets	Cal/cc	mOsm/L	Percentage of Cal pro	Percentage of Cal CHO	Percentage of Cal fat	Percentage of Cal linoleic acid	N:Cal
For maintenance							

Flexical
  orange
  vanilla
  banana
  fruit punch
	1.0	805	8.8	61.1	30.1	2.16	1:264

Precision L-R
  cherry
  lemon
  lime
  orange
	1.08	600	8.8	90.8	.65	.48	1:258

Vivonex
  vanilla
  beef broth
  orange
  tomato
  chocolate
	1.0	550	8.1	90.3	1.3	1.04	1:286

For anabolism							

Precision—HN
  citrus fruit
  vanilla
	1.0	580	16.6	82.9	.42	.33	1:125

Vivonex—HN
  beef broth
  orange
  grape
  strawberry
	1.0	800	16.6	84.1	.78	.62	1:127

Special DFD Aminade	2.02	1050	4	68	28	11	1:418

Protein source	Carbohydrate source	Fat source	mEq Na/L	Function (all DFD are low-residue, clear-liquid diets)
Hydrolyzed protein + Methionine tyrosine tryptophan	Sucrose Dextrooligo-saccharides	MCT Partially hydrogen-ated soy oil	15.2	30% Cal from fat 60% Cal from CHO Protein source require some digestion Usually must be tube fed
Egg albumin	Maltose Dextrins	Safflower oil	27.4	Protein source requires some digestion Can be consumed daily
Crystalline amino acids	Maltone Dextrins	Safflower oil	37.3	High osmolality when flavored Easily absorbed protein source of high bio-logical value Usually must be tube fed
Egg Albumin	Maltose Dextrins	Safflower oil	40.5	Protein source requires some digestion
Crystalline amino acids	Glucose Maltose	Safflower oil	27.4	Easily absorbed protein source
Essential amino acids	Sucrose Dextrins	Soybean oil	2	Provides high-calorie, low-protein diet of high biologic value (only essential amino acids) for use as Giordano-Giovan-etti diet in renal failure Contains no vitamins

Table 14.6 Composition and Indications for Use of Nutritional Supplements

	Cal/cc	mOsm/L	Percentage of Cal pro	Percentage of Cal CHO	Percentage of Cal fat	N:Cal	Protein source
Supplements							
Citrotein	.53		24.1	73.2	2.3	1:93	Egg white solids
Lanolac	.66		21	30	49	1:81	Casein
Lolactene vanilla	.8	670 mOsm/kg	26	52.8	21	1:70	Low lactose non-fat milk
Meritene (liquid) vanilla, chocolate	1.0	640	24	40	30	1:79	Skim milk Casein
Sustacal (liquid) vanilla, chocolate	1.0	638 616	24	41.3	20.7	1:79	Skim Milk
Meritene powder + skim milk	1.0		35.9	62.4	1.7	1:43	Skim milk
Meritene powder + whole milk	1.0		26.4	44.8	28.8	1:48	Milk
Sustagen powder (normal dilution) vanilla, chocolate	1.8	721	24	68	8	1:79	Nonfat dry milk Powdered whole milk
Meal Replacements							
Compleat—B	1.0	468	16	48	36	1:131	Skim milk Beef
Ensure black walnut vanilla	1.06	460	14	54.5	31.5	1:155	Casein Soy protein isolate
Isocal	1.05	350	12.9	49.6	38.5	1:169	Soy protein isolate Casein
Nutri—1000	1.06	400	13	40	47	1:167	Skim milk
Osmolite	1.06	300	14	54.6	31.4	1:156	Casein Soy protein

Carbohydrate source	Fat source	mEq Na/L	Function

Sucrose
Dextrin maltose
	Mono and
	  diglycerides
		23	Contains 50% RDA of
			  protein, vitamins,
			  and minerals

Lactose	Coconut oil	1.1	Protein supplement
			  for low-sodium
			  diets

Corn syrup
Sucrose
	Vegetable oil	36.2	Protein supplement
			  minimal lactose
			  content

Sucrose Lactose Corn syrup solids	Vegetable oil	40.5	Protein supplement

Sucrose
Lactose
Corn syrup solids
	Partially
	  hydrogenated
	  soy oil
		47.1	Protein supplement
			  low lactose
			  content

Lactose Corn syrup solids	Cow milk fat	39.1	Protein supplement utilizing skim milk
Lactose Corn syrup solids	Cow milk fat	39.1	Protein supplement utilizing whole milk
Glucose Lactose Corn syrup solids	Cow milk fat	54.3	Protein supplement

Lactose
Sucrose
	Corn oil
	Beef fat
		59	Tube feeding—
			  unflavored, blenderized
			  house diet for
			  anabolism

Sucrose
Corn syrup solids
	Corn oil	32	Tube or oral feeding
			  lactose-free for
			  anabolism

Glucose
Corn syrup solids
	MCT
	Soy oil
		22.6	Tube feeding—
			  unflavored, isotonic,
			  for anabolism

Glucose Sucrose Lactose Dextrin maltose	Corn oil	23	Tube or oral feeding for anabolism

Glucose
  oligosaccharides
	Corn oil
	Soy oil
	MCT
		23	Tube feeding—isotonic
			  for anabolism
			  Lower potassium
			  of 23 mEq/L

Table 14.6 Continued

	Cal/cc	mOsm/L	Percentage of Cal pro	Percentage of Cal CHO	Percentage of Cal fat	N:Cal	Protein source
Supplements							
Portagen	1.0	354	16	44	40	1:160	Casein
Precision Isotonic vanilla	1.0	300 mOsm/kg	12	60	28	1:183	Egg albumin
Precision Moderate Nitrogen vanilla citrus	1.0	395 mOsm/kg	12	60	28	1:169	Egg albumin

Tube feeding overcomes anorexia and allows for adequate provision of protein and calories.

It is usually best to become familiar with a limited number of products, including one DFD that can be orally or tube fed, such as Precision LR®. Additional calories can be added to these formulas as low osmolar glucose oligosaccharides (Polycose® at 4 cal/g), fat (Lipomul® at 9 kcal/g), medium chain triglycerides (8.3 kcal/g), or protein (Henningsen'® egg albumin).

Patient B, a 47-year-old woman with metastatic breast cancer, developed profound anorexia while receiving radiation therapy during her hospital stay. As her gastrointestinal tract was functional, a nine French silastic nasogastric feeding tube was placed, and 2000 cc per day of Ensure® was given by continuous enteral infusion. The feeding schedule included several hours each day when the feeding tube was plugged to allow free ambulation and trips to the radiation therapy department.

Although limited, the complications of tube feeding can be serious. The most common problem is osmotic diarrhea. If diarrhea persists, antidiarrheal agents, such as Lomotil® syrup, can be used; these work best if mixed with the feeding formula. Most commercial feeding formulas are lactose free, so no problem should occur with primary or acquired lactase deficiency. If a disorder of fat digestion is present, a DFD (one percent fat) can be used.

The DFD are high in carbohydrate, relatively high in potassium, and low in sodium. Care must therefore be taken in monitoring blood glucose concentrations to prevent hyperosmolar syndromes. Serum potassium will often rise to unacceptable levels if a moderate degree of renal impairment exists. In this case either a modular approach (Polycose® and protein and micronutrients without potassium) or an electrolyte-free defined-formula diet designed for renal failure (Aminaid®) with added vitamins and electrolytes can be used.

Feeding through surgical access. Although nasogastric or nasoduodenal feeding is the most practical method of gas-

Carbohydrate source	Fat source	mEq Na/L	Function
Sucrose Corn syrup solids	MCT Safflower oil	27	Oral feeding for malabsorption of long chain fats for anabolism
Glucose oligosaccharides Sucrose	Vegetable oil	34	Tube or oral feeding Isotonic, lactose-free
Maltodextrin Sucrose	Vegetable oil	43.3	Moderate fat content, low osmolality

trointestinal feeding if oral intake is not sufficient, surgical insertion of a gastrostomy or jejunostomy tube may occasionally be necessary for chronic conditions in some patients. Surgical access can be particularly useful in feeding either above a low intestinal fistula such as low ileal or colic or below a high fistula such as gastric, duodenal, or high jejunal. The preferred method for long-term feeding is the gastrostomy because it lends itself to bolus feeding. The major disadvantage is the propensity to aspiration. Jejunostomies limit aspiration problems, but jejunostomy tubes can fall out if a loop of bowel is not tacked to the abdominal wall; the loop can become a nidus for later intestinal adhesions. In addition, jejunostomies require continuous feeding at least part of each day, and may occasionally need pancreatic enzyme supplements.

Patient C, a 38-year-old man, underwent total gastrectomy with esophagojejunostomy for adenocarcinoma of the cardia of the stomach. At operation, a 16-gauge Intracath® was placed as a jejunostomy. The patient developed an anastomotic leak postoperatively, which required drainage and a prolonged period without
oral feeding. Following the drainage procedure, Precision HN® was infused into the jejunostomy until the patient was again able to eat by mouth.

Peripheral parenteral nutrition (PN). Two techniques provide nutrients parenterally; these are standard intravenous hyperalimentation and peripheral vein alimentation with a combination of slightly hypertonic solutions (i.e., 3 percent amino acids in 5 percent dextrose) with 10 percent Intralipid®. While peripheral vein alimentation avoids the use of a subclavian line required for total parenteral nutrition (TPN), it is a temporalizing measure as it maintains nutritional status only for individuals who are not severely catabolic and can only slowly replete malnourished individuals because of volume limitations on total calories and deliverable protein. Table 14.7 shows a sample feeding formula for peripheral vein infusion. Few unique complications exist with this therapy, as the levels of glucose and most electrolytes are similar to those routinely provided. Because this is an anabolic therapy, vitamins and minerals, particularly phosphate and magnesium, must be provided. Intralipid® and Liposyn®, the

Table 14.7 Sample Peripheral Vein Feeding Systems

	Volume (cc)	Source	Protein	Kilocalories	Approximate Osmolarity
I.					
	1500	Intralipid™	0	1500	isotonic
	2000	3% amino acids, 5% dextrose with added electrolytes, minerals, and vitamins	60	580	2–3 × isotonic
Total	3500		60	2080	1½–2 × isotonic
II.					
	1000	Intralipid™	0	1000	isotonic
	2500	3% amino acids, 5% dextrose with added electrolytes, minerals, and vitamins	75	725	2–3 × isotonic
Total	3500		75	1725	1.7–2.4 × isotonic

commercially available fat emulsions, are well tolerated in most patients. Generally, as much as 1500 cc per day can be given. The manufacturer lists relative contraindications that include severe lung and liver disease and hyperlipidemia. The hyperosmolar and irritative property of the amino acid-dextrose component of a peripheral feeding system can often cause phlebitis. This is minimized by infusing the fat emulsion and amino acid-glucose simultaneously through a Y-connector.

Patient D, a 60-year-old man, received combined radiation therapy and chemotherapy for linitis plastica after which he developed persistent gastric bleeding that was exacerbated by eating. A coagulogram showed severe thrombocytopenia, presumably drug induced, which precluded safe insertion of a subclavian "lifeline." Therefore, the patient received isotonic amino acids in five percent dextrose with 500 to 1000 cc per day of Intralipid® through a peripheral line until his clotting picture improved and standard hyperalimentation could begin.

4.0 Total parenteral nutrition (TPN)

Intravenous hyperalimentation has become a safe and effective means of nutritional support of the cancer patient. Hyperalimentation solutions are hyperosmolar (1800 to 2400 mOsm/L) in customary concentrations of 4.25% Freamine® or 5% Aminosyn® in 25% dextrose (Table 14.6). Like Intralipid® and most commercial feeding formulas, hyperalimentation solutions contain one calorie per centimeter. The usual additives are shown in Table 14.8. Each of these nutrients is essential in repleting mal-nourished patients. For example, any re-pletion formula, although adequate in all other respects, will not cause an in-crease in protoplasm if sodium, potassium, or phosphate is absent.

Particular attention should be paid to several of the nutrients. Potassium, mag-nesium, and phosphate will fall dramati-cally and produce serious deficiency syn-dromes in only days if adequate amounts are not provided. Water-soluble vitamins should be provided daily because of the high carbohydrate content of the fluid. Vitamins K, B_{12}, and folic acid must be provided individually, usually weekly. Iron can be added daily. A trace mineral solution containing manganese, chro-mium, iodine, zinc, and copper is rou-tinely provided.

The details of subclavian catheterization are beyond the scope of this chapter. Cath-eter-related complications occur uncom-monly, and only two problems occur with any regularity, even in skilled hands, and these should be mentioned to the pa-tient. The first, pneumothorax, should not occur in more than 1 per 100 catheter-izations. The second is thrombosis of the subclavian vein. Although rarely evi-dent clinically, contrast venograms in asymptomatic individuals show that it is rather common. In patients with cancer-associated hypercoagulability, this poten-tial complication may be accentuated. Heparin appears to minimize this compli-cation, and should be provided (6000 units heparin per day) in the hyperali-mentation solution if not otherwise contraindicated.

Hypertonic intravenous solutions are generally begun at slower rates (40 cc per hour) to allow the pancreas to adapt to the glucose load; full feeding rates are generally achieved in the first two to three days. Insulin can be administered in stat doses when necessary to regulate blood glucose. Insulin need is based on results of capillary blood glucose levels initially

determined every six to eight hours (Table 14.9). After insulin requirements are de-termined it usually is best to add the insu-lin directly to the solutions. Serum elec-trolytes are monitored on Monday, Wednesday, and Friday; a complete blood count, liver function tests, serum albu-min, calcium, phosphorus, creatinine, and magnesium are measured weekly. As the body's responses to nutrient administra-tion stabilizes, frequent blood sugar deter-minations can be discontinued and the electrolyte, urea, and glucose determina-tions reduced to once or twice a week. It is important that hyperalimentation proceed according to a protocol (Table 14.9) and the patient be assessed by a protocol (Table 14.10). Other medication should never be given, and central venous pressure measurements should not be taken through the "lifeline."

Complications of hyperalimentation not due to catheter insertion come under two major headings, catheter sepsis and metabolic complications. Catheter sepsis should occur in less than two to three percent of patients when catheters are placed aseptically and a hyperalimenta-tion nurse cares for the catheter. Septic shock is rare with catheter sepsis, but for the hyperalimented patient whose fever is not explained by a routine fever work-up, the catheter should be changed

---

The TPN subclavian total parenteral nu-trition line should never be used for med-ications and should be monitored by a team.

---

over a guidewire. Cultures are taken from the skin at the insertion site, blood drawn through the catheter, and the catheter tip cultured. In the absence of bacterial growth, the new catheter need not be removed. Metabolic complications are listed in Table 14.11. The importance of prevention by frequent monitoring of

Table 14.8 Concentration*, Amino Acids, and Various Salts of Commercially Available Products

Components	Aminosyn M 3.5% (Abbott)	Aminosyn 5% (Abbott)	Aminosyn 7% (Abbott)
Essential Amino Acids (mg)			
L-isoleucine	252	360	510
L-leucine	329	470	660
L-lysine	252 (as Ac)	360 (as Ac)	510 (as Ac)
L-methionine	140	200	280
L-phenylalanine	154	220	310
L-threonine	182	260	370
L-tryptophan	56	80	120
L-valine	280	400	560
dL-methionine			
dL-tryptophan			
Nonessential Amino Acids (mg)			
L-alanine	448	640	900
L-arginine	343	490	690
L-histindine	105	150	210
L-proline	300	430	610
L-serine	147	210	300
Aminoacetic acid (glycine)	448	640	900
L-cysteine HCl			
L-tyrosine	31	44	44
L-glutamic acid			
L-aspartic acid			
Electrolytes (mEq)			
Sodium	4.0		
Chloride	4.0		
Potassium	1.84	0.54	0.54
Magnesium	0.3		
Acetate	2.7		
Phosphate			
Calcium			

*Per 100 ml
†Reduced by process

serum electrolytes and renal function must be emphasized.

A major theoretical complication of hyperalimentation is the potential for preferentially "feeding" the tumor and promoting tumor growth. As indicated earlier, the qualitative metabolic activities of tumor cells are similar to those of normal cells, and no evidence exists that general distribution of nutrients favors the tumor. No data currently indicate that hyperalimentation promotes preferential tumor growth.

The transition from parenteral to en-

Table 14.8 Continued

Aminosyn 10% (Abbott)	FreAmine II 8.5% (McGaw)	Travasol 5.5% with electrolytes (Travenol)	Travasol 8.5% with electrolytes (Travenol)	Travasol 8.5% (Travenol)	Veinamine 8% (Cutter)
720	590	263	406	406	490
940	770	340	526	526	350
720 (as Ac)	870 (as Ac)	318 (as HC1)	492 (as HC1)	492 (as HC1)	670
400		318	492	492	430
440	480	340	526	526	400
520	340	230	356	356	160
160	130	99	152	152	80
800	560	252	390	390	250
	450				
1280	600	1140	1760	1760	†
980	310	570	880	880	750
300	240	241	372	372	240
860	950	230	356	356	110
420	500				
1280	1700	1140	1760	1760	3390
	20				†
44		22	34	34	†
					430
					400
	1.0	7.0	7.0	0.3	4.0
		7.0	7.0	3.4	5.0
0.54		6.0	6.0		3.0
		1.0	1.0		6.0
		10.0	13.0	5.2	5.0
	2.0	6.0	6.0		†

teral feeding and then to oral food ingestion is an important interim period. Patients are encouraged to eat. Dietary instruction is provided and taste preferences are considered in meal planning. Intravenous feedings alone do not suppress the appetite, and in fact may stimulate it, for repletion of protein stores promotes activity, interest, and a sense of well being. As a patient is gradually able to consume enough protein and calories to meet nutritional requirements, the hyperalimentation is reduced and eventually discontinued.

Table 14.9 Hyperalimentation Orders

Please specify:
  I. Total volume of solution per 24 hours: ___ ml.
      (Please order solutions in multiples of 1000 ml.)
  II. Rate of infusion: ___ ml per hour
  III. Concentration: Crystalline amino acids: ___%; dextrose: ___%.
  IV. 10% Fat emulsion: ___ ml. Piggyback on ___ over ___ hours.
  V. Additives required; please specify amounts/24 h:
      ___ mEQ Sodium chloride (60–150 mEq per day)
      ___ mEq Potassium chloride (60–100mEq per day)
      ___ mEq Calcium gluceptate (9.0 mEq per day)
      ___ mEq Magnesium sulfate (8.1 mEq per day)
      ___ mEq Sodium phosphate (as required)
      ___ mEq Potassium phosphate (30–45 mEq per day)
      ___ mEq Sodium acetate (40 mEq per day)
      ___ mEq Potassium acetate (as required)
      ___ Trace minerals: Cu, Zn, Mn, Cr, and I (2 ml per day)
      ___ ampule vitamins B and C (Tuesday through Saturday)
      ___ vial multivitamins (MVI, Monday)
      ___ mg Folic acid (0.5–1.5 mg per week, Monday)
      ___ mcg Vitamin B_{12} (50–100 mcg per week, Monday)
      ___ mg Iron (1.0–2.0 mg per day)
      ___ units Heparin (6000–8000 units per day)
      ___ units/L regular insulin
  VI. ___ mg Vitamin K (AquaMephyton) IM (10 mg per week, Monday)
  VII. ___ ml Safflower oil (5 ml per day, if not NPO)

5.0 Special applications of nutritional support

Acute renal failure develops commonly in the hospital patient, and mortality averages 50 percent. Mortality rates, however, may be reduced if nutritional support is part of treatment. Nutritional therapy in the presence of renal impairment generally requires fluid, protein, sodium, potassium, magnesium, calcium, and phosphorus restriction. This can be accomplished with intravenous hyperalimentation by using one liter of a 50 percent dextrose, 2 percent amino acid solution containing vitamins, but with electrolytes and minerals only as required. The enteral alternative, represented by one liter of Aminaid®, can be further concentrated to 300 cc and consumed by mouth as a slush.

Patients with cardiac, renal, and liver disease tolerate fluid and sodium loads poorly. Intravenous hyperalimentation solutions can be concentrated using 70 percent dextrose to a final concentration of 35 percent dextrose, 4.25 to 5 percent amino acid, and little added sodium to allow reduction in both total volume and sodium.

The administration of continuous hypertonic dextrose leads to glycogen and fat deposition in the liver, which may cause hepatic dysfunction. For nonstressed individuals who do not require exogenous insulin and who can tolerate changes in fluid rate, administration of intravenous hyperalimentation for 12 to 16 hours per day and plugging of the catheter for 8

Table 14.10 Nutritional Assessment

I. Laboratory Tests:
    ____ Complete blood count
    ____ Chem 6, ____ Chem 18
    ____ Serum transferrin
    ____ Skin tests every 2–3 weeks (Candida, Mumps, and SKSD—call Nurse)
    ____ 24-hour urine for urea N, creatinine, sodium, potassium. Monday and
    Thursday of each week.

II. Routine Patient Care:
    ____ Accurate intake/output
    ____ Weight (daily/every other day)
    ____ Adjustable footboard and trapeze
    ____ Urine test for sugar and acetone daily
    ____ Capillary blood sugar every 8 hours (7A.M., 3P.M., 11P.M.) for ____ days
    ____ Regular Insulin Sliding Scale; administer subcutaneously:
    Blood sugar: 200–250 = 5 units
                    250–300 = 10 units
                     300–350 = 15 units
                     350–400 = 20 units
                     Above 400 = call House Officer

to 12 hours allows mobilization of liver fat and essential fatty acids from adipose tissue and improves liver function.

6.0 Nutritional support in the cancer patient

No strong evidence indicates that nutritional support of the malnourished cancer patient will substantially prolong life in the absence of cancer therapy. Although in some instances quality of life may improve, only the mode and timing of death will be changed in others. For these reasons current philosophy is to encourage voluntary oral feeding for patients with

under special or extenuating circumstances is the invasive technique of intravenous hyperalimentation used.

The most crucial role for nutritional support—whether enteral or parenteral—is as an adjunct to tumor-specific cancer therapy to promote and maintain the patient. The catabolic and anorectic impact of radiation and chemotherapy on the patient may result in substantial malnutrition in spite of a successful antitumor effect. The result of the nutritional loss can be a decreasing tolerance to the therapy. Nutritional support can be crucial to the total therapeutic effort by promoting positive nitrogen balance, and by optimizing tolerance to tumor therapy.

Hyperalimentation is generally not indicated in the cancer patient without tumor-specific treatment.

The major role of hyperalimentation is to promote tolerance to tumor-specific treatment.

---

malignant disease for whom primary tumor treatment is not planned; only

Patient E, a 67-year-old man, presented with a bulky, fixed, rectosigmoid carci-

Table 14.11 Metabolic Complications of Intravenous Hyperalimentation

Complication	Etiology	Treatment
Hyperglycemia, which can progress to hyperosmolar nonketotic coma	Excessive rate of glucose administration; inadequate endogenous insulin; increased insulin needs 2° to glucocorticoids or infection	Stat subcutaneous insulin based on capillary blood sugars every six hours; add insulin to hyperalimentation solution after needs are established
Metabolic acidosis	Excessive chloride content of amino acid solutions or added sodium chloride; excessive base or bicarbonate loss unrelated to solution (i.e., pancreatic fistula)	Decrease sodium chloride in solution, use sodium and potassium as acetate
Hypophosphatemia	Inadequate administration	Add phosphate as potassium or sodium salt
Hyperphosphatemia	Excess phosphorus administration or inability to excrete phosphorus, as in renal failure	Reduce or eliminate phosphorus in solutions
Hyperkalemia	Excess administration or inability to excrete, as in renal failure	Reduce or eliminate potassium
Hypokalemia	Inadequate administration and/or increased losses due to excretion (stool or urine) or anabolism	Add potassium
Hypercalcemia	Excessive calcium or vitamin D administration	Reduce vitamin D and/or calcium

Table 14.11 Continued

Complication	Etiology	Treatment
Hypocalcemia	Inadequate calcium administration or excessive phosphorus administration, particularly in osteomalacia	Increase calcium administration
Hypermagnesemia	Excess magnesium administration, especially with renal impairment	Reduce or eliminate magnesium
Hypomagnesemia	Inadequate provision of magnesium, particularly in anabolic situations	Appropriate supplementation
Essential fatty acid deficiency	Continuous feeding of hypertonic dextrose or true deficiency from prolonged severe malnutrition (rare)	Intralipid or cyclic hyperalimentation for the first, Intralipid™ for the second.
Azotemia	Excessive amino acid administration or reduced renal function	Reduce amino acid load
Elevation in liver enzymes	Continuous infusion of glucose (? essential fatty acid deficiency)	Cyclic hyperalimentation; Intralipid™ daily
Anemia	Excessive diagnostic blood test; inadequate iron, copper, B_{12}, folate, protein replacement	Limit phlebotomies; appropriate supplements
Rare deficiencies (copper, zinc, chromium)	Inadequate administration	Appropriate replacement

noma for which he was begun on radiation therapy. Shortly after beginning treatment he developed anorexia, nausea, and occasional vomiting and was started on intravenous hyperalimentation. He completed his full course of radiation therapy without any further weight loss and maintained positive skin tests. He subsequently underwent successful resection of the primary lesion.

7.0 Summary

Nutritional support can now be safely delivered to all cancer patients. The first step in the treatment of malnutrition is an adequate nutritional assessment for which a simple, sensitive set of objective measurements has been developed. Improved therapeutic response to various modalities of primary cancer treatment can be anticipated, and the potential for increased long-term survival is present in well-nourished individuals. Certainly evidence suggests that short-term reduction in malnutrition-induced infection and mortality can be achieved by adequate nutritional support.

Although it is theoretically possible for one person to perform all the roles of catheter placement, clinical monitoring, dressing change, and solution preparation necessary for hyperalimentation, it is obvious that this practice is not optimal. The team approach with physician, nurse, pharmacist, and dietitian has been much

more effective. Optimal patient care then becomes possible: the pharmacist can provide solutions tailored individually to patient needs; the nurse can care for the catheter and also instruct in physical exercise essential to anabolism; the dietitian can maximize use of enteral nutrition to take advantage of intestinal function; and the physician can attend to the clinical and metabolic monitoring of the patient.

The ultimate role of nutritional support for cancer patients awaits the results of numerous studies now being conducted, but more than preliminary evidence suggests that nutritional support is a major advance in clinical science.

References

Bistrian, B. R. Nutritional assessment and therapy of protein-calorie malnutrition in the hospital. *J. Am. Diet. Assoc.* 71:393–397, 1977.

Blackburn, G. L., and Bistrian, B. R. Curative nutrition: protein-calorie management. In *Nutritional support of medical practice*, Schneider, H. A. et al., eds. Hagerstown, Maryland: Harper and Row, 1977.

Blackburn, G. L., and Bothe, A., Jr. Assessment of malnutrition in cancer patients. *Cancer Bull.* 30:88–93, 1978.

Milder, J. W. Conference on nutrition and cancer therapy. *Cancer Res.* 37:2321–2471, 1977.

Chapter 15

Management of Cancer Pain

J. Lokich

1.0 Background

Although pain is generally considered a common accompaniment to cancer, particularly as metastases develop, the actual incidence of cancer-induced pain is relatively uncommon, and resistance to analgesic therapy is rare. Osler reviewed an extensive group of patients with terminal cancer and found that less than 10 percent required analgesia in the preterminal phase of the disease.

The pain syndromes associated with cancer are classified by nerve distribution or on the basis of organ or visceral invasion site (Table 15.1). In general, cancer pain syndromes are acute and require immediate diagnostic evaluation and therapeutic intervention. Chronic pain syndromes are distinctly unusual in cancer patients although they do occur in patients whose tumors invade regionally. For example, chronic debilitating pain may be observed in patients with rectal or pancreatic cancers.

The diagnostic evaluation of pain associated with malignancy primarily involves radiographic evaluation of the painful areas. Diagnostic tests can identify cancer-related pain, as well as, discomfort from other sources. Confirmation of malignancy often requires surgical biopsy.

Definitive identification of tumor is often not possible, particularly for patients with sacral pain secondary to recurrent rectal cancer or with brachial plexus and shoulder pain secondary to invasion by breast or lung cancer.

Regional pain may or may not be confirmed by biopsy, but is most commonly due to tumor extension and secondary fibrosis.

This chapter will review the pain syndromes that are peculiar to the cancer patient and will examine the therapies of choice for the management of cancer-related pain.

Table 15.1 Classification of Cancer-related Pain Syndromes

Syndrome	Common cancer
Nerve compression syndromes	
Peripheral nerve compression	
Brachial plexus	Breast, lung
Sacral plexus	Rectum, cervix
Paraspinal plexus	Pancreas
Trigeminal plexus	Mouth
Nerve root compression	Breast, lung, myeloma
Visceral lesions	
Osseous metastases	Breast, lung, prostate
Intramedullary tumor, fracture	
Abdominal lesions	Gastrointestinal tumors
ascites, hepatomegaly, obstruction	
Thoracic lesions	Pleural or pulmonary tumors
pleuritis, neuritis	
Special pain forms	
Referred pain	Liver, bone
Phantom limb	Sarcoma
Herpes zoster	Hodgkin's disease
Hypertrophic pulmonary osteoarthropathy	Lung

2.0 Nerve compression syndromes

The nerve compression syndromes can be separated into those developing as a consequence of local or regional tumor extension that entrap peripheral nerves, and those secondary to impingement on nerve roots that may be due to hematogenous dissemination of the tumor or contiguous extension from a metastatic site in a local bone. The three most common peripheral nerve compressions are due to involvement of the brachial plexus, the sacral plexus, and the paraspinal plexus. The clinical syndromes associated with nerve invasion are characteristic, but the tumor is often occult.

Patient A, a 56-year-old woman, developed breast cancer that was controlled initially by mastectomy and local radiation therapy. Three years later shoulder

pain indicated local recurrence in the axilla. In addition, progressive weakness of the arm muscles developed and over 12 months an en cuirasse tumor evolved over the anterior chest wall and shoulder with secondary edema of the extremity (Fig. 15.1).

Patient B, a 72-year-old woman, had a Miles resection for a Duke's C rectal carcinoma and remained well for five years. She complained chronically of tenesmus beginning approximately one year following surgery. At five years she had developed progressive inanition and wasting, and the pain had become intolerable. At laparotomy extensive fibrosis of the pelvis was observed, and local biopsy revealed recurrent rectal cancer.

Pain developing in a patient with a prior history of malignancy, particularly when

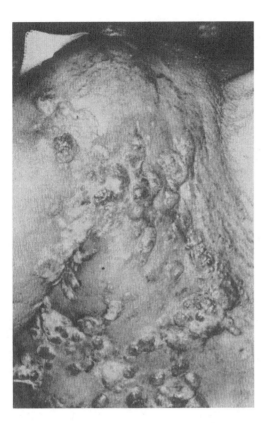

Fig. 15.1 *En cuirasse breast cancer involving the dermis, subcutaneous tissue, and lymphatic channels with secondary edema (Patient A) resulting in narcotic dependent pain.*

localized in the shoulder or pelvis, may be presumed, in most instances, to be a consequence of tumor recurrence.

Pain in patients with a history of prior malignancy should be presumed to be secondary to the tumor.

Another peripheral nerve compression or invasion syndrome is that due to invasion of the trigeminal (V) nerve in the retromolar triangle secondary to intra-oral cancer. Characteristic jaw pain develops that is often associated with hearing loss and trismus of the masseter muscle. This clinical symdrome, often a sign of recurrent tumor, develops some years following the original tumor. Radiation therapy is the principal therapeutic modality.

The root compression syndromes occur as a consequence of impingement on the dorsal nerve roots. These syndromes generally occur in association with osseous lesions and as a consequence of contiguous tumor growth extending outside the bone cortex. Occasionally the tumor simply causes a pathologic fracture, and secondary nerve root compression develops as a consequence of bone compression of nerve. The clinical pain syndrome is often characterized by local pain over the tumor site with radiating pain down the extremity; occasionally a neurologic deficit, either sensory or motor, is observed. Extension of the tumor into the epidural space may result in spinal cord compression characterized by localized pain over the vertebra and secondary neurologic signs (see Chapter 5).

3.0 Organ-related pain syndromes

Tumor-related pain can be categorized on the basis of the site of origin. The five categories of organ-related pain are: osseous, thoracic, abdominal, cephalic, and extremity. In general the pain derived from these sites is a consequence of distention of the organ or interruption of its integrity with secondary hemorrhage and distention of the overlying or enveloping fibrous stroma. For example, osseous pain is due to pathologic fracture with secondary loss of structure; headache due to intracerebral metastases is a consequence of increased intracranial pressure with distention; hepatic pain is derived from distention of the liver and stretching of Glisson's capsule; and pain in the extremities is due to extension and stretching of subcutaneous tissues.

Thoracic wall pain may be a consequence of underlying pleural involvement or may result from direct invasion of intercostal nerves. With a case of superior sulcus tumor, chest wall pain may be referred to the shoulder. The tumor commonly involves the brachial plexus or the intercostal nerves continuous with the primary tumor site. Pain in this area can be chronic and totally resistant to analgesia.

Patient C, a 36-year-old woman, presented with a pleural effusion. Cytologic diagnosis revealed primary adenocarcinoma of the lung. The patient underwent surgical excision of the tumor and was subsequently treated with chemotherapy. Approximately one year following excision, pain in the right anterior chest wall developed. Chest x-ray demonstrated a recurrence of the effusion, and the patient underwent a right pneumonectomy; recurrence of the tumor was found on the pleural surface. Postoperatively the patient continued to complain of pain. This involved the entire chest wall and required narcotic analgesia on an hourly basis. The patient died approximately eight months following the second operation.

Thoracic wall pain can result from direct nerve involvement, secondary bone involvement, or pleural involvement. Local neurosurgical procedures are rarely helpful although central rhizotomy or cordotomy may be useful.

4.0 Special pain syndromes

Four special pain syndromes occur particularly in patients with malignancy. Because these syndromes also occur in patients with benign disease, however, diagnostic evaluation is mandatory. Attributing some forms of pain to nonspecific or benign diseases may delay the diagnosis of a tumor. For patients with previous malignancy, the pain may be attributed to the tumor and benign lesions overlooked.

Referred pain occurs in many diseases. Diaphragmatic irritation from hepatic tumors produces the most common form of referred pain, with discomfort referred to the shoulder through the phrenic nerve.

Patient D, a 59-year-old woman, developed shoulder pain that interfered with her tennis game. A presumed diagnosis of bursitis was made, and the patient received cortisone injections locally for approximately four months. Hepatomegaly was present at her annual physical examination; a liver biopsy revealed adenocarcinoma. A barium enema subsequently demonstrated a lesion of the cecum. The patient's colon cancer had metastasized to the liver and caused the shoulder pain. Intrahepatic infusion therapy resulted in decreased liver size and disappearance of the shoulder pain.

Referred pain is most common in joints (shoulder, hip, knee) and usually is secondary to hepatic or vertebral metastatic lesions, respectively.

Another form of referred pain is due to local bone lesions. The pain may be proximal or distal. Patients with lesions of the vertebrae may present with pain in the knee or hip without a demonstrable lesion at the site. Similarly, patients with lesions in the hip may present with low back pain. Thus, situations exist for which an entire evaluation of the skeletal system is in order even when pain appears to emanate from a local bone source. This is particularly true for patients with a prior history of malignancy. It is most important for patients with primary bone tumors, for whom the early identification of the primary tumor is important to promote cure.

Phantom limb pain is a common syndrome following amputation and is perhaps a form of referred pain. The syndrome often develops in patients with osteogenic sarcoma, particularly if a long period of pain has preceded amputation.

Patient E, a 62-year-old man, developed pain and intermittent weakness of his left shoulder over six months. He initially refused to seek medical attention. Local cortisone injections failed to control the pain and eight months after initiation of the pain syndrome local swelling developed and an x-ray demonstrated a typical osteogenic sarcoma (Fig. 15.2). Amputation was performed, but pain relief was incomplete. The pain syndrome persisted unabated for six months after amputation, and only gradually did the patient improve, although he refused to take narcotic analgesics.

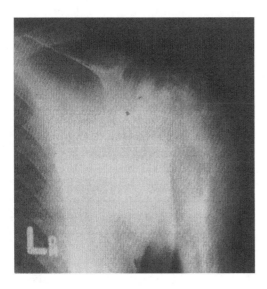

Fig. 15.2 Radiograph of the left humerus demonstrating a typical osteogenic sarcoma of the humeral head with extensive bone destruction and osteoblast formation.

The sensation of the phantom limb persists for a protracted period and may be interpreted either as pain or as a paradoxical awareness of the absent limb. The mechanism of phantom limb sensation is unclear although it is presumed that a reverberating neurocircuit centrally sustains the sensory input. Interruption of the electrical circuit by a constant electrical stimulation peripherally may eliminate the specific syndrome.

Herpes zoster is a characteristic infection for patients with hematologic malignancies, particularly Hodgkin's disease, non-Hodgkin's lymphoma, and chronic lymphocytic leukemia. The zoster infection, or shingles, develops along the dermatome and typically presents as vesicular skin lesions. Occasionally, the pain syndrome develops in the absence of skin lesions; in this situation the diagnosis may be overlooked. Local cutaneous hypesthesia and dysesthesia that can be relieved by ethyl chloride spray or other topical anesthetics may be a useful diagnostic test.

Hypertrophic pulmonary osteoarthropathy (HPO) is a characteristic pain syndrome in patients with primary tumors of the lung, particularly mesotheliomas. In addition, patients with metastatic lung tumors, especially mesenchymal sarcomatous tumors, may develop HPO. Benign diseases such as tuberculosis and hepatitis as well as malabsorption syndromes have been associated with HPO. The mechanism of the periarticular pain is unclear, but in patients for whom the pain is secondary to a pulmonary tumor, surgery or radiation therapy directed at the lung lesions will eliminate the pain syndrome.

5.0 General principles of pain evaluation and control

The primary dictum in the management of cancer-related pain is to define its mechanism. Treatment approaches can then be defined (Table 15.2). When pain is directly related to the tumor, as when pain occurs from invasion of the nerve, tumor-specific therapy may be preceded by localized radiation therapy. When the pain syndrome is diffuse and the tumor disseminated, the additional use of systemic therapy (hormones or cytotoxic drug treatment) is indicated. For patients with tumors that are particularly responsive to systemic therapy, local radiation may be deferred. If clinically feasible, systemic therapy is preferable to radiation, as obliteration of the local osteoblast or fibroblast, common with radiation therapy, is almost always only temporary, or nonexistent with systemic therapy.

Tumor-specific therapy (radiation to regional tumor or systemic chemotherapy for disseminated tumor) is an essential aspect of cancer pain management.

Surgical control of a local tumor with secondary pain is important for achieving maximum palliation and minimal mor-

Table 15.2 General Therapies for Cancer-Related Pain

I.   *Treatment of tumor*
    A. Radiation
    B. Systemic therapy
    C. Surgery (regional resections)
       1. Cryosurgery
       2. Cautery
II. *Diagnostic nerve block*
III. *Drug therapy*
    A. Nonaddictive analgesics
    B. Narcotic analgesics
    C. Psychotropic drugs
IV. *Neurosurgical procedures*
    A. Dorsal rhizotomy
    B. Sympathectomy
    C. Cordotomy
    D. Chemical hypophysectomy

---

bidity. For tumors that result in pain, either because of expanding size and secondary distention of the subcutaneous tissue, because of fixation and invasion of the underlying muscle, or because of local secondary infection, surgical excision may be the treatment of choice regardless of the presence of distant metastases and residual tumor. The two most common situations for which surgery is used are extensive local lesions of the breast and fungating lesions of the extremities. In the former instance, "toilet mastectomy" is performed to eliminate definitively local discomfort and to maximize the secondary application of additional treatment such as radiation therapy and chemotherapy. Fungating extremity lesions are best managed by local surgery involving either cryo- or electrocautery surgery, and by avoiding amputation.

Patient F, an 83-year-old woman, presented with a four-year history of malignant melanoma. Following local excision, the lesion recurred locally with secondary pain and compromised mobility and ambulation (Fig. 15.3). The lesion was associated with multiple satellite nodules, and amputation was initially considered, but because of the patient's age and the presence of obvious dissemination, local electrocautery surgery was performed. Local recurrence did not develop for the duration of the patient's life.

Local surgical excision with tumor debulking may be effectively employed for palliation and may avoid amputation.

Lesions of the extremities with local complications that produce pain, disfigurement, secondary infection, or limited function are candidates for local surgical control. Amputation of such lesions is occasionally necessary, but local cryosurgery or electrocautery surgery may

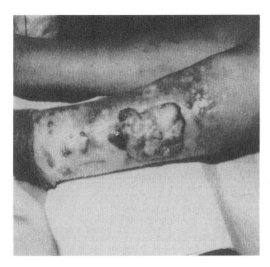

Fig. 15.3 *Extensive exophytic and pedunculated melanoma of the left lower leg with multiple satellite nodules resulting in pain and decreased ambulation (Patient F).*

achieve maximum palliation with minimum morbidity.

A special form of diagnostic evaluation is available for patients with occult pain syndromes, specifically the diagnostic nerve block. The diagnostic nerve block maneuver involves the sequential introduction of an inert substance (placebo) followed by graded doses of Xylocaine® topical anesthesia to the site of local pain. Such graded doses may identify pain emanating as a consequence of sensory irritant to the afferent limb, sympathetic discharge, or motor stimulation of the efferent limb. The diagnostic nerve block also determines the potential effectiveness of a subsequent surgical procedure or application of a neurolytic drug, but it is not uniformly predictive.

6.0 Drug therapy in cancer pain

Analgesia for cancer pain after maximal tumor control involves nonnarcotic antiinflammatory analgesics, a large group of natural and synthetic narcotic drugs, and a variety of psychotropic drugs, all of which individually and collectively may be beneficial in pain management. Specific analgesic drugs may be employed sequentially on the basis of severity of pain and the mechanism by which the pain is induced. Nonnarcotic drugs are generally used at the outset; for the most part, salicylate preparations are comparable or superior to the more complicated and morbidity- associated nonnarcotics such as propoxyphene and indomethacin. The latter may be particularly useful in pain mediated as a consequence of prostaglandin release, but the pathophysiologic mechanism for this pain syndrome is not clear. Salicylate preparations are comparable to low doses of narcotic analgesics; narcotics must be administered in adequate doses to be more effective than salicylate drugs.

The narcotic analgesics can be categorized into natural narcotics derived from the heroin parent compound (including morphine and codeine) and synthetic narcotic drugs (meperidine and pentazocine). Their relative analgesic effect is comparable when equivalent dosage units are employed (Table 15.3). The synthetic narcotics, however, are associated with fewer gastrointestinal symptoms. Major adverse effects of the narcotic analgesics in the cancer patient are disequilibrium and disorientation, common syndromes that often progress to somnolence and withdrawal. In addition, focal neurologic signs may develop, prompting diagnostic evaluation of the central nervous system. An analgesic preparation that has both narcotic and euphoric properties and that does not produce somnolence has been developed. Brompton mixture contains cocaine, alcohol, morphine, with or without, a phenothiazine; the preparation can add substantially to patient comfort and diminish the chronic withdrawal syndrome. The specific advantages over

TABLE 15.3 Relative Potency of Narcotic Analgesics

Drug	Trade Name	Equivalent Dosage Unit
Morphine sulfate	—	10
Heroin	—	3
Hydromorphone	Dilaudid	1–5
Oxycodone	Percodan	15
Meperidine*	Demerol	100
Methadone*	Dolophine	10
Codeine	—	60
Pentazocine*	Talwin	50

*Synthetic narcotic

standard narcotic preparations are controversial. The formula is described in Table 15.4.

Psychotropic drugs can be important additions to analgesic control. They can promote a pharmacologic potentiation of the analgesic drug and ameliorate or alleviate some of the common symptoms associated with the pain syndrome (Table 15.5). Intense anxiety associated with chronic pain may result in depression, which in turn causes the patient to be increasingly aware of pain. Mood elevators and antidepressants may promote control of this ancillary syndrome, allowing for a more satisfactory life style. In addition, such drugs may potentiate the analgesic effect of the narcotic analgesics.

7.0 Unproven methods of pain management

The influence of behavioral conditioning to change the perception of pain (i.e., the threshold, tolerance, and endurance of pain) is well established. The use of mind or behavior modification or deconditioning may therefore have a role in pain control. Hypnosis and acupuncture have been employed in the treatment of chronic pain syndromes and in the induction of anesthesia for dental and other surgical procedures. It is probable that acupuncture

is a form of hypnosis although the issue remains controversial. The mechanism by which hypnosis affects pain perception may be related to the creation of a "nega-

Table 15.4 Brompton Solution #1

Formula

Morphine sulfate	0.5 g
Cocaine HCl	0.5 g
Citric acid	2.0 g
Propylene glycol	100.0 ml
Alcohol U.S.P. 95%	300.0 ml
Sorbitol solution 70%	250.0 ml
Saccharin sodium	0.5 g
Berry-citrus blend	4.0 ml
Water q.s. ad.	1000.0 ml

Procedure

Dissolve morphine sulfate, cocaine HCl, and citric acid in 100.0 ml of water.

Add with mixing sorbitol solution, propylene glycol, and alcohol, in that order.

Dissolve saccharin in 50.0 ml of water. Add with constant stirring to above solution.

Adjust to 900.0 ml. Assay morphine and cocaine. Add flavor.

Q.s. ad. with water to make 1000.0 ml. Filter.

tive" hallucination. A second mechanism of hypnosis is related to the placebo effect achieved by a variety of external suggestions. The latter mechanism is not necessarily dependent upon the capability of hypnotic suggestion for all sensory experiences, but rather may be selective for the sensory experience defined as pain and reinterpreted under hypnosis as a positive stimulus.

Hypnosis should be incorporated with other pain control methods, should orient the patient toward self-hypnosis, and should involve autogenic training to prolong the hypnotic experience and promote its availability whenever the pain stimulus breaks through. It is, however, a delicate decision to employ hypnosis in the treatment of acute and chronic cancer pain, for it may suggest to some patients that their pain is not real. On the other hand, it affords the patient a measure of participation and control and thereby obviates the common withdrawal syndrome. A subject need not be necessarily "hypnotizable," but the "suggestible" subject will benefit more from the hypnosis. Particularly "suggestible" for management with hypnosis are youthful patients and especially those who are cause oriented, or interested in meditation or astrology. Patients involved in commit-

ments to religious cultures or who have been consistent achievers in life are unlikely subjects for hypnosis. The integration of hypnosis with other forms of operant conditioning and behavioral modification under the auspices of psychiatric and psychologic consultation may play an important role in pain management.

Neural stimulation by the application of electrical current to the skin surface is another unproven method of pain control. A variety of electrical devices that can be carried as a battery pack on the body and attached to an area of pain has been developed. For a small proportion of patients, pain relief is provided at least while they wear the stimulator; for a smaller number, complete relief is obtained for long periods after a short period of application. The pain is generally of benign origin, and the application of these devices in the treatment of malignant pain is relatively uncommon.

8.0 Neurosurgical procedures for analgesia

Because neurosurgical approaches to pain control can result in significant morbidity and a compromise in visceral or limb

Table 15.5 Ancillary (Nonnarcotic) Nonanalgesic Drugs

Drug	Use
Phenothiazines	May be synergistic when used concomitantly with narcotics to augment pain control
Antihistamines	Same
Tranquilizers	For patients for whom anxiety decreases the pain threshold
Sedatives or soporifics	For pain-induced insomnia
Mood elevators	For patients for whom depression reinforces the pain syndrome

function, such procedures should be considered only when (1) the pain cannot be controlled by analgesics, or analgesia therapy is intolerable, (2) the patient's life style and performance status are compromised as a consequence of the pain, or (3) disseminated or distant tumor is controlled adequately enough so that substantial longevity can be expected for the patient. The patient should participate in deciding whether to proceed with neurosurgical procedures by considering the potential for neurosurgical control of pain with the potential for neurologic, and therefore functional, compromise. A fourth aspect of the decision regarding the application of a neurosurgical procedure and the type of procedure to be employed is the anatomic distribution of the pain. If the pain presents unilaterally, a neurosurgical procedure will not compromise maintenance of function on the contralateral side.

Dorsal rhizotomy. After disc disease, cancer is the second major indication for pain control by dorsal rhizotomy. Although initial control is not necessarily predicted by the analgesic nerve block, the initial success rate approaches 50 percent. The rate drops to 40 percent for long-term control. The high failure rate of rhizotomy is unexplained, although it seems apparent that multiple dorsal rhizotomies are necessary, particularly if the pain emanates from a site distant from the central spine. Dorsal rhizotomy is infrequently used in the management of cancer pain because of suboptimal long-term responses.

Sympathectomy. Because sympathectomy is most useful when disease is confined to the visceral capsule, it is less likely to be effective for malignant disease. In practice, sympathectomy has been uniformly unsuccessful in the management of visceral cancer pain.

Percutaneous cordotomy. Surgical cordotomy through laminectomy has been employed for more than 50 years, but paralysis and other forms of sensory and motor impairment as well as occasional respiratory arrests have minimized its general application. Percutaneous cordotomy is a more recent development, of perhaps less than 10 years, and because of its ability to define precisely the spinothalamic tract, it is less likely to cause paralysis, sphincter impairment, or death, although occasional dysesthesia may result. In fact, the percutaneous method has made severe dysesthesia the single major complication of cordotomy. This type of surgery does not require anesthesia and permits precise delineation of the pain tract by electrical stimulation of the site.

Cordotomy successfully controls pain in 40 to 60 percent of patients. Because of possible dysesthesia, some surgeons recommend that cordotomy be used only for patients who have intractable pain due to cancer. Pain relief by cordotomy usually lasts only one or two years. Cordotomy should also be reserved for patients who have adequate pulmonary function, particularly if the cord lesion to be induced by neurosurgery is above the C_6 area of the cervical spine.

The use of percutaneous radiofrequency cervical cordotomy for intractible pain has been employed extensively by Rosonmoff. The most common condition for which the cordotomies were employed was malignant disease. More than one-third of the patients required bilateral cordotomy; almost 20 percent required a second cordotomy. Only 25 percent of the patients were available for evaluation after one year. Initial pain relief was achieved for more than 90 percent of the patients, but over the long term only 40 to 70 percent of patients who were alive continued to have pain control.

Hypophysectomy. It has been well established that hypophysectomy is an effective means of treating metastases from breast or prostate cancer. It is less commonly appreciated that hypophysectomy has been employed as a therapeutic modality for bone pain in a variety of tumors that are not hormone sensitive. Moricca has reported on more than 1000 patients in whom "chemical" hypophysectomy was performed by the transsphenoidal injection of a neurolytic agent such as ethanol. In 600 cases treated through 1973, sustained pain relief was achieved in all patients. The mechanism of pain relief is unclear. Opioid receptors are identifiable in hypothalamic tissue and a chemical substance present in the brain has narcotic properties (endorphins). Speculation that hypophysectomy results in an unregulated continuous release of such chemicals or the related enkephalins from the brain substance have been proposed as a mechanism of pain relief. Patients responding to hypophysectomy, however, do not have their pain exaccerbated by the use of endorphin antagonists (naloxone).

Patient G, a 57-year-old woman, had a metastatic cylindroma to bone, lung, and mouth. The primary tumor was treated 10 years prior to the development of lung metastases (Fig. 15.4). She was treated with a variety of chemotherapeutic regimens, in addition to radiation therapy with variable success. Fifteen years after presentation of the primary tumor, she developed thoracic wall pain, which over six months became progressively resistant to narcotic analgesics until she was unable to recline. Local nerve block was unsuccessful, and cordotomy was ruled out because of the extensive lung disease. She underwent transsphenoidal hypophysectomy without major complication except for transient diabetes insipidus. Within seven days she required only a single daily dose of narcotics and for the first time was able to sleep lying in bed.

Pain control has persisted for two months without noticeable regression of the tumor.

This method of pain control is currently investigational.

Thalamic procedures. Surgical and chemosurgical therapies for the thalamic center for pain represent experimental approaches with relatively limited results to date.

9.0 Summary

Intractable pain is the greatest fear of the cancer patient, but many therapeutic modalities are available that ameliorate or eliminate pain for the majority of patients, making intractable pain uncommon if not rare. Occasionally, neurosurgical procedures may be necessary to control pain, but must be cautiously considered. Recently gained information regarding the hypothalamus in relation to endorphin, and the application of hypophysectomy in the treatment of various pain syndromes represent new directions for the future. In addition, a variety of mood-altering drugs and narcotic analgesics with few adverse side effects are being developed.

References

Bonica, J. J. (ed.) *Advances in neurology: international symposium on pain.* vol. 4. New York: Raven Press, 1974.

deJong, R. H. Central pain mechanisms (editorial). *JAMA* 239:2784, 1978.

LaRossa, J. T.; Strong, M. S.; and Melby, J. C. Endocrinologically incomplete transethmoidal trans-sphenoidal hypophysectomy with relief of bone pain in breast cancer. *N. Engl. J. Med.* 298:1332–1335, 1978.

Lipton, S. (ed.) *Persistent pain: modern*

methods of treatment. vol. 1. New York; Grune & Stratton, 1977.

Mehta, M. *Intractable pain.* Philadelphia: W. B. Saunders, Co., 1973.

Moertal, C. G. et al. Relief of pain by oral medications: a controlled evaluation of analgesic combinations. *JAMA* 229:55–59, 1974.

Snyder, S. H. The opiate receptor and morphine-like peptides in the brain. *Am. J. Psychiatry* 135:645–652, 1978.

Steig, R. L. New methods for achieving pain control with transcutaneous nerve stimulation. Presented at the American Academy of Neurology, Toronto, April 1976.

Winnie, A. P. Local anesthetics for chronic pain. *Today's Clinician* 15–20, 1978.

Part V

Systemic Complications of Cancer

Chapter 16

Infectious Complications of Malignancy
J. Pennington

1.0 Incidence of infection

Infection is now the leading cause of death in patients with acute leukemia and lymphoma. This contrasts with the high incidence of hemorrhagic deaths experienced before the advent of modern platelet support systems. The most important factors now limiting the further escalation of doses of antineoplastic chemotherapy are the associated escalation of granulocytopenia and risk of infectious complications. Patients with solid tumors have traditionally received less intensive chemotherapy than patients with hematologic malignancies and have not experienced the high rate of death from infection seen in the latter group. Recent developments in combined chemotherapeutic regimens for various solid tumors, however, will undoubtedly enlarge the group of patients who are granulocytopenic.

Much epidemiologic information has been collected over the past decade, and it is now well established that certain sites are especially vulnerable to infection in immunocompromised patients. Furthermore, certain infectious agents are more commonly encountered than others in this patient population (Table 16.1). Despite specifically vulnerable sites for infection, however, patients with acute leukemia or lymphoma most often exhibit no identifiable source of their bacterial sepsis. Episodes of sepsis are usually associated with gram-negative enteric bacilli and are likely to originate from ulcerated regions in the gastrointestinal tract. Among identifiable sites of origin, however, the respiratory tract is the leading source for infection in both leukemia and lymphoma. The anorectal area, skin, pharynx, and urinary tract are also common locations for infection. All of these regions are characterized by intimate contact with either the external environment and/or high concentrations of opportunistic bacteria.

Table 16.1 Common Sites of Infection in Cancer Patients

Sites	Common Pathogens
Hematologic Neoplasia	
Lung	Staphylococci; E. coli, klebsiella, pseudomonas, aspergillus, pneumocystis carinii, cytomegalovirus
Perirectum	E. coli, klebsiella, pseudomonas, bacteroides
Oropharynx	Fuso-spirochetal, candida, streptococci, gram-negative bacilli
Skin	Staphylococci, gram-negative bacilli
Esophagus	Candida, herpes group virus, gram-negative bacilli
Urine	Gram-negative bacilli, enterococcus, candida
Solid Tumor*	
Gastrointestinal tract	Gram-negative bacilli, clostridia, salmonella, bacteroides
Genitourinary tract	Gram-negative bacilli, bacteroides, enterococcus
Skin	Staphylococci, gram-negative bacilli
Lung (aspiration)	Mixed anaerobes, Staphylococci, Klebsiella

*Infection in necrotic tumor mass is common.

Patients with solid tumors frequently experience localized infections in areas of tumor involvement. Partial obstruction of airways and the urinary tract as well as areas of tumor necrosis in gastrointestinal, genitourinary, or head and neck tumors are particularly common sites of local infection. Thus, it is not surprising that the urinary tract or an intra-abdominal process is the common source of bacteremia in a large group of patients with solid tumors. Many septic episodes in solid tumor patients occur, however, for which no site of origin is found. Also, in contrast to a group of patients with leukemia or lymphoma, Bacteroides sp. accounts for a reasonably high number of septic episodes (10.7%) in patients with solid tumors. This anaerobe is most frequently found in patients with genitourinary cancer.

Because granulocytes are critical in host defense against both the gram-negative bacilli and the staphylococcus and because these organisms are prevalent at skin and gastrointestinal sites, patients with hematologic malignancy are frequently infected with E. coli, Klebsiella, Pseudomonas aeruginosa, or Staphylococcus aureus. Patients with solid tumors also experience frequent E. coli, Klebsiella, or staphylococcal infections, but anaerobes such as Bacteroides sp. and Clostridia sp. are also encountered. This probably relates to the incidence of necrotic tumor mass involving gastrointestinal and adjacent genitourinary tract areas. An increased incidence of Salmonella infections exists for patients with hematologic malignancies and pelvic or rectosigmoid tumors. Other bacterial infections seen with increased frequency in cancer patients are listeriosis, often with meningeal involvement, and Nocardia, especially of the lung; recently, several cases of pulmonary infection with nonanthrax Bacillus sp. have been reported. Bacterial pathogens that are common in the nonimmunosuppressed population (e.g., pneumococcus, Streptococcus pyogenes) are uncommon in most cancer patients. Streptococcus bovis is an unusual pathogen but when observed with bacteremia and endocarditis is suggestive of gastrointestinal malignancy.

Although bacteria continue to be the most frequent pathogens in compromised patients with cancer, fungal infection is increasing in incidence. Disseminated candidiasis, often preceded by colonization of mucosal surfaces, indwelling Foley catheters, or intravenous equipment, is seen with hematologic and solid tumors, and carries a mortality of greater than 70 percent to greater than 40 percent in each group, respectively. Pulmonary infections with Aspergillus, or less commonly mucormycosis, represent the other major fungal pathogens for leukemia and lymphoma patients. Lymphoma patients also occasionally become infected with Cryptococcus. In cancer patients, serious cryptococcal infection may not be limited to the meninges. Rapidly fatal pulmonary cryptococcosis has been seen in a number of of lymphoma patients, especially those with Hodgkin's disease. Compromised patients with invasive or disseminated fungal infection have a much poorer prognosis than those with systemic bacterial infection, but more aggressive methods for early diagnosis and therapy of fungal infections, such as pulmonary aspergillosis, should lead to improved survival.

Also less common than bacteria, but of great frequency in certain cancer centers, is pneumonitis with the opportunistic parasite *Pneumocystis carinii*. Mortality for this infection has exceeded 60 percent in the past, but great improvements in therapy have recently been reported. Survival of 78 percent of patients treated with pentamidine and 79 percent of those treated with trimethoprim and sulfamethoxazole were reported in one study. Patients with lymphomas are particularly prone to both cytomegalovirus and herpes zoster infections. The recent evidence that adenine arabinoside is of value for herpes simplex encephalitis should lend encouragement to further trials of this agent for other herpes group viral infections.

2.0 Immune defects and risk factors for infection

Cancer patients do not have normal defenses against infection. Patients with leukemia have either abnormal granulocytes or lymphocytes, and the resulting defects in phagocytosis, or antibody production, are well known. In addition to functional defects in leukocytes, patients with aleukemic leukemia experience leukopenic states and impaired inflammatory reactions due to their underlying disease. Lymphoma patients, particularly those with Hodgkin's disease, have a tendency to have impaired cell-mediated immunologic reactions. Thus, they are prone to infection with intracellular pathogens that depend upon T lymphocyte-macrophage interaction for clearance. Herpes group virus (cytomegalovirus, herpes zoster, herpes simplex), listeria, nocardia, and cryptococcus are examples of such pathogens. Multiple myeloma and chronic lymphocytic leukemia are noted for either dysgammaglobulinemia or hypogammaglobulinemia. Encapsulated bacteria, such as the Pneumococcus or *Hemophilus influenzae*, depend upon gamma globulin opsonins for effective phagocytic clearance, and thus occur with increased frequency in these diseases. Patients with solid tumors have mechanical problems with postobstruction stasis and with infection in the lungs, genitourinary tract, and head and neck regions. In addition, metastatic tumor invasion of the bone marrow may result in myelosuppression and granulocytopenia. Finally, brain tumors often lead to an impaired mental status and an increased risk of aspiration pneumonia.

Beyond the inherent defects in host defenses associated with the primary tumor is increased immunosuppression secondary to antineoplastic therapy. Various chemotherapeutic agents alter host defenses in different ways, and two recent reviews have correlated specific agents with specific immune defects. In general, the greatest risk for infection comes from myelosuppressive chemotherapy. Peripheral neutrophil counts below 1000/mm^3 are considered particularly dangerous. Whereas many antineoplastic drugs affect marrow function and T and B lymphocyte function simultaneously, adrenocorticosteroids act primarily by altering granulocyte kinetics at sites of inflammation and by suppressing cell-mediated immune functions. The incidence of lung infections in compromised patients is high; a recent report indicates that cyclophosphamide plus glucocorticosteroid drugs in combination lowers the number of alveolar macrophages available in the lung and inhibits the influx of polymorphonuclear leukocytes following a bacterial challenge. In addition to antineoplastic drugs, radiation can also decrease granulocyte numbers and function; Hodgkin's disease patients, for example, have up to a 24 percent incidence of local herpes zoster infection after radiation therapy.

The role of splenectomy for the staging of Hodgkin's disease continues to be controversial. Although some researchers have reported no increased risk of infection for splenectomized lymphoma patients as compared to nonlymphoma patients, a number of fulminating infections have been seen in this group. Recent evidence correlates the highest incidence of infection with splenectomized patients who have received the most aggressive treatment (radiation and chemotherapy) for this tumor. These patients also have lower antibody levels for Hemophilus after more aggressive therapeutic regimens, regardless of splenectomy.

The hospital environment and the equipment used for treating cancer patients are important risk factors for infection. In administering chemotherapy in the out-patient setting, every effort should be taken to reduce colonization of the oropharynx and gastrointestinal tract with hospital-acquired pathogens. Many such organisms are more resistant to usual antibiotic regimens and thus more difficult to treat. Careful attention to in-dwelling urinary and intravenous lines is also critical, as they frequently serve as portals for intractable pathogens such as *Candida species, Torulopsis glabrata,* or bacterial organisms.

The relationship between immune defects and infections is outlined in Table 16.2. No attempt has been made there to distinguish immune defects due to the tumor itself from those secondary to the usual therapy.

3.0 Clinical problems

Diagnosis. The immunosuppressed and leukopenic state of many cancer patients, especially those with leukemia or lymphoma, impairs clinical diagnosis of infection. The decreased ability to mount an inflammatory response at sites of infection alters the usual presentation for a number of infections; for example, neutropenic patients with pneumonia frequently present only with fever and mild dyspnea. A dry cough may or may not be present, and physical signs of pneumonitis (e.g., rales, rub) are often absent.

Patient A, a 34-year-old man with Stage IV Hodgkin's disease, was discharged from the hospital after receiving chemotherapy. He returned after three days complaining of fever, chills, and shortness of breath. Physical examination was unremarkable except for tachypnea and a temperature of 38.7°C. The white blood cell count was 1800/mm^3. Chest roentgenogram (Fig. 16.1) was remarkable for an extensive pulmonary infiltrate despite the lack of findings on physical exam. Lung

Table 16.2 RELATION BETWEEN IMMUNE DEFECTS AND INFECTION IN CANCER PATIENTS

Immune Defect	*Tumor Type*	*Infection*
Granulocytopenia	AML; ALL; CML (blast crisis);* Advanced lymphomas or myeloma. Solid tumors treated with high-dose chemotherapy.	Gram-negative bacilli, *Staphylococcus aureus*, Aspergillus, Candida, *Pneumocystis carinii*
Cell-mediated immunity	Hodgkin's and non-Hodgkin's lymphoma	Cytomegalovirus, herpes zoster, herpes simplex, pneumocystis, listeria, nocardia, cryptococcus, toxoplasmosis
Hypogammaglobulinemia or dysgammaglobulinemia	CLL†; Multiple myeloma	Pneumococcus, *Hemophilus influenzae*, Neisseria meningitis
Splenectomy	Hodgkin's disease	Pneumococcus, *Hemophilus influenzae*
Obstruction and Tumor Necrosis	Solid tumors, occasional lymphoma	*Staphylococcus aureus*, gram-negative bacilli, *Bacteroides* sp., *Clostridia* sp., Salmonella

*AML = acute myelogenous leukemia; ALL = acute lymphocytic leukemia; CML = chronic myelogenous leukemia.
†CLL = chronic lymphocytic leukemia.

biopsy revealed Pneumocystis carinii *pneumonitis.*

Chest x-ray may demonstrate extensive infiltration in spite of minimal physical findings in the neutropenic patient.

Radiographic evidence of a new lung infiltrate may be a surprise during the work-up of fever in leukopenic cancer patients. Sputum production is often minimal or absent, due to lack of purulence in the respiratory tract. The usefulness of routine sputum cultures and stains is thus limited for the leukopenic patient, and more invasive diagnostic techniques may be needed. Furthermore, the usual pharyngeal exudates associated with bacterial pharyngitis are often absent. Sore throats are common, and careful attention should be given to the combination of fever, pharyngeal erythema, and isolation of Streptococcus or gram-negative bacilli from the throat. Neutropenic patients with urinary tract infections may lack dysuria or pyuria, and careful examination and urine culture for evidence of significant bacteriuria are necessary for unexplained fever. Another common problem in leukopenic cancer patients is perirectal infection. Although fever and local pain are common, areas of fluctuation and frank abscess are generally absent until normal numbers of granulocytes reappear.

The infection site may not be identified in the presence of leukopenia; if an inflammatory response is absent, a pulmonary

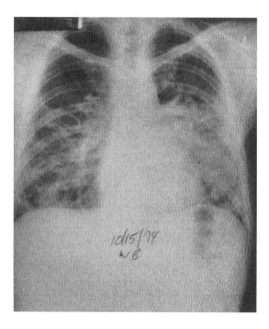

Fig. 16.1 Roentgeongram for patient with normal physical examination of chest. Patient had Pneumocystis carinii pneumonia.

infiltrate or localizing abscess may not develop.

Finally, although central nervous system infection is relatively uncommon in immunosuppressed cancer patients, any subtle evidence of central nervous system disease must be carefully evaluated with spinal fluid examination and culture.

Patient B, a 27-year-old woman with lymphosarcoma, was admitted for fever and personality change. She denied any neurologic symptoms other than an occasional headache relieved with aspirin. Her most recent chemotherapy had resulted in a leukopenia and her white blood cell count on admission was 1500/mm³, with 20 percent neutrophils. Physical examination was normal. A lumbar puncture

was performed, and the spinal fluid grew Listeria monocytogenes after two days.

Infection of the central nervous system is often occult and necessitates lumbar puncture for thorough evaluation for certain febrile patients in whom an infectious source is not established.

Frank nuchal rigidity is less common in immunosuppressed cancer patients. Mild headache, personality changes, or subtle neurologic signs may be the only evidence for listeria or cryptococcal meningitis in lymphoma patients. Toxoplasmosis encephalitis can easily escape detection in these patients, and progressive multifocal leukoencephalopathy must be considered as an explanation for subacute demyelinating disease in the compromised patient with cancer. The clinician may need invasive diagnostic maneuvers such as brain biopsy to make these diagnoses.

Because diagnosis of infection is often difficult for cancer patients, special techniques have been proposed to assist the clinician (Table 16.3). Fever is common in patients with leukemia and lymphoma, yet blood cultures are often negative. Attempts to provide early evidence that bacterial infection is present have been made using the Limulus assay for circulating endotoxin. The lysate of the horseshoe crab gels upon contact with endotoxins and the assay have been used in attempts to provide either a more rapid or a more sensitive test for gram-negative infection than conventional blood cultures. The incidence of false negatives and false positives in blood assays, the variability in sensitivity among lysate batches, and the lack of clinically available testing facilities have, however, made this test less useful than originally hoped. The reduction of nitroblue tetrazolium dye from yellow to black formazen crystals by granulocytes correlates with pyogenic

Table 16.3 Special Tests for Infection in Cancer Patients

Infection	Test	Value
Bacteria	Limulus assay Nitroblue Tetrazolium test	False positives and negatives— unreliable
Fungi		
Candida	Precipitins; agglutinins	False positives and negatives
Aspergillus	Precipitins	False positives and negatives
Cryptococcus	Latex fixation for antigens	Diagnostic if positive
Parasites Pneumocystis carinii	Indirect fluorescent antibodies	False positives and negatives
Viruses		
Cytomegalovirus	Complement fixation	Fourfold rise is highly suggestive. Single high value not diagnostic.

infection and has been helpful in distinguishing fever due to underlying lymphoma ("B symptoms") from fever or infection. But the test lacks sensitivity, and false positives have been reported to be as high as 50 percent. The Limulus assay and nitroblue tetrazolium tests have thus enjoyed only limited popularity for diagnosis of occult bacterial infections and are not routinely available for clinical use. Finally, the use of ^{67}Ga radionuclide scanning has been advocated for occult abscess, but the isotope will localize to pus cells as well as neoplastic cells. Interpretation of results in patients with cancer, especially lymphoma and solid tumors, must therefore be undertaken with extreme care.

Because invasive fungal infection in cancer patients is often associated with negative blood cultures (Candida) or inaccessible lung infiltrates for culture (Aspergillus), serologic tests have been evaluated for these diagnoses. Early evidence that Candida precipitins might be useful has not been confirmed in recent studies, and at present, Candida serology in the patient with neoplastic disease continues to be associated with unacceptable rates of false-positive and false-negative results. Aspergillus precipitins have been evaluated in patients with leukemia and found to convert to positive in 7 of 10 cases of proven *Aspergillus* pneumonia, but a 30 percent false-negative and apparent 50 percent false-positive rate was found in this study. Aspergillus serology thus continues to be inadequate alone to diagnose this infection in the compromised

Ancillary tests to detect and distinguish fever of infection from fever of malignancy are generally suboptimal.

host. Most helpful has been the serologic assay for cryptococcal antigen in blood or spinal fluid. This assay is useful both for lung and central nervous system disease and represents a truly valuable clinical tool. To date, serology for *Pneumocystis carinii* is unreliable.

Therapeutic regimens. This section will discuss only commonly encountered infections in cancer patients and will attempt to emphasize newer approaches to antimicrobial chemotherapy (Table 16.4).

Antibiotic combinations for undefined infection should include anti-Staphlococcus and Pseudomonas regimens in the leukopenic and critically infected patient.

Therapy for gram-negative aerobic rods has become more complicated with an increasing incidence of gentamicin-resistant organisms in many centers. Tobramycin sulfate is a new aminoglycoside similar to gentamicin in spectrum and pharmacokinetics but with better in vitro activity against most isolates of *Pseudomonas aeruginosa*. As mortality from Pseudomonas usually exceeds mortality from other gram-negative bacillary infections, the most potent anti-Pseudomonas agent (tobramycin) should be employed.

Most gentamicin-resistant gram-negative rods are also resistant to tobramycin (with the possible exception of Pseudomonas). The newest aminoglycoside to become available is amikacin sulfate, and this drug generally maintains activity against gentamicin- and tobramycin-resistant gram-negative rods. Therefore, amikacin appears to be the agent of choice when dealing with such infections. In some centers the incidence of gentamicin resistance has reached such levels that amikacin is now used for "empiric" coverage of suspected sepsis (i.e., when cultures are unavailable or negative). This trend must be counterbalanced, however, by the potential for inducing amikacin resistance by overuse of the drug. Each center must evaluate the incidence of aminoglycoside resistance before deciding local policy on this issue. One other new gram-negative drug is ticarcillin. This agent has a

Table 16.4 Therapeutic Regimens for Common Infections in Cancer Patients

Organism	Regimen
Bacteria	
E. coli	Ampicillin + gentamicin or tobramycin
Klebsiella	Cephalothin + gentamicin or tobramycin
Pseudomonas	Ticarcillin + tobramycin
Staphylococcus aureus	Nafcillin (cephalothin, if penicillin allergic)
Nocardia	Sulfonamide (may use trimethoprin-sulfamethoxazole)
Bacteroides fragilis	Chloramphenicol or clindamycin
Fungi	
Candida (local)	Nystatin (low-dose amphotericin B)
Candida (systemic)	Amphotericin B
Aspergillus	Amphotericin B
Mucormycosis	Amphotericin B
Cryptococcus	Amphotericin B (plus 5-fluorocystosine)*
Parasites	
Pneumocystis carinii	Trimethoprim and sulfamethoxazole
Viruses	
Herpes simplex encephalitis	Adenine arabinoside
Disseminated herpes zoster	Adenine arabinoside (if given early)
Cytomegalovirus	Uncertain

*5-fluorocytosine may be contraindicated for patients with severe myelosuppression.

similar spectrum to carbenicillin (including Pseudomonas) but may be used in about two-thirds the dose, thus lowering the sodium load administered.

Much interest in the possible use of carbenicillin for *Bacteroides* fragilis has recently been expressed. If this drug proves clinically successful, it will be possible to avoid using clindamycin or chloramphenicol for this anaerobic infection.

The treatment of staphylococcal infection has produced several new ideas. First, nafcillin has been found to have better in vitro coverage for enterococci than does methicillin or oxacillin. Thus, when using an antistaphylococcal agent empirically, a slightly broader gram-positive spectrum may be covered with nafcillin. Animal studies have also demonstrated synergy between penicillin and gentamicin for staphylococcal endocarditis. Whether this is of clinical importance, however, is uncertain. Our policy has been to employ penicillin or cephalosporin antibiotics without an aminoglycoside for staphylococcal infections other than endocarditis. Finally, the possibility exists for treating Staphylococcus with only an aminoglycoside. One popular empiric antibiotic regimen for febrile neutropenic patients is carbenicillin plus gentamicin, and as carbenicillin is inactive against penicillinase-producing Staphylococcus, the in vitro evidence that gentamicin is active against Staphylococcus is relevant. Two recent clinical studies have demonstrated that gentamicin or amikacin when used alone can at least suppress a staphylococcal infection for short periods of time.

Although 5-fluorocytosine has demonstrated anti-Candida and anti-Aspergillus

Culture-specific confirmation of infection is usually needed for institution of antifungal therapy.

activity, the agent recommended for serious infection with these organisms continues to be amphotericin B. Synergism between amphotericin B and 5-fluorocytosine has been shown in vitro, but the potential for bone marrow suppression in cancer patients makes this combination less attractive. Amphotericin B has been administered in low intravenous doses (e.g., 5 to 10 mg per day for 10 days) for symptomatic relief of candidal esophagitis.

Patient C, a 62-year-old man with chronic myelogenous leukemia, developed severe dysphagia while receiving chemotherapy for a blast crisis. The patient had extensive oropharyngeal monilia infection and was receiving Nystatin mouthwash and swallows to no avail. A barium swallow revealed a typical picture of candidal esophagitis in the lower one-third of the esophagus. Intravenous amphotericin B, 5 mg per day, was administered for 10 consecutive days. By day five, the patient noted marked relief and was able to take food and liquid well. No sign of drug toxicity was noted. Although oral patches of Candida persisted, the dysphagia did not recur.

A 10-day course of 5 mg per day of amphotericin B is relatively nontoxic, and produces dramatic relief for many patients who fail to improve with oral nystatin therapy. One setting in which a combination of 5-fluorocytosine plus amphotericin B (in about one-half the usual dose) appears to be clinically synergistic is cryptococcal meningitis. Studies are underway to evaluate this therapy fully. A new antifungal agent, miconazole, has been associated with a number of treatment failures and to date has not assumed a significant role in treating fungal infections in cancer patients.

Pneumocystis has, until recently, been treated with intramuscular pentamidine isethionate. This agent, however, is

Trimethoprim-sulfamethoxazole is the treatment of choice for suspected or culture-confirmed Pneumocystis infection. It should be administered intravenously in patients requiring respiratory support.

associated with a high incidence of toxicity. Trimethoprim-sulfamethoxazole (TMP-SMX) has recently been shown to be effective for treatment. It must be used in high doses (TMP 20 mg/kg/day; SMX 100 mg/kg/day) but may be given orally for many patients. Several critically ill patients have developed paralytic ileus and failed to absorb this medication, however, and treatment failures have been correlated with poor absorption of the drug. It may be advisable to use parenteral TMP-SMX (currently available as an investigational drug) unless serum drug levels can be followed. A study comparing the efficacy of TMP-SMX to pentamidine showed equal cure rates (> 70%) for both agents. Thus it would appear that the least toxic agent (TMP-SMX) should now be used for Pneumocystis infection.

Several antiviral agents have been evaluated for serious herpes-group infections. Cytosine arabinoside and idoxuridine

Antiviral agents have rarely been effective and should not be empirically applied for suspected infection.

have been both toxic and unsuccessful in controlled trials. Recent reports, however, indicate that adenine arabinoside produces significantly better results than does placebo for both herpes encephalitis and disseminated herpes zoster. This agent is employed at a dosage of 10 to 15 mg per day intravenously and is relatively nontoxic at these doses. Excessive fluid load however can present problems.

Although cyclic courses of antineoplastic chemotherapy form the basis of treatment for many types of cancer, it is common for these protocols to be interrupted because of concurrent infection. The myelosuppressive nature of many anticancer drugs, plus the suppression of humoral and cellular immune responses to infection, often make therapy impossible during serious infection. Nevertheless, patients with non–life-threatening infections, such as well controlled and clinically responsive tuberculosis, may occasionally receive concurrent antineoplastic and antimicrobial therapy. In addition, patients with fever of uncertain cause may respond to tumor chemotherapy when empiric antimicrobial therapy has failed. Clinical judgment must prevail in deciding when to reinstitute treatment for underlying malignancy during periods of fever or infection.

Fever and neutropenia. Cancer chemotherapy frequently results in neutropenic states, and the clinician may be frequently confronted with a neutropenic cancer patient (granulocyte count less than 1000/mm^3) with new onset of fever. Many of these patients have fevers of undetermined origin at the onset of illness. Past reports have shown that in 50 to 60 percent of these patients, infection, usually bacterial, is the cause of the fever. Because the patient may succumb in 72 hours if not properly treated, prompt administration of empiric antibiotics for fever and neutropenia has become standard procedure.

It is clear that the febrile, neutropenic patient should receive empiric antibiotics, but exactly which drugs are most appropriate is of some debate (Table 16.5). The spectrum to be covered must include Staphyloccocci (penicillinase-producing) and the full range of aerobic gram-negative bacilli, including Pseudomonas. Coverage for *Bacteroides* fragilis is less important for patients with hematologic neoplasia, but patients with gastrointestinal or genitourinary tract solid tumors should be treated for this anaerobe. Several

combination of cephalothin plus gentamicin resulted in a 12 percent incidence of
azotemia, while the other combinations
had only 2 to 4 percent nephrotoxicity. In
another recent trial, carbenicillin plus
either gentamicin or amikacin were compared, and no difference in efficacy or
toxicity was noted between the regimens.

The question of drug synergy for gram-
negative infections also is important.
As the combination of cephalothin plus
gentamicin may cover staphylococcal
infections better than carbenicillin and
gentamicin but is more nephrotoxic, some
researchers have advocated empiric coverage using a specific narrow spectrum
antistaphylococcal agent such as nafcillin
plus gentamicin. Recent evidence that

combinations of antibiotics have been
evaluated for fever and neutropenia. By
and large, two-drug combinations, such as
carbenicillin plus gentamicin, tobramycin, or amikacin, have been as effective as
three-drug combinations, such as cephalothin, carbenicillin, and gentamicin, with
overall survival reported of 70 to 82 percent (Table 16.5). The largest comparative
trial of empiric antibiotics is the recently
completed E.O.R.T.C. study, in which
either cephalothin plus gentamicin, carbenicillin plus gentamicin, or cephalothin
plus carbenicillin were randomly as-
signed for treatment of fever in neutropenic cancer patients. No significant difference existed in clinical response among
regimens (all were excellent), but the

Table 16.5 Past Trials of Empiric Combinations of Antibiotics for Fever of
Undetermined Origin and Neutropenia

Trial	Drug combination	Number treated	Success (percentage)
Schimpff et al. 1971	Gentamicin Carbenicillin	75	51
Tattersall et al. 1972	Methicillin Gentamicin Carbenicillin Clindamycin Cephalothin	27	59
Bloomfield et al. 1974	Cephalothin Gentamicin Carbenicillin	51	82
Lau et al. 1977	Gentamicin (or Amikacin) Carbenicillin	157	75
E.O.R.T.C. 1977	Gentamicin Carbenicillin or Gentamicin Cephalothin or Carbenicillin Cephalothin	625	70

neutropenic patients treated for gram-negative infection with two synergistic drugs have lower mortality than those covered with a single active agent makes empiric coverage with two agents active against gram-negative bacteria highly desirable. Our current position based on these studies and on our own experience is that gentamicin or tobramycin plus carbenicillin is effective, well tolerated, and appropriate for neutropenia with fever of undetermined origin.

Duration of treatment is as important as initiation of treatment. Past studies have found that in more than 50 to 60 percent of febrile episodes in neutropenic patients, some microbiologic evidence of infection can be obtained. This has not been confirmed in a recent report, however, in which 43 such febrile episodes revealed documentation of a specific pathogen in only 21 percent. Despite this low yield from cultures, 23 of 43 patients had a prompt response to antibiotics and appeared to benefit from treatment. The emphasis on early empiric treatment of febrile episodes has thus resulted in many situations in which the clinician must prescribe an entire course of therapy without knowing the exact etiologic agent of the infection. If the culture-negative patient is promptly defervescent, the situation is less complex and therapy should be continued for about five days. If, however, the fever remains and cultures are negative, the choices are either to stop therapy and risk sudden deterioration from undiscovered infection or to continue empirical antibiotics and risk fungal superinfection.

Patient D, a 51-year-old woman with acute myelogenous leukemia, developed a fever while neutropenic from chemotherapy. There were no other signs or symptoms with the fever, and blood and urine cultures were negative. The patient received cephalothin and gentamicin but the fever persisted. Except for daily temperatures of 39°C, *the patient was stable, with no signs of hypotension or toxicity. During the third week of antibiotics, mild liver function abnormalities were noted, and a liver biopsy was performed. Biopsy material revealed yeast microscopically, and cultures grew Candida albicans. The patient then received intravenous amphotericin B and became afebrile within five days. Blood and urine cultures were never positive for Candida.*

Empiric antibiotic therapy should continue for at least four days but not more than seven if fever persists, and at least seven days if fever abates.

The exact duration for empiric antibiotic coverage depends upon the clinical condition of the patient. If the patient deteriorates with negative cultures, consideration of empiric amphotericin B should be given. If the patient is stable and normotensive, however, antibiotics may provide more risk of superinfection after seven or more days of coverage than benefit for an occult bacterial infection. It appears that stopping antibiotics at less than seven days is not advisable. With this information a scheme has been devised for approaching the febrile neutropenic patient who has no obvious source for fever (Table 16.6)

Fever and pulmonary infiltrates. The leading site of infection in patients with hematologic neoplasia is the lung, and this site carries the highest mortality. Several factors conspire to make fever with a new pulmonary infiltrate one of the most frustrating clinical problems in the management of cancer patients. First, the syndrome can have a wide variety of etiologies, both infectious and noninfectious (e.g., tumor; radiation pneumonitis; drug reactions to bleomycin, busulfan, or methotrexate; hemorrhage; pulmonary embolus or infarct). These various causes

Table 16.6 Clinical Approach to Fever and Neutropenia in the Cancer Patient

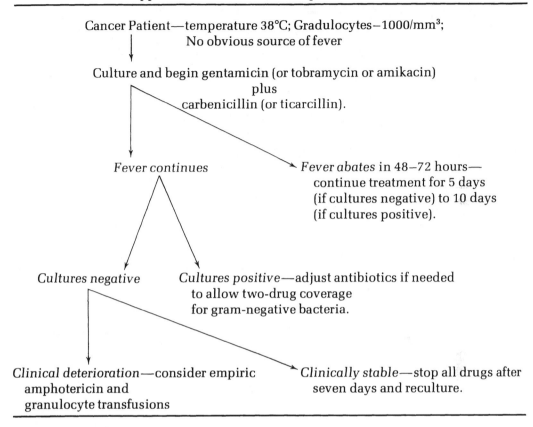

Cancer Patient—temperature 38°C; Gradulocytes–1000/mm³; No obvious source of fever

Culture and begin gentamicin (or tobramycin or amikacin) plus carbenicillin (or ticarcillin).

Fever continues

Fever abates in 48–72 hours— continue treatment for 5 days (if cultures negative) to 10 days (if cultures positive).

Cultures negative

Cultures positive—adjust antibiotics if needed to allow two-drug coverage for gram-negative bacteria.

Clinical deterioration—consider empiric amphotericin and granulocyte transfusions

Clinically stable—stop all drugs after seven days and reculture.

all require different therapy or perhaps no therapy at all. Second, the high mortality, up to 45 percent, necessitates rapid diagnosis and proper therapy. Third, sputum is not generally helpful for making the diagnosis, and invasive diagnostic techniques such as transbronchial brushing, percutaneous needle aspiration of lung, forceps biopsy through a fiberoptic bronchoscope, or even open-lung biopsy are often required. Fourth, these patients are often hypoxic and thrombocytopenic and are poor candidates for invasive lung biopsy. Finally, the radiographic appearance of the infiltrate can not assure the clinician of the diagnosis.

Patient E, a 74-year-old woman with lymphoma, developed a fever after receiving chemotherapy. The white blood cell count was 550/mm³, and a roentgenogram of the chest revealed localized infiltrates in the upper lobes (Fig. 16.2). The patient did not respond to broad-spectrum antibiotics, and the infiltrate became cavitary. The clinical impression was that of fungal pneumonia, but a transbronchial biopsy demonstrated Pneumocystis carinii (Fig. 16.3). Cultures of the bronchial washing later grew Aspergillus fumigatus.

Patient F, a 56-year-old woman with chronic myelogenous leukemia, developed a fever while leukopenic from chemotherapy. Despite the use of broad-spectrum antibiotics for two weeks, her fever persisted and a new infiltrate was noted on chest roentgenogram (Fig. 16.4). The bilateral interstitial and reticulonodular pattern, plus severe dyspnea led

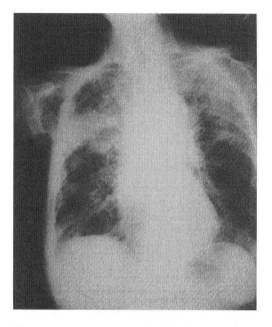

Fig. 16.2 Roentgenogram showing bilateral upper-lobe infiltrates. Confluence and air bronchograms are prominent on right.

to the empiric use of pentamidine for suspected Pneumocystis carinii. An open-lung biopsy performed three days later revealed widespread Aspergillus and no sign of Pneumocystis on specially stained lung sections.

Pulmonary infiltrates are nonspecific and can develop with any class of opportunistic infection. All fungal infections are not nodular and all Pneumocystis infections are not interstitial.

Thus, empiric therapy is often incorrect or even unneeded in these patients.

The general rule in approaching a febrile cancer patient with a new lung infiltrate should be to obtain lung tissue or at least deep bronchial washings as soon as possible. The exact diagnostic technique used will vary from center to center depending on local expertise. If bleeding is of utmost

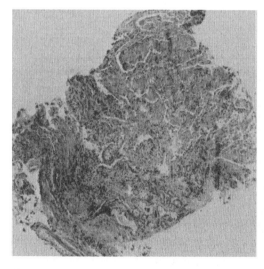

A

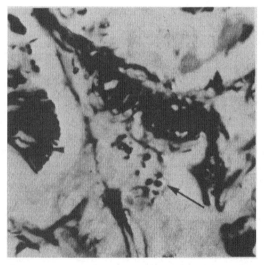

B

Fig. 16.3 Low-power microscopic view of lung tissue specimen (1 × 2 mm) obtained by forceps lung biopsy using flexible fiberoptic bronchoscope. Note availability of lung parenchyma for tissue examination (A). High-power view of same specimen, stained with methanamine silver. Several cysts, diagnostic for Pneumocystis carinii are seen (arrow) (B).

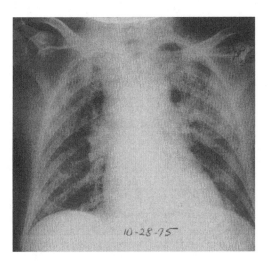

10-28-75

Fig. 16.4 Diffuse bilateral lung infiltrates with predominantly reticulonodular-interstitial pattern. Disseminated aspergillosis was found on open-lung biopsy.

concern (e.g., platelets less than 50,000/mm³), the safest procedure appears to be open-lung biopsy. Biopsy procedures allow histologic tissue examination while aspirations do not. This is of value when considering the large number of patients with nonspecific interstitial pneumonitis. In these cases, potentially toxic empiric therapy may be discontinued when infection is ruled out. Bronchial brushing has been much less helpful for diagnosis than either transbronchial biopsy or open-lung biopsy. The value of biopsy through the fiberoptic bronchoscope is, of course, the avoidance of chest tubes, anesthesia, and local pain from thoracotomy.

One approach to cancer patients with fever and new lung infiltrates is depicted in Table 16.7. A word of caution is needed. Because TMP-SMX is much less toxic than pentamidine and is now employed for empiric coverage of Pneumocystis, the temptation is to simply cover all bilateral pneumonias with this agent and avoid trying to make a specific diagnosis. This is not recommended, however. A wide vari-

ety of conditions mimic Pneumocystis, including drug reactions, viral infection, and even fungal pneumonia. The recent evidence that invasive Aspergillus can be cured in immunosuppressed patients if treated early makes every effort to obtain the exact diagnosis necessary. Finally, Pneumocystis may not present with typical bilateral interstitial infiltrates but may mimic the usual bacterial or fungal pneumonia. Nevertheless, our general rule in approaching febrile cancer patients with infiltrates is to assume a localized process to be bacterial or fungal, and a diffuse process to be Pneumocystis or a viral or drug reaction until proven otherwise (Table 16.7).

Other local infections. Mucosal fissures commonly allow gram-negative rods and anaerobic organisms access to the perirectal soft tissue in cancer patients. When patients are neutropenic and immunosuppressed, these areas rarely fluctuate and drain. Therefore, little benefit will result from incisions in the infected area until an adequate inflammatory reaction can occur. It may even be hazardous surgically or manually to manipulate this area during neutropenic states as sepsis could result. Treatment with antibiotics, sitz baths, and granulocyte transfusions, if available, is recommendable.

Mucositis, oral candidiasis, mixed anaerobically infected ulcers (Vincent's angina), and bacterial pharyngitis are all common in immunosuppressed cancer patients. Staphylococcal infection in the mouth rarely occurs. Thus, a regimen of penicillin, usually with gentamicin, is recommended for oral bacterial infection. Nystatin mouthwash may suppress thrush but is frequently ineffective during neutropenic states.

The lower one-third of the esophagus appears to be another vulnerable site for infection in cancer patients. Candida, herpesvirus, and rarely, gram-negative rods have all been found at this site. Our policy

Table 16.7. Clinical Approach to Fever and Pulmonary Infiltrate in Cancer Patients

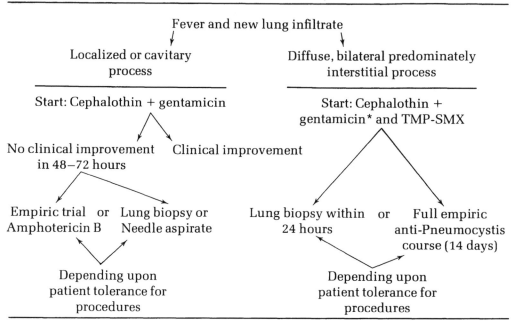

*Usually not bacterial, and empiric antibiotics often may be stopped in 48–72 hours if cultures negative.

is to obtain barium swallow x-rays in cases of severe dysphagia but to avoid endoscopy and biopsy if possible. If nystatin swallows are unsuccessful, low-dose parenteral amphotericin B is used.

Staphylococcal and gram-negative rods are common pathogens in skin ulcers in cancer patients. A relatively small and seemingly inconsequential skin process such as erythema around a finger stick or bone marrow puncture site may progress to fatal septicemia in patients undergoing intensive chemotherapy.

Patient G, a 24-year-old woman receiving intensive chemotherapy for acute myelogenous leukemia in relapse, developed pain and erythema at the site of a finger stick. Within 24 hours she became febrile and blood cultures were obtained. White blood cell counts were in the 300–500/mm³ range during this period. Antibiotic coverage was begun with cephalothin and gentamicin, but the patient failed to re- *spond. Blood cultures and cultures of material draining from her infected finger both grew Klebsiella. The patient expired five days after noticing the painful finger.*

Careful skin care, including such measures as avoidance of unnecessary intravenous equipment and care of nail beds, cannot be overemphasized.

4.0 Newer methods for prophylaxis and therapy for infection in cancer patients

Vaccines. The high incidence of gram-negative infection in cancer patients has led to consideration of either vaccination against gram-negative bacteria or the use of hyperimmune serum for patients infected with gram-negative rods. To date, the only commercially produced vaccine for gram-negative bacteria is a *Pseudomonas aeruginosa* vaccine made from antigenic lipopolysaccharide cell wall components. Although not approved for general distribution, several clinical trials with this vaccine have been conducted in cancer patients. The largest randomized trial showed a significantly lower incidence of Pseudomonas-associated deaths among a group of 170 vaccinated cancer patients. A smaller trial in children with leukemia was not able to confirm this, however. Although such endotoxinlike side effects as fever and local pain are common with this vaccine, a recent study showed that a small local dose of corticosteroid would improve patient tolerance without significantly decreasing antibody response. At present, the role of Pseudomonas vaccine or hyperimmune serum therapy for cancer patients is unsettled. It may prove particularly helpful in hospitals with high rates of nosocomial Pseudomonas infection.

Other attempts to vaccinate for gram-negative infections have used the concept of cross-reacting antibodies. For example, immunization of rabbits with a core glycolipid from *Salmonella minnesota* protected from challenge with a wide variety of non-Salmonella gram-negative rods. Cross-reacting antigen vaccines or antisera are being studied in humans.

Prophylactic antibiotics. To date, several successful uses of absorbable oral antibiotics (TMP-SMX) for prevention of bacterial infections in neutropenic patients have been reported. Furthermore, a recently completed randomized study of prophylactic oral TMP-SMX designed specifically to prevent Pneumocystis in a high-risk population has produced positive results.

Oral, nonabsorbable antibiotics have been used to decrease the number of potential pathogens in the gastrointestinal tract. It is hoped that these antibiotics will also decrease opportunistic infection during periods of neutropenia. In one randomized study, the use of oral gentamicin, vancomycin, and nystatin signfi-ciantly reduced the number of infections, even when patients were not put into reverse isolation quarters although a separate, randomized study was unable to confirm these findings. Because the incidence of diarrhea, foul tastes, and general patient intolerance of oral, nonabsorbable antibiotics is high (20% or more) it is difficult to use them in clinical practice. It has not been standard at our institution to employ these drugs unless a totally sterilized (e.g., laminar air flow room, or "Life Island,") environment has also been provided.

Sterilized environments. It has been shown in randomized studies that leukemia patients undergoing chemotherapy will have fewer infections if they are kept in a sterilized environment and given nonabsorbable antibiotics for gut decontamination. This is a considerable undertaking both psychologically and economically, and it does not guarantee success. A recent review of the large number of studies of sterile environment protection for neutropenic cancer patients is noteworthy for the conflicting data among these reports. Until the cost and effort can be justified for all cancer patients receiving chemotherapy, the use of sterile environments on a routine basis will likely not take place.

Granulocyte transfusion therapy. One of the most exciting developments in treating sepsis in neutropenic cancer patients has been the increasing availability of granulocyte transfusion therapy. Several methods for collecting granulocytes from normal donors are now available, and cells need not be HLA matched to the recipient for effectiveness. Two recent randomized trials of granulocyte transfusion therapy in neutropenic cancer patients have shown benefit for patients who have proven sepsis during prolonged periods of neutropenia. The use of granulocytes for fever without proven infection was of no benefit. In most neutropenic patients, it is impossible to predict at the onset of fever whether blood cultures will be positive; the question that remains is whether to administer granulocytes and then to stop them if cultures are negative. In one study, transfusions were only begun after positive cultures were obtained. Even with this delay in therapy, the transfusion group had better survival rates.

Among the side effects from granulocyte transfusion therapy are fever, hypotension, pulmonary infiltrates, and even death. Granulocyte transfusions are clearly not without risk, nor are collection techniques or blood bank facilities adequate to provide these cells on a routine basis for all patients who appear to need them. It also is not known whether granulocyte transfusions affect long-term survival. Nevertheless, this technique for replacing the most critical cell in host defense against gram-negative infection is quite promising and deserves continuing investigation.

5.0 Summary

Infection is now seen as the single most important complication for patients with hematologic neoplasias and is also a growing problem in patients with solid tumors. Intensive and potentially curative chemotherapy is limited primarily by neutropenia rather than by thrombocytopenia. Thus, current investigative efforts to develop better methods for prophylaxis and therapy of infection in this high-risk population are well directed.

Several encouraging advances in dealing with infection in cancer patients have been made in recent years. Newer aminoglycosides that are active against highly resistant strains of gram-negative bacteria are becoming available. Granulocyte transfusions also appear valuable for gram-negative infections in neutropenic pa-

tients. Gram-negative (Pseudomonas) vaccines are currently studied in cancer patients. Aspergillus pneumonia, hitherto believed to be uniformly fatal in immunosuppressed cancer patients, has now been successfully treated at several centers. A new and less toxic therapy for Pneumocystis is also available, and mortality from this infection appears to be decreasing. More effective and earlier use of invasive diagnostic techniques for patients with fever and lung infiltrates has at least partially accounted for this improvement in treating opportunistic lung infection. The recent success of adenine arabinoside for herpes simplex encephalitis offers the possibility that this agent may be of value for other herpes viral infections in cancer patients. Probably most helpful for clinicians, however, has been the large number of excellent clinical papers appearing over the past seven years describing the epidemiology of infection in cancer patients. These studies alllow an enlightened approach to the empiric therapy of fever in immunocompromised patients when no microbiologic information is available.

The most important advances in preventing infection in cancer patients will likely be made when the defects of host defenses are exactly defined for each clinical setting (e.g., tumor and drugs) and when specific immunologic protection (e.g., immuno-enhancing agents, specific cell-type transfusions) can be given.

References

Alavi, J. B. et al. A randomized clinical trial of granulocyte transfusions for infection in acute leukemia. N. Engl. J. Med. 296:706–711, 1977.

Armstrong, D.; Young, L. S.; Meyer, R. D.; and Blevins, A. H. Infectious complications of neoplastic disease. Med. Clin. North Am. 44:729–745, 1971.

Bloomfield, C. F., and Kennedy, B. J. Cephalothin, carbenicillin and gentamicin therapy for febrile patients with acute nonlymphocyte leukemia. *Cancer* 34:431–437, 1974.

Bode, F. R.; Pare, A. P.; and Fraser, R. G. Pulmonary diseases in the compromised host. *Medicine* (Baltimore) 53:255–293, 1974.

Bodey, G. P. et al. Quantitative relationships between circulating leukocytes and infection in patients with acute leukemia. *Ann. Intern. Med.* 64:328–340, 1966.

Chang, H. Y. et al. Causes of death in adults with acute leukemia. *Medicine* (Baltimore) 44:249–268, 1976.

E. O. R. T. C. International Antimicrobial Therapy Project Group. Infection in febrile granulocytopenic patients with cancer. *J. Infect. Dis.* 137:14–29, 1978.

Fauci, A. S.; Dale, D. C.; and Balow, J. E. Glucocorticosteroid therapy: mechanisms of action and clinical considerations. *Ann. Intern. Med.* 84:304–315, 1976.

Feld, R.; Bodey, G. P.; Rodrigues, V.; and Luna, M. Causes of death in patients with malignant lymphoma. *Am. J. Med. Sci.* 258:97–106, 1974.

Feldman, N. T.; Pennington, J. E.; and Ehrie, M. G. Transbronchial lung biopsy in the compromised host. *JAMA:* 1377–1379, 1977.

Gurwith, M. et al. A prospective controlled investigation of prophylactic trimethoprim-sulfamethoxazole in hospitalized granulocytopene patients. Amer. J. Med. 66:248, 1979.

Herzig, R. H. et al. Successful granulocyte transfusion therapy for gram-negative septicemia: a prospectively randomized controlled study. *N. Engl. J. Med.* 296:701–705, 1977.

Hughes, W. T.; Feldman, S.; and Chandhary, S. Comparison of trimethoprimsulfa-methoxazole and pentamidine in the treatment of *Pneumocystis carinii* pneumonitis.

Pediatr. Res. 10:399A, 1976.

Hughes, W. T. et al. Successful chemoprophylaxis of pneumocystis carinii pneumonitis. *N. Engl. J. Med.* 297:1419–1426, 1977.

Lau, W. K. et al. Comparative efficacy and toxicity of amikacin/carbenicillin versus gentamicin/carbenicillin in leukopenic patients. *Am. J. Med.* 62:959–966, 1977.

Leventhal, B. G.; Cohen, P.; and Triem, S. C. The effect of chemotherapy on the immune response in acute leukemia. *Isr. J. Med. Sci.* 10:866–887, 1974.

Levine, A. S. et al. Protected environments and prophylactic antibiotics. A prospective controlled study of their utility in the therapy of acute leukemia. *N. Engl. J. Med.* 288:477–483, 1973.

Levine, A. S.; Robinson, R. A.; and Hauser, J. M. Analysis of studies on protected environments and prophylactic antibiotics in adult acute leukemia. *Eur. J. Cancer* 11:Supplement 57–66, 1975.

Levine, A. S.; Schimpff, S. C.; Graw, R. G.; and Young, R. C. Hematologic malignancies and other marrow failure states: progress in the management of complicating infections. *Semin. Hematol.* 11:141–202, 1974.

Pennington, J. E. Aspergillus pneumonia in hematologic malignancy: improvements in diagnosis and therapy. *Arch. Intern. Med.* 137:769–771, 1977.

Pennington, J. E. Bronchoalveolar cell response to bacterial challenge in the immunosuppressed lung. *Am. Rev. Respir. Dis.* 116:885–893, 1977.

Pennington, J. E. Fever, neutropenia and malignancy. A clinical syndrome in evolution. *Cancer* 39:1345–1349, 1977.

Pennington, J. E. Infection in the compromised host: recent advances, and future directions. *Semin. Infect. Dis.* 1:42–168, 1978.

Pennington, J. E.; Reynolds, H. Y.; and Carbone, P. P. Pseudomonas pneumonia: a retrospective study of 36 cases. *Am. J. Med.* 55:155–160, 1973.

Pennington, J. E. et al. Use of a pseudomonas aeruginosa vaccine in patients with acute leukemia and cystic fibrosis. *Am. J. Med.* 48:629–636, 1975.

Pennington, J. E., and Feldman, N. T. Pulmonary infiltrates and fever in patients with hematologic malignancy. *Am. J. Med.* 62:581–587, 1977.

Rodriguez, V.; Burgess, M.; and Bodey, G. P. Management of fever of unknown origin in patients with neoplasms and neutropenia. *Cancer* 32:1007–1012, 1973.

Schimpff, S. C. et al. Origin of infection in acute nonlymphocytic leukemia. *Ann. Intern. Med.* 77:707–714, 1972.

Schimpff, S. C.; Satterlee, W.; Young, V. M.; and Serpick, A. Empiric therapy with carbenicillin and gentamicin for febrile patients with cancer and granulocytopenia. *N. Engl. J. Med.* 284:1061–1065, 1971.

Schimpff, S. C. et al. Infection prevention in acute nonlymphocytic leukemia: laminar air flow room reverse isolation with oral, nonabsorbable antibiotic prophylaxis. *Ann. Intern. Med.* 83:351–358, 1975.

Shaefer, J. C.; Yu, B; and Armstrong, D. An aspergillus immunodiffusion test in the early diagnosis of aspergillosis in adult leukemia patients. *Am. Rev. Respir. Dis.* 113:325–329, 1976.

Sickles, E. A.; Greene, W. H.; and Wiernik, P. H. Clinical presentation of infection in granulocytopenic patients. *Arch. Intern. Med.* 135:715–719, 1975.

Singer, C.; Kaplan, M. H.; and Armstrong, D. Bacteremia and fungemia complicating neoplastic disease. *Am. J. Med.* 62:731–742, 1977.

Tattersall, M. H. N. Aggressive cancer treatment and its role in predisposing to infection. *Eur. J. Cancer* 11:Supplement 9–19, 1975.

Tattersall, M. H. N.; Speirs, A. S. K.; and Darrell, J. H. Initial therapy with combination of five antibiotics in febrile patients with leukemia and neutropenia. *Lancet* 1:162–166, 1972.

Walzer, P. D. et al. *Pneumocystis carinii* pneumonia in the United States: epidemiologic, diagnostic, and clinical features. *Ann. Intern. Med.* 80:83–93, 1974.

Weitzman, S., and Aisenberg, A. C. Fulminant sepsis after the successful treatment of Hodgkin's disease. *Am. J. Med.* 62:47–50, 1977.

Williams, D. M.; Krick, J. A.; and Remington, J. S. Pulmonary infection in the compromised host. *JAMA*: 1377–1379, 1977.

Young, L. S.; Meyer, R. D.; and Armstrong, D. Pseudomonas aeruginosa vaccine in cancer patients. *Ann. Intern. Med.* 79:518–527, 1973.

Young, L. S.; Stevens, P.; and Ingram, J. Functional role of antibody against "core" glycolipid of enterobacteriaceae. *J. Clin. Invest.* 56:856–861, 1975.

Young, R. C.; Bennett, J. E.; Geelhoed, G. W.; and Levine, A. S. Fungemia with compromised host resistance. A study of 70 cases. *Ann. Intern. Med.* 80:605–612, 1974.

Chapter 17

Psychologic Complications of Malignancy

C. Gates

P. Hans

1.0 Background

A diagnosis of cancer is catastrophic both to the patient and to the patient's family. Cancer can strike people of all ages, from the youngest infant to the oldest grandparent, but all cancer patients are faced with a sudden shocking threat to mortality. The threat to a young person's life is usually considered more devastating and tragic than is the threat to an elderly person whose life has been lived and who is more susceptible to other life-threatenting illnesses. Still, stress for all cancer victims is severe.

Stress. The major variables are how patients handle stress and what it means to them. Each person who has had experience with stress in the past has developed a style for handling it and so has an established automatic response when new stresses occur. Part of the evaluation of cancer patients should be a careful inquiry as to what stresses have afflicted the patient in the past, how he or she has dealt with them, and what support has been available from important family members.

The stress of cancer includes not only the diagnosis, but the possibility that the disease will not respond to treatment, or even if it does respond, the likelihood of recurrence and eventual threat to life. Cancer causes chronic stress both from the disease itself and from the various treatments. These stresses are additional burdens in the daily lives of cancer patients.

Cancer therapy generally involves surgery, radiation therapy, chemotherapy, or combinations of these. Obviously, surgery to remove a breast or a leg is traumatic to the patient. While the patient is relieved that the disease may have been cured, the amputee must endure an irreparable cosmetic or functional change. Similarly, the stress of radiation therapy and chemotherapy compounds the morbidity of the treatment.

Self-esteem. Cancer has a devastating emotional impact on the patient's self-esteem. Cancer and its treatment are severe assaults on the person's body, and attitudes toward the body are components of self-esteem. A person's life style includes those activities and attitudes that coincide in forming and maintaining self-esteem. This can be viewed as a kind of emotional hematocrit for which such injuries to self-esteem as cancer and its treatment are metaphors for blood loss. If blood is not properly regenerated, symptoms develop to compensate for the loss and preserve homeostasis.

The final common issue for dealing with stress is maintaining self-esteem.

The process for handling stress provides a mechanism for preserving optimal self-esteem. Part of the process involves restitution, if possible, and compensation. For example, a breast or limb prothesis, reconstructive plastic surgery, and organ implantation, all help to repair the injury to self-esteem. Patients often plunge into new activities or address their old ones with renewed vigor, thereby compensating for losses sustained to their bodies. Cancer patients and their families frequently lead their lives with a renewed drive and energy after the assault of the disease and its treatment.

Some reactions to stress are not helpful to patients and cause further emotional stress and damage. These are the all-too-familiar situations of patients who work too hard, withdraw from their friends and families, attempt new activities, affairs, or marriages, all of which end badly and generate additional stress. While injuries

to self-esteem cause patients to respond with hostility, this anger can either stimulate energy for renewed efforts, or if handled inappropriately, can lead to negative activity and further injury. Therefore, how patients have handled anger in the past, their awareness of hostility, and their usual mechanisms for handling stress are important to understand. In this sense, it is necessary both to deal with actual injuries and to encourage responding to the injuries in an adaptive way.

The patient-family interaction. The diagnosis of cancer is a blow to the patient's immediate family as well as to the patient. Clearly, a mother with breast cancer, a father with lung cancer, a brother with Hodgkin's disease, or a son or daughter with leukemia will affect everyone in the family. Feelings of guilt, of regret, and of wanting to be "special" often influence how family members feel and act toward each other.

Sometimes the illness can bring family members closer together, deepen relationships, and promote growth. Unfortunately, the opposite also occurs, and family members often are driven apart when one family member is seen as a scapegoat. This increases emotional distances.

The psychopathology of cancer as well as its psychotherapeutics involves the entire family/friend/patient structure.

For example, a cancer patient can put his or her spouse in an impossible position, and in many ways the partner may feel unable "to do anything right." This ambiguity has a negative impact on the relationship since spouses often misunderstand the patient's efforts to handle stress and so find themselves withdrawing from the relationship.

In addition, the enormous emotional problems of cancer are accompanied by financial burdens. Expenses often accrue for direct medical care, medicine, and institutional services that even the best insurance does not fully cover. Additional costs may arise for transportation, houseworkers or other assistants, protheses, dressings, and other equipment.

It is obvious that both the patient's emotional state and those of the spouse and family should be considered when cancer is diagnosed. The family should be evaluated periodically to see whether its members are responding in the most productive way.

Evaluation of personal and interpersonal psychologic support systems. The clinician providing the primary therapy interacts with the patient intuitively to evaluate the psychologic systems the patient uses to sustain self-esteem. Thus, psychologic assessment is a crucial part of patient care. The physician must understand the patient's reaction to the diagnosis of cancer, to treatment, to the health care team, to family and friends, and to the environment. The family structure must be considered in addition to the patient's activity and life goals.

The past medical history can also help in understanding reactions to stress and resolutions of previous stressful situations, such as loss of a family member, job failure, or other personal trauma. The physician should evaluate the appropriateness of the interaction with the health care team as well as the perspective of the other members. For the most part, the physician accomplishes the evaluation intuitively and develops a "subjective gestalt," which helps to determine an approach to the patient. Objective assessment by such formal psychologic testing as the Minnesota Multiphasic Personality Inventory (MMPI) has been used to predict and evaluate a patient's reactions to cancer.

Time influences the overall resolution of internal and interpersonal conflicts.

Sufficient time is needed to recognize life's value and to develop a sense of proportion. Acceptance of the realities permits the patient and family to share their grief, and expressing remorse allows growth and transition to a subsequent stage. Rapid transition from apparent health to a terminal state precludes time for emotional evolution and often provokes the family's guilt and hostility toward the medical care team. Similarly, prolonging the dying process may accentuate the patient's fear of dependence and loss of dignity, while the family members become increasingly intolerant of the interruption to their lives. Thus, a critical factor in developing psychologic support systems is an understanding of the course of the disease.

2.0 Psychologic reactions to cancer diagnosis

The first hurdle the patient confronts is the diagnosis, and here preconceived and erroneous notions about cancer influence the patient's reaction. Previous defenses against stress are equally important. The three major psychologic reactions to a diagnosis of cancer are denial, withdrawal, and anger.

Denial. Emotional defenses are unconsciously motivated regulatory processes that help a person deal with emotional trauma too overwhelming to be accepted on a fully conscious level. For example, denial is operating when one sees a disaster and responds with shock, numbness, or inability to believe. Denial prevents awareness of overwhelmingly painful feelings when they are a part of everyday life, and it can be very healthy. It is the most common initial reaction to a diagnosis of cancer and protects all patients from intensely emotional reactions to any severe emotional stress.

Denial, to preserve the patient's sense of immortality, is the most common reaction to a diagnosis of cancer.

Denial involves both awareness of the facts and awareness of feelings surrounding the facts. Patients, often demonstrating a biologic developmental urge toward specificity, have varying capacities to handle denial. Denial allows the patient to be aware of the diagnosis and to pursue the optimal treatment method, but prevents him or her from constant awareness and preoccupation with the illness. Healthy denial does not block other areas of emotional response, thus permitting the patient to respond in other situations not related to the cancer treatment.

Most denial, however, is nonspecific. The process that blots out awareness and responsiveness to the cancer reduces responsiveness and awareness in other areas of life. This is particularly true for a patient whose cancer is thought to be under control but who has a recurrence or develops metastases. Denial often blankets the patient's emotional life, or as one physician put it, the patient "pulls down the shade." This is why patients who show strong emotional reactions to the diagnosis, to initial treatments, and to amputations and mutilations sometimes exhibit a blasé attitude about the same losses when the disease recurs.

Withdrawal. Withdrawal, both emotional and physical, is another common reaction to the diagnosis and treatment of cancer. It is similar to denial in that patients simply draw into themselves and become less responsive to their environment. As with denial, the process can be either adaptive or maladaptive depending on its use. Some withdrawal from peripheral activities and reinvestment in human relationships is very healthy.

Patient A, a 62-year-old chronic schizo-phrenic, developed an intra-abdominal malignancy of unknown primary tumor site that disseminated rapidly within the abdominal cavity. The patient complained bitterly of secondary symptoms, including abdominal pain, nausea, and vomiting. Because of her psychiatric history, the patient was isolated and became progressively withdrawn. She refused to eat or to sleep and finally refused to leave her bed. She gradually assumed a fetal position and became totally uncommunicative. She died within three weeks of both the initial diagnosis and the withdrawal syndrome.

Withdrawal is unhealthy when a person withdraws from family and friends, stops performing usual activities, and loses the self-esteem that might have helped compensate for the injury sustained from the illness and treatment. Withdrawal, like denial, should be diagnosed and monitored with both the patient and the family members.

Anger and hostility. Such writers as Kubler-Ross have noted that hostility is part of the reaction to cancer, severe stress, and thoughts of death (1970). Hostility is not a phase through which one passes, but shows inner feelings without the patient's emotional defenses. Hostility is a response to the injuries inflicted by the illness and its treatment and is expressed in many ways by patients who continue their activities. In cancer patients, the threshold for hostility is often slowly eroded so that minor stresses of daily life become irritating. Traffic jams, disconnected telephone calls, or a child's refusal to do something are more likely to provoke an angry response than they might have otherwise.

Hostile reactions among patients are as varied as they are in the general population and include everything from temper outbursts and physical violence to such subtle forms of withdrawal as depression and passive-aggressive behavior.

Patient B, a 37-year-old woman with primary lung cancer, presented with superior vena cava syndrome and was treated initially with radiation therapy; her symptoms resolved rapidly. When informed of her diagnosis, she was somewhat sullen. She began to smoke more frequently and was secretive about her home life. It was subsequently learned that her husband had left her. She required intermittent hospitalization, and on each occasion she would ask her physicians to wait while she prepared herself with her morning ablutions. With each encounter she distanced herself further and further from the medical team.

Anger is the most destructive reaction to a cancer diagnosis and creates alienation from the health care team, thereby perpetuating the anger.

The physician should specify how the patient handles hostility, to what degree it is put to productive use, and whether it serves to increase the distance between the patient and others. Disharmony between the patient and the medical personnel interferes with treatment.

3.0 Psychologic reactions to cancer therapy

The impact of cancer treatment can be both temporary and permanent. Patients' reactions to therapy depend on a complex interaction between the physical stress of treatment and the impact on self-esteem.

Therapy may compromise self-esteem when it causes a cosmetic or functional disability.

Temporary side effects of treatment can include nausea and vomiting secondary to chemotherapy or radiotherapy. For most patients, these effects pass in 24 to 48 hours after treatment, but the severity and duration of reactions differ. A patient's anxiety can aggravate and prolong an otherwise normal physiologic reaction to chemotherapy, causing nausea and vomiting in anticipating or remembering treatment.

Alopecia is another side effect that occurs with a variety of chemotherapeutic agents and usually lasts for the duration of treatment. Good wigs are available and provide a temporary solution for many patients, but even with a wig, hair loss may be traumatic for both cosmetic and symbolic reasons. One woman was afraid of sleeping on an airplane for fear her wig would slip off and people would know her condition. A man was very upset with his hair loss, fearing that since the hair was dead the same thing would soon happen to him. In this case, his denial of illness was compromised by the physical reality of the hair in his comb, on his shoulders, and in the bathtub.

Surgical intervention can bring permanent changes. Probably the most difficult surgery to adjust to is maxillofacial disfigurement from head and neck cancers. Dramatic emotional accommodation is required by the patient; no hiding under a wig or behind a prosthesis is possible. Support from the family and the medical staff is essential in providing such patients with enough confidence to go out in public and continue their daily activities. It is remarkable that most patients adapt emotionally both to the cosmetic injury and to the functional losses involved.

Mastectomy for breast cancer is generally well tolerated biologically. The experience, however, is traumatic to most women and the few men who undergo the operation. Feeling like a freak, sexless, or deformed are frequent reactions. The considerable interest in reconstructive surgery and in excision or radiation as alternatives to mastectomy speak for the efforts patients make to avoid disfigurement when their survival is not jeopardized. Reactions to mastectomy vary, but maladaptive reactions to mastectomy occur in about 20 percent of cases. For example, one patient who had a caring and supportive husband and family and a stable home life, underwent the operation and returned to her previous life style within several weeks. Another patient, who also had a loving husband and family, had trouble sleeping and moderately severe postoperative depression. She had suffered polio as a child and walked with a leg brace and cane and therefore had expected herself to handle the stress of mastectomy well. The opposite occurred because the mastectomy stirred up many unresolved feelings about her previous illness, which added to the burden of her current stress and contributed to her depression.

Colostomy, while hidden from the public, is a recurrent reminder of disease to the patient. The continuing burden of having to empty the bag daily, to keep an adequate supply of bags on hand, and to care properly for the stoma are borne remarkably well by most people. Colostomy clubs in which participants discuss their experiences, their problems, and their solutions for living with a colostomy attest to the value of ongoing support, but times of particular anxiety include sexual contact and public showers. When patients report problems keeping the bag in place, stoma irritation, or other physical symptoms, an emotional difficulty often exists as well. A careful history of the physical problem and its interference with daily life, activities, and relationships usually points to these emotional difficulties.

Amputation, for which lower limb loss is the most common form, is generally well tolerated by most patients. Patients require considerable contact with others for rehabilitation and for fitting and use of a prosthesis. This interpersonal contact provides considerable emotional support. As with colostomy and, to a lesser extent, mastectomy prostheses, patients are constantly reminded of their illness. Their emotional lives are changed, and they must accommodate to limb loss and prosthesis use.

Support systems to deal with therapy-induced self-esteem deterioration must deal with the psychologic as well as physical effects of the cancer.

4.0 Psychologic reactions to the terminal stage

Virtually any type of response is possible for cancer patients during the terminal phase of illness. It is usually not a single response that occurs when a person faces the prospect of death, but rather a complex and changing pattern of thoughts, moods, and behaviors. How an individual acts and reacts during the late stages of cancer depends on the interaction of many factors, including earlier reactions to crisis, the nature of the illness and its specific psychologic significance, the degree of physical debility, the psychosocial context, and the degree to which the patient has accepted death.

All people use psychologic mechanisms and maneuvers, both conscious and unconscious, in an effort to tolerate, accept, and overcome stressful events in their lives. Valliant, in describing these mechanisms, has attempted to link them to stages of psychosocial development (1977). It must be emphasized that these mechanisms are universal and that their mere presence does not imply either mental health or psychologic illness. The behavior exhibited by a dying person should not be viewed as absolutely adaptive or maladaptive. Only when a particular mechanism is used exclusively or inflexibly should it be ascribed to psycho-

pathology. In addition, behavior that
may initially seem bizarre, in fact, may be
highly adaptive.

*Patient C, a 69-year-old woman who was
unmarried and a retired executive secre-
tary, had breast cancer for 15 months. She
had been hospitalized with extensive
bone metastases that caused excruciating
pain and rapid deterioration. Because
curative measures were no longer feasible,
she was treated palliatively with potent
analgesics. While in the hospital, she
became disoriented in the evenings and
described richly elaborated delusions
in which she was in an foreign land. The
delusions were accompanied by vivid
visual hallucinations. Whenever medical
or nursing staff came to see her, she
would engage them in protracted conver-
sation having to do either with her illness
or her personal reminiscences.*

*In psychiatric consultation, it became
evident that she feared losing all that was
familiar and dear. She yearned for her
relationship with her family doctor rather
than with her oncologist. She tried des-
perately to maintain her affective grasp on
people and memories of what had been
a gratifying earlier life. She repeatedly
expressed the wish for someone to rely on.
She and a younger sister were the only
remaining members of her family and she
often spoke of being the last of her line.*

*Although her demands for attention
were often counter-productive because
staff felt that they were exploited, became
annoyed, and withdrew, her behavior
was an attempt to make a human connec-
tion and to hang on to it while her world
was unstable and rapidly slipping away.*

Certain psychologic responses manifested by fatally ill persons are encountered commonly. As discussed earlier, denial is both a conscious and an unconscious process by which anything too
painful or unacceptable is erased from
awareness. It is one of the most important,

valuable, and common self-preservative
devices used during the terminal phases of
cancer.

*Patient D, a 53-year-old divorced woman
with three adult children, presented in
the final stages of widespread ovarian
carcinoma. A colostomy, which had been
performed to allow normal feeding and
maintain the patient at home, had become
obstructed, but no further anticancer
therapy was considered. The prognosis
was explained in detail to the patient and
to her family. Despite knowledge of her
disease state, realization of the uncomfortable measures that would be required
to sustain her and the obvious severe
physical inanition, the patient maintained
a cheerful countenance, avoided talking
about death, and expressed the hope
that she would soon improve and attain
her previous level of functioning.*

This tenacious denial of a confirmed prognosis helped the patient to sustain an
image of courageous independence that
had always been her style. Denial is common in those who have been lifelong
optimists. It also enabled her to maintain
a posture toward her family that made
them willing to care for her at home and
therefore kept her attachment to them
very strong. Denial, however, should not
be reinforced by the physician, nor should
the patient be ceremoniously reminded
of the prognosis.

A second defense mechanism and
source of strength is intellectualization,
which enables a person to replace anxiety-
producing feelings with rational thought
processes. Thus, the recognition that
death is near may be avoided or made eas-
ier by a preoccupation with such things
as minute details of daily events, objective
discussions of drug side effects, or read-
ings about statistical studies of cancer.
Another defense mechanism is displacement, the process by which feelings
aroused by a person or situation are redi-

rected toward relatively less important people or things. The effect is to help the individual avoid or to decrease the discomfort associated with the original source of the feelings.

Patient E, a hospitalized 59-year-old man, who was a retired Marine Corps officer, presented with inoperable and untreatable metastatic lung carcinoma. He expressed acceptance of his disease, stating that he had led a full and satisfying life, had accomplished most of his goals, had enjoyed his family and his work, and felt he had made a positive contribution to society. He saw his cancer as one of a series of hardships people had to endure in life, believed he had managed far more disturbing stresses in the past, and thought he could tolerate this one.

The patient entered the hospital for investigation of a small, seemingly unimportant cyst on his scalp. Although he was relatively unconcerned about his carcinoma, he showed intense feelings about the cyst. He bitterly complained that the doctors were not paying enough attention to his lesion, and felt frustrated and angry about the relative indifference of the medical and nursing staff.

This patient displaced his concern over his terminal illness to worry about an inconsequential scalp lesion. His anger was not directed at the carcinoma, and his own impotence to do anything about it, but rather at the failure of his physicians to take adequate care of his cyst.

Reaction formation produces thoughts and/or behavior directly opposite to what the person is experiencing consciously. Therefore, patients frightened by a growing sense of weakness and helplessness may attempt in exaggerated ways to prove their strength and independence.

When seeking gratification of needs, patients often revert to forms of behavior associated with an earlier level of psycho-

social development. The behavior is called regression.

Patient F, a 58-year-old man, was unmarried and had always lived alone and taken pride in his ability to care for himself. He developed inoperable laryngeal carcinoma and had radiation therapy following tracheostomy to relieve airway obstruction. Throughout almost one year of out-patient treatment, he was able to function well on his own. Shortly after radiation therapy ended and despite no objective worsening in his condition, he appeared at the emergency room demanding that he be admitted to the hospital. After an intense argument with the patient, the emergency room staff decided to admit him briefly so that an adequate evaluation could be made and an appropriate disposition worked out. Once in the hospital, the patient rapidly regressed. He insisted that someone else shave him and he claimed he could not clean and maintain his tracheostomy, demanding that a nurse do it for him even though he had done it for months at home. Although he had no physical restrictions, he denied that he could perform even routine tasks and withdrew to his bed. Only when he was given an absolute deadline for leaving the hospital did he change this behavior and secure appropriate living arrangements with a relative.

Everyone facing imminent death needs to adapt to what is essentially a painful and usually dreaded situation. Integrating the many physical and psychologic traumas associated with dying requires time, effort, capacity to change, and acknowledging and accepting loss. To the extent that this can be accomplished, a person may achieve some level of equanimity.

The fear of mutilation or pain, not death itself, creates the greatest potential for psychopathology.

Weisman and Hackett suggest that death can lose much of its terror if it is viewed as appropriate (1972). Weisman elaborated on the idea of an "appropriate death."

Appropriate deaths are those which suffering is at a low ebb, conflict is minimal and behavior has been maintained on as high a level as is compatible with physical status. Moreover, the dying patient indicates that what has already been done corresponds to what he expected of himself, of the people who matter most, of those to whom he turned for relief, and finally of the world in general. Literally and metaphorically it is time to die. Relief of anguish and resolution of remaining conflicts join in a harmonious exodus. The patient both accepts and expects death and is willing albeit ruefully to die. It is the ultimate of successful coping!!

A critical aspect of patients' psychological adaptation is the way they die. Patients will accept death as ultimate peace if they can be reassured of an absence of pain, availability and commitment of professional care, and freedom from becoming a burden to loved ones.

The adaptation process is often more difficult for the family than for the patient. A critical therapeutic ingredient is time, time to grieve and to share grief, thus allowing an acceptance of the inevitable. This essential and universal process dictates the need in most patients for knowing the diagnosis and the prognosis.

The patient and family who are mutually aware of the dying state may be able to communicate more effectively and to resolve their individual anxieties.

Weisman has suggested a series of responses that people may have when faced with the threat of catastrophic illness or death and has linked these responses with the capacity to cope (1972). He defines coping as "a goal directed process related to defined problems and intended to bring about relief, reward, quiescence and equilibrium." Using the work of Sidle and co-workers (1969), Weisman has a list of approaches that are helpful for estimating how well an individual is adapting to the prospect of death. In this process, a person may:

1. Find out more before acting (rational investigation).
2. Talk it over with someone to relieve distress (share concern).
3. Laugh it off, see humor in the situation (reversal of affect).
4. Try to forget, don't worry, wait and see (suppression/isolation/attachment).
5. Put mind on other things, do something for distraction, carry on business as usual (displacement/diversion).
6. Carry out positive action based on present understanding (confrontation/negotiation).
7. Rise above it, accept the situation, find something favorable or encouraging, make virtue out of necessity (redefinition/rationalization/reinterpretation).
8. Submit to the inevitable, stoic acceptance of the worst (passivity/fatalism).
9. Do something, anything, however ambiguous, impractical, reckless, irrelevant or magical (acting out/impulsive acts/compulsive rituals).
10. Consider alternatives based on past situations (rigid or uncorrected repetition).
11. Drain off or reduce tension with eating, smoking, drinking, drugs (tension relief by physiologic means).
12. Get away from it all, fantasize or pretend (social withdrawal/stimulus reduction/avoidance).
13. Blame someone or something, disown responsibility, get angry (projection/externalization).

14. Comply, yield to authority, seek direction (adopt a role/obediance/compliance).
15. Blame self, atone, sacrifice (masochistic surrender).

These various maneuvers may facilitate adaptation. By keeping these options and responses in mind and evaluating them in the context of the patient's illness, treatment, and interpersonal relationships; the physician, family, and patient may better maximize strengths and help one another through this most difficult period.

5.0 Role of spouse

The spouse has a key role in the care of the cancer patient. It is most important that the spouse be taken into routine evaluation and ongoing care and that reports of a spouse's disinterest or unavailability be investigated carefully. Patients frequently provoke distance between themselves and their spouses, rendering each other helpless at times of stress. The patient feels lonely, and the spouse feels useless.

When patients are in distress, they can create situations that put spouses in a helpless position. An extreme example was a terminal cancer patient who accused her husband of infidelity. The husband was not unfaithful but could not convince his wife of that. Careful investigation of the situation revealed that because the patient felt inundated, she created a situation that overwhelmed her husband. After identifying the problems, it became possible to help the patient become aware of her outrage and helplessness. Treatment was effected through the spouse, who recognized that his wife was depending on him for this kind of help.

The wife of a 35-year-old lymphoma patient was greatly concerned about her husband. He had been active both professionally and socially in the community, but his illness forced him to stay at home, caused discomfort, and changed his activities. He made increasing demands on his wife and would ask her for assistance and reject it when it was offered. The patient's wife was able to withstand the rejection and able to discuss the problem with her husband. They agreed that he would no longer make inordinate demands on her. A careful balance between support and definite limits allowed her to stay with her husband and provide him great support.

The 39-year-old husband of a terminal breast cancer patient was not able to accept his wife's illness. In previous times of stress, he would leave the house, overindulge in alcohol, and go to the dog races. This pattern was repeated when his wife's illness became worse. He bet heavily on the races and lost household money that was needed for the patient's care. When he took money from his children, outside intervention was required to limit his activities. He had previous emotional losses and was clearly unable to cope with the stress of his wife's illness.

6.0 Role of the family

Like the spouse, the total or extended family is very important in the emotional support of cancer patients. Although it is generally not possible to evaluate the emotional configuration of cancer patients' families, every member of the patient's immediate family is emotionally involved.

Consequently, patients often ask physicians what they should tell their children about their cancer. The implication is that if they say nothing, the children will not know and will thus be spared the sadness and heavy emotional burden of the illness. Physicians should remind patients that since 70 percent of communication is nonverbal, it is impossible for a family not to communicate to children that something is radically wrong. Depending on the age of the child, the parents should acknowledge that an illness exists, that they are concerned, but that care has been undertaken. Frequently, young children will then ask, "Is Mommy (or Daddy) going to die?" This can be alarming both to patients and to spouses because death is utmost in their own minds, and they usually do not want to think about it.

In general, children can tolerate thoughts of death and mutilation if their parents and families can draw closely together through common concern. If parents cannot tolerate these feelings, but rather try to hide them, the children will sense the confusion, will soon realize that discussion is not allowed, and will not talk about it. Children who are not given the facts, however, will manufacture explanations for inconsistencies they see. However frightening and gruesome the actual facts are, the child's fantasies are usually more terrifying and therefore more devastating.

It is well for the physician to realize that if family functioning is compromised when one of its members has cancer, the emotions aroused by the illness and treatment may be responsible. Some of the obvious symptoms are deteriorating performance in school or on the job, alcoholism, drug abuse, gambling, and other self-destructive activities. Family dynamics are complex and not easy to clarify, but the physician can be alert when family members show signs of distress. This is a time for diagnostic intervention by a social worker, psychologist, or psychiatrist.

Patient G, a 39-year-old woman with advanced breast cancer, had a 16-year-old daughter and a 19-year-old son. Within six months of diagnosis of her recurrent cancer, the daughter became pregnant out of wedlock, and the son had a serious motorcycle accident. The family situation was out of control. The patient consulted many different doctors; the husband was unable to set limits; and the children acted out in ways that were self-destructive and clearly revealed their distress.

As with individual patients, families have a self-esteem that represents the combined self-esteem of its members. This value is obviously assaulted in cancer, but the response can be productive, spurring all family members on to closer communication and heightened awareness of life and its opportunities. It is often difficult to stabilize a family, but the alert physician can at least monitor family functioning.

7.0 Psychotropic drug therapy

Three major symptom complexes that might require the use of psychotropic drugs for cancer patients are anxiety, depression, and toxic psychosis. Psychotropic medication should be considered whenever the patient's capacity to function becomes seriously impaired at work or in social situations and when psychologic factors pose a major threat to the patient's safety or to the safety of others. Recognizing that depression, for example, is an appropriate response to impending death, does not preclude the prudent use of drug therapy if the psychologic reaction is overwhelming.

Psychotropic drug therapy should be considered whenever the excessive reaction interferes with life style, regardless of the qualitative appropriateness of the reaction.

Anxiety. Although anxiety may manifest itself at any time during the course of a neoplastic illness, it is strongest at the time of diagnosis, at initiation of treatment, and at realization of treatment failure. It may take many forms including feelings of apprehension or dread, tension, worry, and restlessness, or such somatic symptoms as hyperventilation, sweating, palpitations, and lightheadedness. Mild to moderate anxiety is a universal and normal response to stress. In these situations, it is usually self-limited and may not require any specific measures. A patient's emotional resources and reassurance from supportive people are sufficient. It can be a great relief to a patient simply to know that what he or she is experiencing is normal and will pass. Allowing patients to ventilate feelings, discussing any fears they may have, helping to clarify ambiguous situations, and answering any questions that may arise enables most people to tolerate and to overcome most of the emotional obstacles encountered during the course of the illness.

The three potentially critical stress times to the cancer patient are presentation of the diagnosis, initiation of treatment, and failure of treatment.

When the intensity of feeling is disabling, or when the anxiety becomes pervasive, it may be necessary to use medication to alleviate the patient's symptoms. Work, social activities, sleep, and sexual performance all may be adversely affected by excessive anxiety. In most instances, the drugs of choice are the benzodiazepines (Table 17.1). They are safe, effective, and have few side effects. Within this family of drugs, flurazepam hydrochloride (Dalmane) is the only compound designated as a hypnotic, although all drugs in this class can induce sleep. For patients whose anxiety is not reduced with a benzodiazepine, low doses of a neuroleptic, a major tranquilizer, may be helpful. The selection depends not so much on the drug's effectiveness, as all are effective in equivalent doses, but rather on the presence or absence of side effects. For example, where the goal is relief of anxiety without sedation, such high potency drugs

Table 17.1 Sedative-Hypnotics: Benzodiazepines

Generic Name	Trade Name	Dosage Range MG/Day	Duration of Action
Tranquilizers			
Chlordiazepoxide	Librium, generic	15–100	Long 12–24 hours
Chlorazepate	Trenxene	15–60	Long
Diazepam	Valium	6–40	Long (> 40 hours)
Oxazepam	Serax	30–120	Short 8–15 hours
Lorazepam	Activan	25–30	Short 8–18 hours
Hypnotics			
Flurazepam	Dalmane	15–30	Long

as trifluoperazine hydrochloride (Stela-
zine) or haloperidol (Haldol) may be used.
If, in addition to decreased anxiety, sedation to aid sleep is desired, the choice
might be chlorpromazine (Thorazine) or
thioridizine (Mellaril).

Organic psychoses. Organic psychoses
are common in patients with carcinoma,
especially the elderly. The mental disorders may result from systemic effects of
the primary illness, medications used
in treatment, or from brain metastases. Delirium, by far the most common clinical
problem encountered, usually consists of
disorientation or memory disturbance;
disturbance of attention; perceptual disturbances manifested either by simple
misinterpretation of the environment, by
delusions and hallucinations, by increased
or decreased psychomotor activity, or by
sleep disturbance. The clinical features
usually develop rapidly and characteristically fluctuate over time. No matter what
the cause, the patient's symptoms are
always secondary either to destruction of
brain tissue or to general cerebral dysfunction. Treatment with medication
should therefore be used cautiously as
most psychoactive drugs will either intensify central nervous system depression
or produce powerful effects on neuro-
transmitters, which may only worsen or
confuse the clinical picture. Before initiating any drug therapy, it is necessary to
rule out other treatable causes of a disordered central nervous system such as
electrolyte disturbances, hyper- or hypocalcemia, uremia, hepatic failure B_{12} or
folate deficiency, drug intoxications, and
the various endrocrinopathies. Correction
of these metabolic abnormalities, discontinuance of unneeded medications, or
revision of the tumor-specific therapy are
the most important initial steps.

Another important measure in treating
organic psychoses involves placing the
patient in a suitable environment and
providing protection with frequent or

constant observation. The patient should
be cared for in a quiet, well-lighted room
where there is a minumum of activity.
The use of consistent personnel, family
members, or other familiar people is very
important. Calm reassurance, help in
maintaining orientation, and the slow,
clear repetition of instructions for procedures or changes in location are helpful in
avoiding problems. Where drugs are to
be used, the choice should depend on the
presenting symptoms, the desired results,
and a thorough knowledge of the medication used.

Sedative hypnotics are generally contraindicated because all cause central
nervous system depression and are therefore potentially more dangerous than
helpful. The barbituates, chloral hydrate,
glutethimide, methyprylon, ethchlorvy-
nol, and methaqualone all interfere with
REM sleep and induce enzyme activity
in the liver. Barbiturates can have such
paradoxical effects as causing excitement
in the elderly. Chloral hydrate and other
chloral derivatives interfere with protein
binding. Other drugs, such as the antihis-
tamines, probably interfere with REM
sleep and potentiate the action of anticholinergic drugs.

The neuroleptic agents can be very effective if used judiciously (Table 17.2).
Where agitation or violence is especially a
problem, low doses can control symptoms
without undue sedation. Severe anxiety or
panic can also be effectively managed.
Where disturbed sleep patterns and ex-
haustion are prominent, an appropriate
choice might be one of the low-potency
drugs such as chlorpromazine. These
have significant sedative effects and when
given at night can help to produce calm
and to induce sleep. These drugs, however, also cause orthostatic hypotension
and have powerful anticholinergic effects;
consequently, they should be used only
when these properties will not produce
serious problems. The high-potency drugs
such as trifluoperazine, haloperidol, and

Table 17.2 Neuroleptic Agents: Dosage Potential Side Effects

Drug	Initial dose	Sedation	Ortho-static hypo-tension	Anticho-lingergic effects*	Extrapy-ramidal effects†	Cardio-vascular effects	Genitouri-nary effects
			Side Effects				
Phenothiazines Aliphatics Chlorpromazine (Thorazine)	50–150 mg PO 25–50 mg IM	+ + + (80 %)	+ + +	+ + +	(1) + (2) + + (3) + +	+	+ +
Piperidines Thioridazine (Mellaril)	25–100 mg PO	+ + +	+ + +	+ + +	(1) + (2) + + (3) +	+ +	+ + +
Piperazines Trifluoperazine (Stelazine)	2–4 mg PO		+ +	+ +	(1) + + (2) + + + (3) + + +	+	+
Butyrophenones Haloperidol (Haldol)	1–2 mg PO/IM		+	+	(1) + + (2) + + + (3) + + +		
Thioxanthenes Thiothixene (Navane)	2–4 mg PO		+	+ +	(1) + + (2) + + + (3) + + +		

*Dry mouth, mydriasis and cycloplegia, tachycardia, decreased intestinal mobility, urinary retention, and delirium in high doses
†Extrapyramidal side effects (15% overall)
  1. Dystonias (5–10%)
  2. Akathesia (50%)
  3. Parkinsonism (40%)
  + + + = severe reaction; + + = moderate reaction; + = mild reaction

thiothixene can significantly decrease agitation, hostility, and severe anxiety; in low doses these drugs do not produce sedation, orthostatic hypotension, or significant anticholinergic effects.

Depression. Depression is an endemic response to major illness and ordinarily does not require intervention in the form of psychotherapy or medication. Most depressive episodes are mild and temporary and can be managed by the patient alone. At times, others can help in this process by attentive listening, sympathy, and emotional support. The person's symptoms can, however, intensify and take on the character of a true depressive syndrome. The patient becomes depressed or irritable; insomnia occurs, often with early morning wakening, and the patient becomes anorectic. Psychomotor retardation may markedly slow movement and thinking; agitation may be shown by pacing, hand wringing, or severe restlessness. A significant decrease in interest in activities the patient ordinarily enjoys may affect work, social, or sexual functions. The patient often feels unusually fatigued, even with adequate rest; diurnal variation may occur so that a patient feels more depressed in the morning. Marked feelings of hopelessness, worthlessness, and pessimism are common. Feelings of guilt may be pervasive and intense, at times reaching delusional proportions. For example, some patients unreasonably blame themselves for hardships imposed on others, or they see themselves as causes of misfortunes such as floods or fires. Patients often experience difficulty concentrating and may be bothered by wandering thoughts or indecisiveness. Suicidal thoughts often intrude into conscious thinking and may become pervasive. About one-fourth of all depressed people complain of somatic symptoms, particularly of the gastrointestinal tract and musculoskeletal system. Once this syndrome develops, it can become autonomous (i.e., unresponsive to the environment), and the patient becomes unable to take pleasure in situations or in people who ordinarily would bring them happiness.

This set of symptoms makes a patient an excellent candidate for antidepressant medication. The tricyclics are generally the drugs of choice and can be effective in 70 to 90 percent of cases (Table 17.3).

Psychotropic drugs for the elderly. For patients over 60 years of age, there are significant changes in the ways medications are absorbed, metabolized, and excreted. Psychotropic medication should, initially and maximally, be one-quarter to one-third of the usual dose, and the medication should be increased much more gradually than for younger individuals. This is especially true of the antidepressants. The neuroleptics and benzodiazepines have a broad therapeutic range

with relatively benign side effects. The tricyclic antidepressants are far more dangerous especially because of their cardiac toxicity, anticholinergic properties, and orthostatic hypotension, and careful observation and caution in their use is advised.

8.0 Psychotherapy

The indications for psychotherapy are similar to those for drug intervention. In both cases, the individual has symptoms that have not been responsive to support, reassurance, or clarification; have persisted beyond a reasonable length of time; or interfere significantly with the patient's capacity to function in a reasonably normal way.

The problem may be obvious, with the physician, patient, and family all acknowledging that psychologic factors are having a substantial and deleterious effect on the individual's life. A more complicated situation exists when the patient denies any difficulty and maintains a happy and trouble-free facade contrary to other evidence of dysfunction. This false posture may take various and often subtle forms. The person may stop working or may take increasing numbers of sick days with little justification. Patients at home may spend longer periods of time in front of television or lying in bed. They may

Table 17.3 Tricycle Antidepressants

Generic name	Trade name	Dosage range mg/day
Amitriptyline	Elavil	50–300
Nortriptyline	Aventyl	50–100
Protriptyline	Vivactil	15–60
Imipramine	Tofranil	50–300
Desipramine	Norpramin, Pertofane, Pamelor	75–300
Doxepin	Adapin, Sinequan	75–300

gradually lose interest in activities that had been attractive and exciting. Mood changes with periods of crying or marked irritability may ensue. Sleep patterns may be disrupted. The physician becomes aware of an increasing number of telephone calls or visits but cannot find any physical changes to account for these. The patient may become preoccupied with relatively minor physical problems that do not respond to medical intervention, or may worry over minor details of the treatment regimen. Whenever the patient uncharacteristically increases contact with the physician or has complaints that are incompatible with the physical findings, the doctor should suspect an underlying emotional problem and consider psychiatric evaluation.

Choice of individual counseling, group psychotherapy, or a combination of the two will depend on the situation and availability of resources. For patients who feel that they are the only people ever to experience cancer and who seem to be especially isolated, a group setting can be extremely helpful. Groups are also valuable for families of cancer patients and for couples whose otherwise good relationship is severely stressed by the distorting influences of a chronic, intense, and often fatal illness. Individual psychotherapy might be more appropriate when the onset or course of the illness precipitates, exacerbates, or intensifies an internal conflict that can best be handled by the patient alone. It might also be the treatment of choice for the patient who feels too embarrassed or shy to share other feelings with a group.

9.0 Summary

The psychologic complications of malignancy are characteristic and develop in a consistent and chronological pattern in all patients. The intensity and duration of the psychologic reaction to the diagnosis, to therapy, or to the terminal stages determines pathology. The maintenance of self-esteem is crucial in sustaining normal functioning despite adverse effects of therapy. The management of emotional complications depends on an awareness of and sensitivity to the patient's psychologic reactions and interpersonal relations and on the capacity to support the patient's stability. The primary care physicians, nurses, social workers, and other health care professionals together with the patient's family should be aware of the potentialy overwhelming psychologic experience that cancer is to the patient.

References

Aronson, J. *The realization of death: a guide for the psychological autopsy.* Boston: Little, Brown and Co., 1974.

Baldessarini, R. J. *Chemotherapy in psychiatry.* Cambridge, Mass.: Harvard University Press, 1977.

Barton, D., ed. *Dying and death: a clinical guide for caregivers.* Baltimore: Williams and Wilkins, 1977.

Dunphy, E. J. Annual discourse on caring for the patient with cancer. *N. Engl. J. Med.* 295(6):313–319, 1976.

Holland J., and Frei, E., III. *Cancer medicine.* Philadelphia: Lea & Febiger, 1973.

Krant, M. The role of a hospital-based psychosocial unit in terminal cancer illness and bereavement. *J. Chronic Dis.* 29:115–127, 1976.

Kubler-Ross, E. *On death and dying.* New York: Macmillan, 1970.

Mastrovito, R. D. Cancer: awareness and denial. *Clin. Bull.* 4(4):142–146, 1974.

Norton, J. *Treatment of a dying patient: the psychoanalytic study of the child.* London: International Universities Press, 1963.

Rosenbaum, E. H. *Living with cancer: a*

guide for the patient, family and friends. New York: Praeger Publishers, Inc., 1975.

Schmale, A. H. Psychological reactions to recurrences, metastases or disseminated cancer. *Int. J. Radiat. Bio.* 1:515–520, 1976.

Shader, R. I., ed. *Manual of psychiatric therapeutics.* New York: Little, Brown and Co., 1974.

Sidle, A. et al. Development of a coping scale. *Arch. Psychiatry* 20:226–232, 1969.

Vaillant, G. E. *Adaptation to life.* Boston: Little, Brown and Co., 1977.

Weisman, A. D., and Hackett, T. P. Predilection to death: death and dying as a psychiatric problem. *Psychosom. Med.* 23:232–256, 1961.

Weisman, A. D., and Worden, J. W. *Coping and vulnerability in cancer patients.* National Cancer Institute research report. Boston, 1977.

Weisman, A. D. *On dying and denying: a psychiatric study of terminality.* New York: Behavioral Publications, 1972.

Weisman, A. D., and Worden, J. W. The existential plight in cancer: the significance of the first 100 days. *Int. J. Psychiatry.* 7:1–15, 1977.

Chapter 18

Complications of Cancer Therapy

R. Weichselbaum
R. Goebbels
J. Lokich

1.0 Background

The cancer cell represents uncontrolled growth of a normal cell population secondary to either mutation or a carcinogenic stimulus. Cancer therapy involves two modalities, radiation and cytotoxic drugs, that lack specificity for the cancer cell. As a consequence, a narrow therapeutic index is observed for the majority of treatment regimens. Tumor-cell kill is a dose-response phenomenon based on first-order kinetics; therefore, substantive therapeutic effect on the cancer cell results in major compromise to normal cells exposed to the therapeutic agent. In contrast, immunotherapy may be selective for tumor cells. Complications of immunotherapy are theoretically important nonetheless and include the potential for augmentation of cancer growth.

The mechanism by which chemother-apy or irradiation induces adverse host effects may be classified on the basis of either organ site or chronology (whether the effects are acute or chronic).

Acute reactions to therapeutic modalities are due either to immunologic (allergic) mechanisms or to interruption of DNA synthesis at the cell level.

Acute reactions are generally a consequence of a direct effect of the therapeutic modality on DNA synthesis with secondary interruption of a regenerative capacity. Chronic adverse effects are a consequence of a cumulative effect on the tissue with a secondary host reaction. Systemic reactions to therapy, particularly the constitutional symptoms such as lassitude, are classified separately, generally developing

during therapy. Their severity is unpredictable, but they are uniformly transient.

**Chronic reactions to therapeutic modali-
ties are due to a cumulative reaction to
therapy and may appear months to years
after treatment is discontinued.**

This chapter will consider the acute,
long-term, and systemic effects of chemotherapy and irradiation as well as the
adverse effects of combined modalities.
Systemic and organ-related complications
of immunotherapy, although currently
investigational, will also be described.

2.0 Acute effects of chemotherapy

The three general categories of acute complications secondary to cytotoxic drug
therapy are hematologic and immunologic
suppression; gastrointestinal effects including nausea, vomiting, and bowel
function abnormalities; and cutaneous or
epithelial changes including effects on
the integument, nails, hair, and mucosal
surfaces. Such effects are generally dose
related and reversible.

Bone marrow suppression. With few
exceptions, the cytotoxic drugs uniformly
inhibit the bone marrow stem cells to
produce anemia, leukopenia, and thrombocytopenia. The degree of bone marrow
suppression is variable and depends on
the drug, dose, and schedule of administration. Marrow suppression is an important monitor of the biologic effectiveness
of drug therapy and assures the adequacy
of the therapeutic dosage. Assuming a
dose-response relationship for tumor-cell
kill, the concomitant effect on the formed
elements to produce leukopenia and
thrombocytopenia attests to the adequacy
of the cytotoxic drug dose.

**Marrow suppression is generally dose
related. Nadir and risk intervals are pre-
dictable and are related to dose, cumulative drug effect, and marrow reserve.**

The quantitative nadir level of the white
blood cell or platelet count and the chronology of the peripheral manifestations of
marrow suppression similarly depend
on the drug, dose, and schedule. Generally, the nadir blood counts are achieved
at 10 to 14 days after initiation of therapy,
and the duration of leukopenia (defined as
white blood cell count < 3500 cells/mm^3
and platelets $<$ than $100,000$ cells/mm^3)
persists for 5 to 7 days. Many therapeutic
programs involving multiple-drug chemotherapy are based on these chronologic
variables so that drug schedules involve
treatment at three- or four-week intervals.
Some drugs, particularly the nitrosoureas
and mitomycin C, induce leukopenia
and thrombocytopenia in a delayed fashion with nadir achieved at 21 to 28 days;
the intermittency of therapy is therefore
extended to six- or eight-week intervals.

The principles for monitoring patients
receiving cytotoxic drug therapy and the
use of blood products including platelets,
granulocytes, protein fractions (hyperimmune globulin), and bone marrow reconstitution by transplantation are reviewed
in Chapter 11. Blood product support
during the nadir period, either prophylactically or therapeutically, can effectively control the secondary complications
of hemorrhage and infection while marrow restitution and regeneration are
achieved. Bone marrow transplants may
occasionally be employed, but these are
generally reserved for patients whose
diseases primarily affect the bone marrow,
such as leukemia. Such bone marrow
stimulants as androgens have been used
with chemotherapy to minimize the peripheral cytopenias. In some studies androgens have also been effective in pre-

venting the anemia associated with cytotoxic drug therapy, but such methods have not generally been successful.

Immunosuppression. Drug therapy affects the immunologic system as well as the bone marrow. Immunosuppression can be consistently demonstrated in a variety of in vitro and in vivo assays of immunologic function, and like the peripheral cytopenias, may be expressed to a variable extent depending upon the drug, dose, and schedule. A major rationale for intermittent therapy has been the observation that chemotherapy acutely compromises immunologic function, and that with immunologic restitution various parameters of immune function are exaggerated. Potentiation of this exaggerated immunologic system with such immune stimulants as bacillus Calmette-Guerin has been studied in a variety of therapeutic trials. Restitution of immunologic function by bone marrow transplantation, thymic transplantation, provision for passive transfer by sensitized lymphocytes, transfer factor, and immune RNA are areas of intense investigation.

Gastrointestinal effects. Adverse effects of cytotoxic drugs on the gastrointestinal tract are extremely difficult for the patient and physician to control. Fear of nausea and vomiting is one of the major deterrents to therapy and is the basis for therapy withdrawal in many instances. Although this effect is categorized as an acute-phase reaction, the pathophysiologic mechanism is not related to interference with the replicating mucosal cells of the gastrointestinal tract. The two most prominent mechanisms for the induction of nausea and vomiting are a direct effect on the emesis center in the thalamus and the secondary conditioning effect that develops and is reinforced as therapy continues. The emetic stimulus directly mediated

The gastrointestinal effects of chemotherapy are compounded by the behavioral conditioning effect, which becomes more prominent than the direct drug effect.

through the central nervous system develops approximately 1 hour following drug administration and may persist for 6 hours to 8 hours, after which mild anorexia may be present for an additional 24 hours. In some treatment programs, initiation of emesis is delayed for 5 hours, such as with the common combination chemotherapy program of cyclophosphamide and Adriamycin, but the duration of the gastrointestinal effect is similarly transient, lasting only 6 to 8 hours. A unique effect of the drug imidazole carboxamide (dacarbazine, DTIC) is tachyphylaxis, in which the drug's emetic stimulus decreases with time.

The treatment of drug-induced emesis with phenothiazines and sedation is suboptimal, but new antiemetic drugs including phenothiazine congeners and marijuana derivatives such as tetrahydrocannabinol are under investigation. Table 18.1 lists common antiemetic drugs and their uses in the management of chemotherapy-induced nausea and vomiting.

The quantitative measurement of the adverse gastrointestinal effects of cytotoxic drugs is variable; a small proportion of patients will experience either minimal gastrointestinal effects or none at all. As treatment continues, a conditioned response to emesis accentuates the intensity of the vomiting as well as its duration. Patients may, in fact, experience vomiting even before the administration of therapy. The interruption of conditioning may be accomplished by prophylaxis, such as inducing behavior modification through a variety of mechanisms including hypnosis. Although hypnosis may be effective after a conditioned response is established, deconditioning is difficult. A potentially

Table 18.1 Antiemetic Programs for Chemotherapy

Antiemetic drugs Generic name	Trade name	Dose units	Recommended dose
Cyclizine	Marezine	50-mg tablets	50 mg t.i.d. or q.i.d., up to 200 mg/day
		50-mg ampules	50 mg t.i.d. or q.i.d., IM only, up to 200 mg/day
		100-mg supplements	100 mg t.i.d. or q.i.d., up to 400 mg/day
Benzquinamide	Emete-con	50-mg vial	0.5–1.0 mg/kg IM. First dose may be repeated in 1 hour, and every 3–4 hours thereafter. First dose only may be given IV (0.2–0.4 mg/kg).
Perphenazine	Etraton Triavil	2-, 4-, 8-, or 16-mg tablets	Up to 30 mg/day in divided doses
	Trilafon	5 mg ampules	5–10 mg IM up to 30 mg/day
			5 mg IV, single dose only
Prochlorperazine	Combid Compazine Eskatrol	5-, 10-mg tablets	10 mg t.i.d. or q.i.d.
		10-, 15-mg "spansules"	15–20 mg/day
		10 mg ampules	5–10 mg IM every 3–4 hours, up to 40 mg/day
		25 mg supplements	25 mg b.i.d.
Thiethylperazine	Torecan	10 mg tablets	10–30 mg/day
		10 mg ampules	10–30 mg/day, IM only
		10 mg supplements	10–30 mg/day
Trimethobenazmide	Tigan	250 mg capsules	250 mg t.i.d. or q.i.d.
		200 mg ampules	200 mg t.i.d. or q.i.d., IM only
		200 mg supplements	200 mg t.i.d. or q.i.d.
Haloperidol	Haldol	0.5-, 1-, 2-mg tablets	1–2 mg
Sedatives			
Secobarbitol	Antora-B Seconal	200–400 mg po or ½ IM and ½ po	
Diazepam	Valium	10 mg	

Timing	Combined Therapy
Evening or morning prior to visit	Tranquilizer or antiemetic
1 hour before anticipated emesis	Sedative and antiemetic
Every 4–6 hours, to 24 hours thereafter	Antiemetic

more effective prophylactic measure may be the use of anamnestic drugs for sedation at the time of cytotoxic drug administration.

Ulceration of the mucosal lining is commonly observed with the antimetabolites, particularly with 5-fluorouracil and methotrexate. Symptomatic stomatitis or oral mucosal ulceration and proctitis are tran-sient effects that may be managed locally with topical anesthetic agents. Diarrhea may develop as a consequence of or in association with mucosal ulceration with hypermotility of the bowel. An uncommon effect on the gastrointestinal tract is observed with the periwinkle alkaloids. Vincristine particularly compromises the neurogenic supply to the bowel and re-

Table 18.2 Cutaneous Reactions to Cytotoxic Drug Therapy

Dermatologic Manifestation	Associated Drug	Comment
Bullous eruption (hives)	Methotrexate L-Asparaginase	Allergic mechanism
Desquamation	Bleomycin Methotrexate 5-Fluorouracil	Dose related and idiosyncratic
Pustules	Actinomycin D	Dose related, radiation recall
Pigmentation	Adriamycin Busulfan	Dose related

sults in secondary constipation that may progress to obstipation. This effect is transient but may persist for an extended period.

Cutaneous effects. The integument including the skin, hair, nails, mucosal lining, and conjunctiva can all be affected by cytotoxic drugs. A classification of the dermatologic manifestations of a variety of cytotoxic drugs is indicated in Table 18.2 (see also Chapter 12). The cutaneous reactions are relatively uncommon as a group and for the most part are dose related. Desquamative skin reactions associated with bleomycin therapy can be correlated with pulmonary toxicity for the drug (Fig. 18.1). The extreme desquamative reaction associated with methotrexate therapy can be life threatening and is typically manifested as the "scalded skin" syndrome. Although 5-fluorouracil rarely causes a skin reaction, idiosyncratic reactions to it are generally desquamative and associated with significant alopecia. The actinomycin skin rash is often acneiform with pustular formation. The rash may develop in an area of previous radiation and may arise in part because of the radiation-sensitizing effect of actinomycin D.

Hyperpigmentation is common with Adriamycin; particularly in the pigmented races, and develops on mucosal surfaces as well. Such pigmentary effects are generally not reversible and are observed in the nail beds as discrete horizontal lines. These lines represent a secondary manifestation of growth arrest.

Hair loss is a common accompaniment to the administration of many but not all cytotoxic drugs. Adriamycin, cyclophosphamide, and vincristine are the most potent inducers of alopecia; the anthracycline derivatives generally produce total scalp alopecia as well as loss of eyebrows, eye lashes, and axillary and pubic hair. Other drugs, predominantly the alkylating agents, induce partial alopecia. Regeneration of hair, particularly in the scalp, is often not complete until two or more months following completion of chemotherapy although hair growth may be observed even during treatment. Scalp hair generally begins to recede within 3 weeks, and hair loss reaches a maximum by 6 to 10 weeks. Prevention or amelioration of scalp alopecia has been reported in anecdotal cases through the use of the scalp tourniquet technique. In one randomized trial, the scalp tourniquet, which

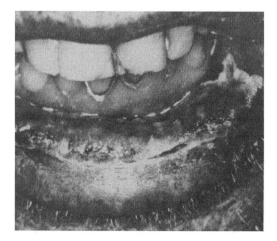

Fig. 18.1 Ulceration up to but not beyond the vermilion border of the lip in the patient receiving methotrexate. The precise border delineation along the transition zone between mucosal and the dermal epithelium is dramatic and diagnostic of drug-specific effect.

necessitates maintenance of pressures more than 40 mm Hg above systolic arterial pressure for at least 20 minutes, decreased the likelihood of scalp alopecia. The tourniquet presumably excludes drugs from the hair follicle area but may also exclude drugs from tumor implants present in the subcutaneous scalp.

The mucous membrane component of the integument, which includes the vaginal mucosa, glans penis, anus, and oral cavity, is directly affected by many of the chemotherapeutic agents, especially by the antimetabolities. The effect on the integumentary mucosa is similar to that of the gastrointestinal mucosa. In addition, the antibiotics, particularly actinomycin D and Adriamycin, may induce mucosal ulcerations. Reconstitution of the mucosal surface is generally achieved by five to seven days after the maximal effect, which develops at five to seven days following drug exposure. A related effect on surface epithelium is observed in the conjunctiva,

particularly with methotrexate, Adriamycin, and 5-fluorouracil. The conjunctival effect is compounded by the loss of eyelash protection and a change in the lacrimal fluid secretion, which functions as a lubricant. Thus, antitumor drugs can produce a clinical conjunctivitis that is manifested as inflammation. This effect is transient, and supportive therapy with artificial tears and topical decongestants is employed although the effectiveness of these products is limited.

Cutaneous necrosis secondary to extravasation of sclerosing drugs at the injection site represents the most devastating cutaneous complication of cytotoxic drug therapy. A number of cytotoxic drugs are topical irritants and must be administered intravenously to avoid necrosis (Table 18.3). The nonsclerosing drugs may be administered orally or intramuscularly without adverse effects on the tissues. Sufficient dilution of drug concentration and meticulous attention to and monitoring of the intravenous infusion are important prophylactic procedures, but the drugs often affect the veins by inducing local endothelial sclerosis of the vein wall. With time, the risk of extravasation increases as adequate vein access becomes more difficult.

Patient A, a 72-year-old obese woman with metastatic breast cancer, was treated over a prolonged period with a variety of chemotherapeutic regimens. When the bracheoplexus syndrome and edema of the right arm developed, venous access was restricted to the left arm. Treatment with Adriamycin infusion in this patient resulted in extravasation, which was unrecognized at the time of injection. Two days following the injection, erythema and pain developed at the local injection site (Fig. 18.2). The erythema increased over the next five days, and a cutaneous septic process was suspected. Central pallor developed, and subsequent necrosis

Table 18.3 Classification of the Cytotoxic Drugs According to Irritant Effect
on Veins*

Sclerosing Drugs	Nonsclerosing Drugs
Adriamycin	5-Fluorouracil
Actinomycin D	Methotrexate
Mitomycin C	Cytosine arabinoside
Vincristine	Bleomycin
Nitrogen mustards	Cyclophosphamide
Imidazole carboxamide dacarbazine (DTIC)	

*Mechanism unknown, but these drugs may lead to thrombosis of veins with continuous use
and to ulceration and necrosis if extravasation occurs.

*required debridement of the entire area
and skin grafting. The necrotic process involved tendons as well as vacular
channels.*

Extravasation may not be recognized immediately but should be suspected in
patients who complain of pain at the injection site during the injection procedure.

**Extravasation of sclerosing or irritating
drugs may not result in clinical effects for
two to three days.**

The pain may be a consequence of venous vein wall irritation, and if it is not
diminished by slowing the rate of injection, or if adequate blood return is not
achieved, the infusion should be discontinued. If extravasation is established
clinically, tissue binding of drugs such as
Adriamycin may be diminished by instill-
ing an 8.4 percent bicarbonate solution
(5 cc) along the same needle tract. The
secondary administration of corticosteroids, predominantly decadron, through
the needle in place or by a multipuncture
gun, may be applied additionally. The
success of such treatment has not been
established, but empiric application has
suggested that the technique decreases

evolving necrosis. The surgical approach
requires debridement of the entire area
as well as grafting, depending upon the
extent of the necrosis.

3.0 Chronic effects of chemotherapy

The chronic adverse effects of cytotoxic
therapy can be classified according to
organ system. These are neurologic and

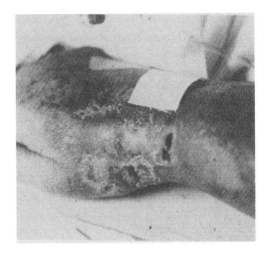

*Fig. 18.2 Depigmentation and scaling
approximately five days following extravasation of Adriamycin into the subdermal and subcutaneous tissues.*

muscular effects, pulmonary effects, cardiac effects, hepatic effects, and urinary tract and genital function effects. The mechanisms by which the drugs induce organ-specific toxicity are variable and in some instances unknown, but the quantitative effect is generally dose related and cumulative. In contrast to the reversibility of acute adverse effects of chemotherapy, many of the chronic effects are prolonged and sometimes permanent.

Neurologic toxicity. A number of cytotoxic chemotherapeutic agents are associated with neurologic toxicity (Table 18.4). These can be classified as effects of the central nervous and peripheral nervous systems, and are generally reversible. The peripheral neuropathies are the most common, and the prototypical drug is vincristine. The related periwinkle alkaloid, vinblastine, rarely causes neurologic effects. Vincristine is an inhibitor of the microtubular substance in cells and affects the tube-sheathing structure in motor and sensory sheathing nerves as well as the autonomic nervous system. Early mani-

Table 18.4 Cytotoxic Drugs Associated with Neurologic Toxicity and Myalgia Syndromes

Central Nervous System Toxicity
  Procarbazine
  L-Asparaginase
  Methotrexate
  5-Fluorouracil
  Mithramycin

Peripheral Nervous System Toxicity
  Vincristine
  Procarbazine

Myopathic Toxicity
  Periwinkle alkaloids
  Corticosteroids
  Imidazole carboxamide (dacarbazine, DTIC)

festations of vincristine neurotoxicity are sensory parasthesias of the peripheral extremities. These parasthesias are experienced by virtually 100 percent of patients treated with the usual therapeutic doses. The agent is discontinued, however, only if motor function is compromised. Restitution of neurologic function may develop only after a protracted period of weeks to months.

The second most common drug associated with peripheral neuropathy is procarbazine, a methyl hydrazine derivative employed almost exclusively for the treatment of Hodgkin's disease in the combination chemotherapy regimen, MOPP [Mechlorethamine (nitrogen mustard) + Oncovin (vincristine) + Procarbazine + Prednisone]. The mechanism of peripheral neuropathy may be related to an interference with pyridoxine metabolism. The peripheral neuropathies that develop in association with drug therapy may be accentuated in patients with an underlying neuropathic disease such as diabetes.

Drug-induced neuropathy may be accentuated in patients with underlying neuropathy.

The less common central nervous system effects of chemotherapeutic agents are generally manifest as a nonspecific encephalopathy associated with somnolence or disorientation. These manifestations are often transient, although methotrexate-induced encephalopathy associated with intrathecal administration or high doses of the drug may produce permanent neurologic effects. A unique form of cerebellar ataxia and dysfunction has been associated with 5-fluorouracil and may be a direct consequence of a metabolic breakdown of this drug into fluorocitrate. L-asparaginase, which is employed predominantly for acute leukemia, is associated with an encephalopathy of varying severity in more than 25 percent of patients, and may be accentuated in patients with hepatic abnormalities.

The myopathic effects of cytotoxic drugs may or may not be related to the neuropathic effects. The periwinkle alkaloids may induce a diffuse myalgia five to seven days following drug administration; in 20 percent of patients imidazole carboxamide (DTIC) produces a flulike syndrome that is associated with muscle aches. Steroid withdrawal may lead to diffuse myalgia and is common in such intermittent treatment programs as MOPP or COP [Cyclophosphamide + Oncovin (vincristine) + Prednisone]. Corticosteroid-induced myopathy is a common secondary effect of chronic daily use of the drug.

Pulmonary effects. A number of cytotoxic drugs have been associated with pulmonary side effects. The most common, drug-induced pneumonitis, occurs with bleomycin therapy (see Chapter 9). In addition to bleomycin pneumonitis, which results in an acute interstitial pneumonia and a mortality of more than 50 percent, chronic interstitial fibrosis develops in a dose-related fashion beyond 200 mg/M^2 cumulative dose. Busulphan has also been associated with an interstitial pneumonitis that is progresssive and chronic. Cyclophosphamide, nitrosoureas, and methotrexate induce similar pulmonary changes in function as well as radiographic alterations; the pathophysiologic mechanism for these changes is unclear. Methotrexate in particular has been associated with a pleurisy-type reaction in addition to alveolar consolidation. Cyclophosphamide-induced lung toxicity has invariably been associated with extremely high doses of the drug and with patients receiving cyclophosphamide prior to bone marrow transplantation.

Cardiac toxicity. Although 5-fluorouracil and cyclophosphamide have been

implicated as agents inducing cardiomyopathy, the protocotypical drugs associated with cardiac toxicity are the anthracycline compounds daunomycin and Adriamycin. In approximately 10 percent of patients, cardiac arrhythmias, predominantly sinus tachycardia and abnormalities of the electrocardiogram, are observed acutely but are not associated with secondary clinical effects and are always reversible. The major dose-related form of cardiac toxicity developing in association with the anthracyclines is a cardiomyopathy characterized clinically by progressive congestive heart failure.

Patient B, a 38-year-old woman with metastatic breast cancer, was treated with a combination of cyclophosphamide and Adriamycin to a maximum cumulative dose of 450 mg/M^2. Because of continuing remission of her disease, therapy was continued beyond the usual maximum cumulative dose. At 700 mg/M^2 cumulative dose, the patient was clinically well, but an endocardial biopsy revealed Grade III changes characteristic of Adriamycin toxicity (Fig. 18.3). Therapy was continued nonetheless, and at 850 mg/M^2 the patient developed acute congestive heart failure. She died 36 hours following presentation of the first symptoms.

The mechanism of pathologic alteration of the myocardium may be mediated as a consequence of Adriamycin-DNA complexes with secondary dropout of muscle fibers. The effect is dose related and rarely occurs below a maximum cumulative dose of 550 mg/M^2. When Adriamycin is employed in association with cyclophosphamide or is used for patients with limited myocardial reserve, the clinical syndrome may develop at a lesser dose. Pathologic changes have been observed in patients with a maximum cumulative dose as low as 200 mg/M^2. Recent studies have suggested that when Adriamycin

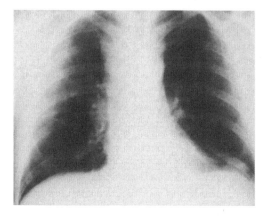 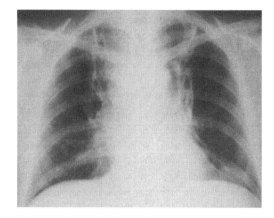

Fig. 18.3 Chest radiographs of right paratracheal tumor treated with mediastinal
radiation (A). Paramediastinal fibrosis
developed three months following radiation and conformed to the treatment port
(B).

is administered on a weekly schedule and
at a slower dose rate than prescribed by
the usual therapeutic programs, patients
are less likely to develop cardiac myopathy and may tolerate as much as 1 g/M²
cumulative dose. Approximately 30 percent of patients given anthracycline drugs
beyond the maximum cumulative dose
will develop clinical cardiomyopathy and
a mortality rate of 10 percent has been
observed, although the majority of patients
can be managed with drug withdrawal
and administration of digitalis. The clinical syndrome develops most commonly
while patients are on therapy but may
be delayed from one to three months. Prophylaxis has been possible in animal
model systems using such oxidizing
agents as tocopherol, but clinical trials
have not been initiated. Monitoring of the
cardiac effects by noninvasive measurements such as the presystolic ejection
time, the electrocardiogram, or the ratio of
the preinjection period to the left ventricular ejection time have been variably
successful in predicting subsequent heart
failure. Anthracycline therapy should
be withdrawn in patients when the maximum cumulative dose has been reached.

Hepatic toxicity. Liver function abnormalities, particularly enzymopathy, are
commonly observed with only two agents:
methotrexate and the mercaptopurines.
A drug-associated hepatitis and hepatic
fibrosis are observed in a major proportion
of patients treated with these drugs, but
generally the hepatitis syndrome is transient. The fibrosis-cirrhosis syndrome develops in less than 10 percent of patients
and only in those on long-term maintenance therapy. The drug, 6-mercaptopu-
rine, and a parent compound, azathioprine, induce clinical and pathologic
changes that are relatively infrequent as
compared with methotrexate, and the
syndrome is generally observed early.
These compounds have been employed in
the treatment of autoimmune diseases
including chronic active hepatitis. Although the nitrosoureas cause acute hepatitis less commonly, hepatic toxicity can
be observed. Liver abnormalities occur
consistently on radionuclide scans in
patients receiving nitrosoureas.

*Patient C, a 69-year-old man with colon
cancer metastatic to cervical lymph nodes,
the abdominal cavity, and peritoneal*

surfaces, was treated with 5-fluorouracil in association with the bischlorethyl nitrosourea (carmustine, BCNU). Three weeks following a five-day course of combined therapy, the patient developed jaundice and fever. On examination the cervical masses had disappeared completely. Liver scan demonstrated a shift in the radiocolloid to the spleen and bone marrow and, in general, diminution in the radionuclide absorption within the liver reticuloendothelial system. At autopsy, diffuse hepatic necrosis was observed and all tumor had disappeared.

Hepatic toxicity of drug therapy and hepatic metabolism of drugs are important considerations in treatment. For example, Adriamycin is metabolized in the liver and secreted into the biliary system. Obstruction or compromised hepatic function may therefore prolong the half-life of the drug and potentiate the general systemic toxicity of Adriamycin therapy. Another example is cyclophosphamide, which requires activation by the mitochondrial enzymes in the liver. Alterations in enzyme function and quantitative levels may result in a decreased or increased systemic toxic effect of cyclophosphamide therapy.

Urinary tract. Renal or genitourinary toxicity is often reversible; the three types are glomerular, tubular, or epithelial lesions (see also Chapter 10). The hemorrhagic cystitis associated with cyclophosphamide is a particular example of epithelial toxicity; the alteration of the bladder's mucosal epithelium is often severe enough to appear cytologically as anaplastic cell architecture. The management of hemorrhagic cystitis can be facilitated by the use of antiinflammatory drugs such as corticosteroids, but for persistent or overwhelming hemorrhage local bladder sclerosis with formalin or cystectomy may be necessary.

Gonadal function. Cytotoxic drugs predominantly affect spermatogenesis in men and the ovarian cycle in women. Chemotherapy spares Sertoli and Leydig cells in the testis so that potency and testesterone levels remain normal. Azospermia, however, occurs consistently, particularly in patients treated with alkylating drugs. These effects may last more than two years and are probably permanent in a large proportion of patients. The use of sperm storage has been recommended for patients treated with chemotherapy for potentially curable malignancies if these men have not completed their families. Unfortunately, many such patients have oligospermia as a consequence of the disease, and obtaining adequate sperm for storage may not be possible.

Sperm bank facilities are available for patients on therapy that may induce sterility.

Primary ovarian failure or disruption of estrogen secretion develops in most patients receiving alkylating drugs, and secondary abnormalities of menses, amenorrhea, and premature menopause may develop in patients who are perimenopausal. The primary determinants of ovarian failure are the drug, dose, duration of therapy, and proximity to menopause. Unlike azospermia, ovarian function in women often returns following discontinuance of therapy. It is common for younger patients completing MOPP chemotherapy or combination chemotherapy for acute leukemia to conceive and give birth.

4.0 Systemic effects of chemotherapy

The major systemic effects of chemotherapy are mutagenesis, carcinogenesis, and the general category of constitutional and psychological effects of therapy. The nonspecific effects of cytotoxic chemotherapy on a state of well being, including motivation and performance status, are difficult to assess. The metabolic imbalances and abnormalities induced by cancer chemotherapy may be subclinical or subtle, and the psychologic effects are difficult to dissect from those directly due to the tumor and the patient's premorbid psychologic standing. Nonetheless, the impact of chemotherapy on the patient's self-image, and a conglomerate of noxious insults to a variety of visceral organs may result in a secondary syndrome of withdrawal, disinterest, weakness, and lassitude. These "tertiary" effects of chemotherapy may be mitigated by education and by providing motivation for the patient and the patient's family.

Mutagenesis. The development of fetal abnormalities as a consequence of the antineoplastic drug is well established in humans. The antipurine drugs, methotrexate, and the alkylating agents have all been implicated as inducers of abortion; furthermore, a multiplicity of fetal abnormalities have been ascribed to these drugs. The periwinkle alkaloids and procarbazine have been associated with teratogenesis in animal systems. The most commonly used drug that frequently induces fetal abnormalities is methotrexate. The mutagenic effect may result in abortion if the induced anomaly is severe, or the fetus may survive to birth with a variety of structural abnormalities. The severity of the mutagenic effect depends upon the drug and the time of fetal exposure; more severe effects develop if exposure occurs during the first trimester. The effect of cytotoxic drugs on a fetus conceived after completion of therapy is unknown.

Carcinogenesis. Cytotoxic drugs, particularly the aklylating agents, have been implicated in the induction of second malignancies in patients treated for a variety of primary cancers. Of the 80 or more cytotoxic drugs in current use, only the alkylating agents have been strongly associated with second malignancies. The true incidence of second malignancies is generally unknown, and because the cytotoxic drugs have in the past been employed predominantly for patients with advanced disease and a limited prognosis, the numbers of cases of second malignancy are relatively small.

A related experience is that of renal transplants in which immunosuppressive therapy with azathioprine and prednisone is administered to patients with a substantially longer life expectancy. The incidence of primary malignancy in this population is 5 percent. The predominant neoplasm in renal transplant patients is epithelial tumors of the skin and mucosa (e.g., cervix) as well as the lung. Approximately 40 percent of the tumors, however, are mesenchymal neoplasms and histiocytic lymphomas with a predisposition to the central nervous system. De novo tumors also develop in patients treated with cyclophosphamide for autoimmune diseases. Bladder cancers are predominant in these patients. Presumably, a metabolic breakdown product of cyclophosphamide affects the transitional epithelial lining of the bladder, which is bathed by the urine containing a carcinogen.

A common second malignancy in patients treated with alkylating drugs is acute myelogenous leukemia. An increased incidence of leukemia has been associated with phenylalanine mustard therapy for multiple myeloma, breast cancer, and ovarian cancer. Although the mechanism of leukemogenesis is unclear, such patients characteristically endure prolonged periods of pancytopenia.

Another increased incidence of second malignancy, and particularly of acute leukemia, has recently been identified in patients with Hodgkin's disease who have received therapy. These patients, however, have invariably received radiation therapy in addition to chemotherapy, and the use of chemotherapy alone has not as yet been reported to increase the likelihood of the development of the second malignancy.

Distinguishing the factors involved in the development of a second malignancy is difficult. It is well known that second malignancies increase in incidence as a consequence of a first malignancy and that a genetic predisposition to multiple tumors exists. As the number of cancer patients who live long enough to develop second malignancies increases, more data about the variables involved in second tumor induction will become available.

5.0 General concepts of radiation hazard

Two general types of therapeutic radiation hazards are whole-body and localized exposure. Whole-body irradiation is employed for non-Hodgkin's lymphoma therapy, and less commonly, for other malignant diseases. This type of hazard is therefore more an environmental problem than a therapeutic one. Clinical radiotherapeutic practice concerns itself more with the complications of localized radiation treatment. For radiation therapy, as for systemic chemotherapy, both tumor control and normal tissue damage follow a sigmoid dose-response curve. For certain tumors, such as early-stage seminoma, doses of radiation having a high probability of local tumor control can be administered with low probabilities of causing normal tissue complications. In most cases, however, the dose-response curves for tumor control and normal tissue complications are close to one another and have steep slopes in the therapeutic range. Practically, this means that for many tumors a small increase in the probability of control is attended by a much greater

increase in the risk of normal tissue complications. An important part of the radiotherapeutic management for a given patient thus is the evaluation of the risks to normal tissue to which the therapist is willing to subject the patient for maximum tumor control expectation. Decreasing risk to the patient is the basis for much of modern radiotherapeutic clinical research: hypoxic cell sensitizers, radioprotectors, heavy particle therapy, and dynamic treatment planning to minimize the dose to critical tissues while maximizing the dose to tumors. Another way of improving the therapeutic index is to implant radioactive materials into tumors to localize the treated area and spare normal tissue. This technique has been especially effective in the treatment of breast and prostatic neoplasms.

Radiation complications can develop chronologically and can be categorized mechanistically as acute or chronic radiation effects. The percentage of the organ irradiated (field size) and the fractionation scheme (total time and total number of treatments required to give the total dose of irradiation) are important considerations in the development of secondary complications. In general, for a given dose of irradiation and for a larger portion of the organ irradiated, the more quickly the dose is given and the larger the dose per treatment (fractionation), the more likely are radiation complications.

Radiation complications are related to the total dose, fractionation or dose rate (schedule), and the volume of tissue irradiated.

Rubin has divided dose-limiting tissues into classes of organs grouped according to their life-threatening potential (1975). Class I organs are those in which radiation lesions are fatal or result in severe morbidity. These include the bone marrow, liver, intestine, brain, spinal cord, heart, lung, kidney, and fetus. Class II organs are those in which radiation lesions result in moderate to mild morbidity but in which permanent sequelae are usually compatible with survival. These include the oral cavity, pharynx, skin, esophagus, rectum, salivary gland, bladder, ureter, testis, cartilage, eye, endocrine glands, peripheral nerves, and ear. One can then ascertain the minimal and maximal tissue tolerance doses (TTD) that give either 5 percent or 50 percent complications within five years of radiation treatment. These are abbreviated $TTD_{5/5}$ and $TTD_{50/5}$, respectively, and are commonly used as guidelines for clinical practice.

6.0 Acute effects of radiation therapy

Acute and intermediate effects of radiation therapy occur during therapy or up to one year thereafter. Acute effects are the result of depletion of actively proliferating cells in otherwise homeostatic cell renewal systems. These include the bone marrow, skin, and the epithelium of the upper aerodigestive tract and bladder. Typical reactions include bone marrow depression, mucositis, epithelialitis, epilation, and gastrointestinal upset. Bloomer and Hellman suggest that acute effects are dose rate- and fractionation-dependent (1975). Although acute effects of radiotherapy are occasionally severe enough to warrant an interruption in treatment, they should not be used as criteria for terminating treatment. A 10 percent reduction in the daily dose increment from 200 to 180 rad per day is often adequate modification for amelioration of acute effects and will often alleviate excessive mucosal reaction and unacceptable gastrointestinal symptoms.

Symptomatic treatment alone is often adequate for acute reactions to radiation. Antispasmodics, opiates, and other analgesics often suffice for gastrointestinal

and urologic symptoms. Local anesthetics (Viscous Xylocaine® and Oxaine®) are employed for symptoms in the mouth, pharynx, and esophagus. In skin reactions secondary to supervoltage radiation, mild lubricants can be used for dry desquamation. For moist desquamation, scrupulous hygiene, including removal of excessive crusting by soaking and topical antibiotics should infection occur, is usually sufficient. Such reactions usually resolve shortly after radiation treatment is completed. In general, thick layers of petroleum-based lubricants and metallic powders must be avoided during radiation, as they can destroy the skin-sparing advantages of supervoltage beams.

Intermediate radiation reactions are related to the total effective dose, as well as time-dose fractionation characteristics, and appear to result from injury to cells in a slowly proliferating cell-renewal system, possibly epithelial or connective tissue. Clinically, the most important syndromes include acute radiation pneumonitis, pericarditis, hepatitis, and nephritis.

Acute radiation pneumonitis. Acute radiation pneumonitis follows a latent period of one to three months after completion of radiation therapy. It may be asymptomatic, particularly if the radiation was directed primarily to the upper lobes where pulmonalry perfusion and aeration are markedly reduced. Frequent symptoms, however, include a dry, hacking cough, which may progress to a purulent sputum if secondary bacterial infection supervenes; dyspnea on exertion; shortness of breath; and fever, particularly if larger lung volumes are irradiated. If both lungs have been irradiated and are involved in the pneumonitis, severe respiratory distress, cyanosis, and cor pulmonale with death from cardiorespiratory failure can occur. Roentgenographic findings frequently outline the treatment portal, do not follow normal pulmonary anatomic distributions, and are readily distinguished from recurrent or progressive disease. The hisopathologic picture is one of atypical epithelial cells, congested capillaries, and mononuclear cell infiltrates in the alveolar septa. In humans, hyaline membranes line the alveolar spaces. Consequently, the diffusion capacity, total viral capacity, and compliance are reduced.

The tolerance of the lung depends on the total dose of radiation, the number of fractions, the overall time, the portion of the lung volume irradiated, and any modifying effects of drugs. In particular, the total number of treatment fractions and the volume of lung irradiated are most important. Well-defined small volumes in mantle therapy for Hodgkin's disease tolerate relatively high doses in the range of 4000 to 4500 rad, with whole-lung tolerance more restrictive. In particular, the $TD_{5/5}$ and $TD_{50/5}$ for the entire lung for radiation pneumonitis are 1500 and 2500 rad. Fields of 100 cm² are felt to have $TD_{5/5}$ and $TD_{50/5}$ of 3000 and 3500 rad. Lung tolerance is further compromised by concomitant actinomycin D, which is frequently given for Wilms' tumor. Antibiotics are recommended in radiation pneumonitis when superimposed infection is present. Steroids are probably best reserved for the patient with symptomatic cough and dyspnea and should not be used for patients with only radiographic findings without symptoms. If steroids are instituted they should be tapered slowly, as rapid cessation of steroid has been reported to lead both to reappearnace of prior symptomatic pneumonitis and to the development of new infiltrates in both irradiated and nonirradiated areas of the lung.

Acute radiation-induced heart disease. In acute, radiation-induced heart disease, symptoms usually occur within 12 months of the initiation of thoracic radiation. Patients present with fever, chest pain, and pericardial friction rub, the signs and symptoms of which are indistinguishable from acute pericarditis of any etiology. Electrocardiogram changes compatible with pericarditis, including a low QRS voltage, abnormal T waves, and ST elevations are found. Approximately one-half of the patients develop mild to severe tamponade, which usually subsides with conservative management alone. $TD_{5/5}$ and $TD_{50/5}$ for 60 percent of the heart are considered to be about 4500 and 5500 rad, respectively, dependent also on fraction size. For smaller areas, such as those involved in internal mammary irradiation, higher doses may be acceptable, depending upon the volume of heart treated. Most clinicians, however, hesitate to give more than 3000 to 3500 rad to the entire heart if it is included in the field. With potentially cardiotoxic drugs such as Adriamycin now used in a variety of multidisciplinary programs, the heart is probably more important as a dose-limiting structure; treatment plans minimizing cardiac volume irradiated and total cardiac dose may need to be devised.

Acute radiation hepatitis. The liver is commonly irradiated in the treatment of Wilms' tumor, abdominal lymphoma, neuroblastoma, pediatric hepatoblastoma, testicular cancer, esophageal carcinoma, and metastatic ovarian carcinoma, with dosages from 1000 to 5000 rad. The usual presentation of acute radiation hepatitis is the asymptomatic development of liver dysfunction as measured by biochemical parameters several weeks after completion of radiation therapy. Elevation of alkaline phosphatase, generally to less than 30 Bodansky units, may be present, but the clinical picture may be considerably more severe, with gross liver enlargement and ascites. Liver scan may show defects of liver imaging corresponding to the radiation field areas. Unlike most other types of acute radiaton injury, the histopathologic lesion is venous in origin, with dilatation of hepatocytes at the pericentral sinusoids, and edema about the central vein.

Radiation hepatic changes begin to occur at total doses above 3000 rad ($TD_{5/5}$). Above 3500 rad the incidence increases sharply, and the $TTD_{50/50}$ level is reached at 4000 rad. Children may develop severe thrombocytopenia with or without leukopenia when radiation to the liver is associated with actinomycin D therapy. The thrombocytopenia is promptly reversible with drug and irradiation withdrawal, but the mechanism of this effect has not been established.

The large size of the liver, which occupies an area in proximity to various internal viscera, makes it vulnerable to damage when many tumors are irradiated. In addition, para-aortic node radiation for testicular tumors, Hodgkin's disease, and other tumors of the genitourinary tract exposes the liver. General guidelines for such treatment include the exclusion of at least 25 to 39 percent of the total liver volume and doses exceeding 2500 rad in 150 to 200 fractions. If higher doses than these are contemplated, such maneuvers as shrinking field techniques, lateral fields, or other specially designed fields to minimize liver dose, must be designed. Liver shielding should be required at appropriate times when either large abdominal fields or strip field technique is used.

Acute radiation nephropathy. Acute radiation nephropathy appears at the 5 percent level at 2000 rad and achieves a 50% level at 2500 rad when both kidneys are included in the treatment field. The delivery of 2800 rad in five weeks is associated with a 10-year mortality rate of 70 percent. A 2300-rad dosage to both kidneys can cause hypertension and renal failure. In the first few months following radiation to the kidneys, it is difficult to predict from clinical findings the extent of renal injury that may have occurred. Starting 4 to 12 months after treatment, the patient may develop a benign essential hypertension syndrome, malignant hypertension, or asymptomatic proteinuria. It is believed that these effects are mediated by radiation-induced changes in the microvasculature of the kidney.

The most important factor in preventing radiation nephropathy is the segmental protection of one-third of the total renal mass from dosages of radiation above 1500 rad. This level may be somewhat lower for children, and is important for children and infants undergoing unilateral nephrectomy; the dosage to the remaining kidney from either primary or scattered radiation should be below 2000 rad. When structures contiguous to the kidneys must be irradiated to high doses, maneuvers such as reducing fields with tumor regression, small boost fields, or reducing the kidney dose by multiple portals or rotational techniques should be attempted.

Spinal cord complications. An early, generally reversible syndrome termed "acute transient radiation myelopathy" is usually indicated by electric-shock-like sensations (Lhermitte's sign), pain, and parasthesias, most often distributed about the lower lumbar nerves, are brought on by neck flexion. It is usually self-limiting, lasts 2 to 37 weeks, and has a peak onset from 2 to 24 months after radiation.

7.0 Chronic effects of radiation

The primary determinant of late radiation effects is the total effective dose received by limiting normal tissue within a treatment portal. Usually these complications are chronic and do not necessarily correlate with prior acute or intermediate tissue reactions. In patients for whom treatment is planned with a high expectation for cure, these tissue effects ultimately limit the total effective dose that may be safely delivered to a tumor. The common target organ of these effects appears to be epithelium or connective tissue, and common late findings such as tissue necrosis, fistulas, and dense fibrosis are consistent with this hypothesis. In many cases the vascular supply following surgery in these areas is tenuous, and conservative management is preferable.

Chronic radiation pneumonopathy. With sufficiently high doses, acute radiation pneumonitis is irreversible and will progress into a chronic phase. When pneumonitis involves all of both lungs, it progresses to death or reverses completely. With smaller volumes of exposure (i.e., one lung or less) the patient survives long enough for progression from acute to chronic pneumonitis. In some cases with a small volume of irradiation, a patient who never experienced clinically significant acute radiation symptoms may develop chronic changes that may be noted only on x-rays. The basic lesion shows progression from an acute capillary obstructive exudative phase into a chronic phase and is accompanied by a loss of pulmonary volume as the alveolar spaces are obliterated and no longer aerated. This happens because of cell proliferation. Pulmonary function is lost in the involved volume, and, as blood flow may decrease less than ventilation, a decreased arterial oxygen saturation may develop. A dense consolidation and loss of lung volume are seen on x-ray. This may cause a shift in the mediastinum when a large volume of lung is involved. Chronic changes usually begin about four months after radiation and stabilize at about one year, with the lung becoming recanalized by small vessels. A chronic cough may develop, and the lung becomes more susceptible to infection, especially to fungal infection.

Chronic radiation heart disease (pericarditis and pancarditis). Chronic radiation pericarditis usually occurs within the first year after irradiation and is often asymptomatic and observed only on a routine follow-up chest x-ray after radiation therapy. In one-half of the cases, the acute effusion will clear spontaneously after as long as two years. Constrictive pericarditis is much less common and appears later, usually 6 to 30 months after treatment. It is heralded by chronic effusion or episodes of acute pericarditis; often both effusion and construction are present. Pericardiectomy may be required if construction is present.

Pancarditis is the most serious late complication and is characterized by pericardial and myocardial fibrosis. Clinically, the patient may present with intractable heart failure, usually after having received 6000 to 9800 rad to the heart, often in repeated courses of therapy. It is believed that the chronic changes result from failure of microcirculation, which causes ischemia and leads to diffuse irreversible fibrosis of the myocardium.

Chronic radiation nephropathy. Chronic radiation nephritis due to progressive vascular sclerosis usually develops two or more years after radiation treatment. The spectrum of clinical presentation is wide, varying from the asymptomatic patient, whose kidneys are found to be scarred at postmortem examination, to others with steadily progressive renal failure leading to uremia. Symptoms can vary from benign proteinuria to malignant hypertension. The intravenous pyelogram may show bilaterally or unilaterally shrunken kidneys, and individual kidney function studies should be obtained to assess the functional reserve of the involved kidneys. In the case of unilateral renal irradiation, a later-appearing syndrome of benign hypertension can occur as the result of a development of Goldblatt kidney. This can be corrected by excising the previously irradiated organ.

Chronic radiation-induced liver disease. This occurs from six months to several years after hepatic radiation and correlates with severe luminal narrowing of the central veins with perivenous sclerosis. Usually there are no significant signs of liver cell failure; rather, patients are likely to present with ascites and complications of the esophageal varices. Liver function tests are usually normal or slightly elevated.

Radiation-induced gastric damage. At dosages to the stomach of greater than 4500 rad, gastric radiation ulceration may appear, usually six months to one year after completion of treatment. At 5000 rad, 50 percent of the patients are symptomatic, which implies that this is a significant dose level for tolerance. The $TTD_{5/5}$ and $TTD_{50/5}$ for supervoltage therapy are estimated to be 4400 to 5500 rad, respectively. A portion of the stomach is included in fields in which aortic nodes are treated for Hodgkin's disease and for occult metastases from genitourinary neoplasms; the prescribed doses are usually below 5000 rad. On the microscopic level, occlusion of veins and associated connective tissue proliferation and scarring compromise the normal blood supply so that the normal mucosal epithelium cannot be supported and ulceration results. The presence of gastric acidity does not rule out radiation ulceration, as the fundus and body of the stomach may not be in the treatment fields to cause achlorhydria. Achlorhydria may result four to six weeks after the administration of 1600 to 2000 rad to the entire stomach. The 50 percent reduction in the secretion of acid may persist for a year or more in 40 percent of patients given such therapy.

Radiation-induced chronic small bowel disease. The intestine is the preeminent dose-limiting organ in abdominal radiation. Roswit has linked the intestinal segments in order of increasing radiosensitivity to radiation effects as follows: ileum, transverse colon, sigmoid colon, esophagus, and rectum (1972). From 6 months to 5 years after therapy, chronic radiation syndromes including obstruction, and in some cases ulceration and perforation can develop. These depend on the total dose and on the volume of tissue irradiated. For a small (100 cm square) field, the $TD_{5/5}$ and $TD_{50/5}$ are 5000 and 6500, respectively. For larger fields (400 cm square) the dose is decreased to 4500 and 5500 rad, respectively. This corresponds pathologically to vascular epithelial proliferation and to thrombosis in the vessels of the muscularis propia. The resulting hypoxia can lead to ulceration and possibly to proliferation. The differential diagnosis is usually between radiation changes and recurrent tumor. Previous laparotomy and previous instillation of intraperitoneal radioisotopes can increase the small intestine's susceptibility to injury. Repeated irradiation and overlapping of fields are also hazardous, as radiation tolerance dose levels can be readily exceeded.

The severity of previous acute intestinal radiation symptoms is not well correlated with late chronic effects. The symptoms of diarrhea result from intestinal hypermotility. The proliferating epithelial cells of the intestinal crypts are damaged by irradiation, but after a period of compensation by the intestine, especially with fractionated treatment, crypt stem cells recover because of their capacity to repair sublethal injury. This recovery tends to restore the damaged epithelium. Occasionally, with very large doses, ulceration or infarction is encountered in the acute stage.

When diarrhea persists after the initial radiation course has ended, the syndrome of cholic enteropathy resulting from impairment of absorption of bile salts from the terminal ileum should be suspected. This condition is corrected by cholestyramine, a nonabsorbable anion exchange resin that binds and inactivates bile salts.

Radiation-induced central nervous system damage. In the period between one and five years after brain radiation, recrudescence of neurologic symptoms may be due either to recurrent tumor or radiation-induced necrosis. Pneumoencephalography will often show atrophy in patients with brain damage due to radiation. Histopathologic changes in the small arteries lead to a transudation of fluid that separates the brain parenchyma from the vessels. The resulting ischemia may cause focal parenchyma necrosis beyond the field of irradiation as well as within it. This results in a clinical picture akin to vascular occlusive disease with infarction, and patients may present with neurologic deficits involving sensory and motor distributions compatible with those expected from atherosclerotic occlusive events.

On the basis of the best clinical data available, the $TD_{5/5}$ and $TD_{50/5}$ for whole-brain radiation therapy for infarction and necrosis are 6000 and 7000 rad, respectively, and for smaller volumes (25% or less of brain) are 7000 and 8000 rad, respectively. If irradiation of deeply lying tumors or of large areas of brain to high dose is contemplated, the use of techniques such as multiple portals or rotational techniques, which minimize inhomogeneities outside of the tumor volume, should be considered.

Radiation myelopathy is a long-term neurologic complication that can accompany excessive irradiation to the spinal cord during aggressive radical radiation therapy. It is especially tragic for those patients, usually those with head, neck, or lung tumors, and lymphoma, in whom radical irradiation controls the tumor, but progressively severe debilitation and death result from spinal cord degeneration. The syndrome may take one of several forms. Most common is chronic progressive myelopathy, developing over weeks or months and usually confined to the lateral columns. The other syndromes are acute paraplegia or quadriplegia developing over a few days, and more rarely,

degeneration of lower motor and peripheral nerves after lumbar irradiation. The syndromes may begin as early as four months or as late as 30 months after radiation, but onset is usually between 11 and 24 months.

Clinically, the apparent level of injury appears initially below the level of the irradiation and subsequently proceeds upward. The upper level of the sensory or motor deficit eventually localizes within the irradiated volume. The axons traverse several cord segments before joining a nerve root. Consequently the vertebral level of injury usually corresponds to a dermatome two segments lower. The neurologic deficits are usually progressive and unremitting. They commonly include spastic paraplegia or quadriplegia, loss of sphincter control, and diaphragmatic breathing with cervical lesions. A typical Brown-Séquard's syndrome may appear. With thoracic and lumbar lesions paraplegia and sphincteric involvement are common. Mortality is high for cervical and thoracic lesions, with an average survival of about 10 months after symptoms begin.

Differential diagnosis includes extramedullary metastases from the original tumor or compression from a collapsed vertebral body due to metastases or trauma. To support the diagnosis of myelopathy it is first necessary to elicit a history of irradiation in sufficient doses to cause myelopathy. The segment of cord irradiated must be at least slightly above the dermatome of the symptom. In radiation myelopathy, routine spinal fluid tests are within normal limits. Myelography may show either focal diminution of cord size or no change. In most cases Lhermitte's sign is absent. Histologically, the picture is one of the slow evolution of vascular sclerosis with secondary tissue ischemia and finally circumscribed areas of necrosis that are frequently large enough to provide functional cord transaction.

The cord's tolerance to irradiation depends mainly on the radiation dose but is also influenced adversely by large fraction size and irradiation of long segments of cord. The 5 percent incidence dosage for myelitis in a 10-cm length of irradiated cord is 4500 rad, and the 50 percent dosage is 5500 rad. In general, accepted clinical practice dictates that the maximally acceptable dose that the cord should be allowed to receive in 25 fractions over five weeks is 5000 rad. Most treatment plans introduce spinal cord shielding after 4500 rad in 200-rad fractions.

Careful attention to treatment planning can aid in decreasing this complication. Care should be taken to calculate accurately the maximum cord dose for any plan, as relatively small changes in the contour of the patient may shift the point of maximum inhomogeneity in the treatment plan closer to the cord or may otherwise raise the dose to the cord. In the treatment of thoracic tumors, delivery of part of a radical dose of irradiation by oblique portals, in which the tumor is treated but the spinal cord is blocked, is preferable to using other methods that may inadvertently overdose the cord. For obvious reasons, care must be taken to avoid overlapping the long field (e.g., mantle and para-aortic fields in Hodgkin's treatment). With close attention to technical radiation therapy, the incidence of radiation myelitis should decrease considerably.

Radiation effects on bone marrow. The bone marrow is affected by whole-body and segmental irradiation. After whole-body radiation the clinical potential for survival is as follows: for dosages greater than 600 rad—nearly impossible; for 200 to 600 rad—survival possible; for 100 to 200 rad—survival probable; and for less than 100 rad—survival nearly certain. Death, when it occurs, is usually from infection or hemorrhage secondary to bone marrow effects. The kinetics of the peripheral blood cells after whole-body irra-

diation reflect the relative insensitivity to radiation of mature nonlymphocytic peripheral cells. This contrasts to radiation to the marrow stem cells and to all lymphocytes that are exquisitely sensitive to x-rays. The picture is thus dominated largely by the half-lives of the circulating cells—for erythrocytes, 120 days; for granulocytes, 66 hours; and for platelets, 8 to 10 days—and their different radiosensitivities. The radiation dosages to reduce the number of cells to 50 percent of their basal levels are as follows: for lymphocytes, 40 rad; for reticulocytes, 100 rad; for granulocytes, 150 rad; and for platelets, 575 rad. In addition to strictly kinetic considerations, after whole-body irradiation nearly immediate lymphopenia and a transient granulocytosis occur within 48 hours; these conditions are probably hormonally mediated.

Segmental irradiation affects acute marrow depopulation in the same way that whole-body irradiation does (i.e., ablation of the stem cells within the irradiated field). After high doses of local field fractionated irradiation, bone marrow regeneration appears to be accomplished by local conversion of uncommitted mesenchymal cells to stem cells. With standard segmented irradiation, depopulation of the marrow is evident at 500 rad, and complete depopulation occurs with 1000 rad. After 2000 rad, significant recovery of the marrow occurs by one year, but by 4000 rad, long-term severe depopulation occurs. This is apparently due to radiation damage to the vasculature in the sinusoids, making them less able to support stem cell growth and differentiation.

For planning aggressive multidisciplinary therapy, the bone marrow is probably the most crucial limiting organ, and the administration of adequate therapeutic doses of radiation and/or chemotherapy may be prevented because of therapy-induced thrombocytopenia and leukopenia.

If less than 50 percent of bone marrow

is irradiated, minimal and transient depression of blood counts usually occurs. If more than 50 percent is irradiated, as in total nodal irradiation, total abdominal irradiation, or abdominal radiation with "cone down" radiation to the pelvis, moderately severe depression of the white blood counts and platelet counts is likely to occur. Regeneration after large field treatment for Hodgkin's disease may require two to three years for full recovery.

Morbidity-associated effects. The previously discussed tissues may cause fatal complications if the organs indicated are improperly irradiated. Other tissues can also experience severe morbidity. Several of these, including the eye, salivary glands, mandible and similar bones, middle ear, thyroid, and esophagus, are commonly at risk when head and neck tumors are treated radically to high dose. Similarly, the bladder, rectum, and ureters may be damaged when pelvic tumors are treated. Other tissues in this category include the skin and the gonads.

Skin damage. Skin damage is the most frequently observed reaction following radiation therapy and usually appears two to three weeks after the onset of treatment, because the cells take time to migrate from the basal layer to the keratinized layer of skin. The stages of damage with increasing doses include erythema and both dry and moist desquamation. At higher doses the skin may slough, and the cutaneous adnexa, including hair, sebaceous glands, and sweat glands, may be destroyed. Unless severe damage occurs, full healing of the skin within two to three weeks is the rule. Time-dose ratios relating skin dose for necrosis to field size, total dose, and duration of treatment have been derived and tabulated graphically for reactions from erythema to necrosis. Similar graphs exist for tumor kill for skin cancer. Safe fractionation schemes for the treatment of skin cancers of different

sizes can be obtained from these graphs. The erythema dose varies with the type of radiation used from about 300 rad with low-energy radiation to about 900 rad with cobalt 60. The $TTD_{5/5}$ and $TTD_{50/5}$ for high-energy beams and consequent ulceration are about 6000 and 8000 rad, respectively. Beginning three months after irradiation, chronic reactions, including thinning of the skin, visible telangiectasia, loss of skin adnexa, and dermal fibrosis, may appear. This can lead to future ulceration and enhanced scarring secondary to minor trauma.

In general, chronic skin reactions, including dense fibrosis, can best be avoided by choosing treatment plans that minimize the subcutaneous dose. Rotational plans are best for this, and in general, parallel opposed and single portal plans are inferior. Acute skin reactions are seen least in treatments with megavoltage machines, which, unlike orthovoltage and low-energy electron beams, allows the maximum dose to occur from several millimeters to several centimeters below the skin surface. The "skin-sparing" effects of megavoltage beams, however, may be negated by covering the skin with artificial material such as wax, or "bolus," or by applying metallic powders.

Damage associated with head and neck irradiation. The oropharyngeal mucosa reacts similarly to the skin; but reactions appear earlier than in the skin, generally at about two weeks. This is presumably due to the more rapid turnover of the nonkeratinized epithelium of the mucosa. Accompanying destruction of accessory mucous glands in the submucosa adds to dryness. Healing almost invariably progresses rapidly during treatment and is often aided by a small decrease in fraction size of 200 to 180 rad. The $TTD_{5/5}$ and $TTD_{50/5}$ for necrosis are 6500 and 8500 rad and are slightly higher than for skin. Later damage includes recurrent ulceration and necrosis, which usually heals with conservative management, involving good oral hygiene, removal of ill-fitting dentures, and discontinuance of smoking and ethanol ingestion.

Modification of salivary gland function by irradiation begins at low doses. At about 2000 rad, salivary function may be temporarily suppressed, and acutely painful swelling of the gland with elevations of serum amylase may occur. The serum amylase may be elevated after as little as 100 to 400 rad. Above dosages of 4000 rad, at which recovery may be complete, markedly permanent impairment of salivary function may occur. A 50 percent reduction in secretion occurs in 5 percent of patients receiving 4500 rad and in 50 percent of those receiving 5500 rad. The most common chronic change, occurring months to years after irradiation, is xerostomia, a chronic dryness of the mouth brought on by a decrease in the amount and a relative decrease in the serous portion of saliva. Secondarily, an increase in dental caries develops.

Although attempts are being made to treat xerostomia pharmacologically using artificial saliva, the only adequate cure remains prevention, using treatment plans that spare one parotid or maintain the low dose. Acceptable treatment plans include "wedged pairs" of portals, anterior–posterior and posterior–anterior portals missing one parotid, and unilateral electron beams with rapid dose fall-off. Unfortunately some tumors, such as those of the soft palate and base of tongue, require high-dose parotid irradiaton.

Radiation effects on special organs of the head. The eye may be at risk for damage in treating several head and neck tumors; the lens is the most sensitive structure. Radiation-damaged cells in the lens are retained, causing a cataract because of the absence of a cell-removal system. The 50 percent level for clinically troublesome cataracts occurs at 3000 rad. If neutrons are employed rather than x-rays, these levels are considerably lower. Although radiation cataracts are managed in the same way as ordinary cataracts, the procedures of choice are those treatment plans that spare the lens.

Less vulnerable structures in the eye include the cornea, retina, lacrimal gland, and optic nerve. Dosages above 3000 rad can cause chronic corneal ulceration and keratitis, necessitating enucleation. Dosages of 5000 to 6000 rad can cause lacrimal gland injury with xerophthalmia and corneal injury. Retinal hemorrhages, possibly leading to blindness, occur at above 5500 rad, with a 50 percent level at 6500 to 7000 rad to the entire retina. Optic nerve damage, with blindness in some cases, has been seen in the treatment of tumors of the paranasal sinuses and of the pituitary. The use of decreased fraction size sometimes appears to have decreased the rate of these complications.

Hypothyroidism may result in adults after 6000 rad to the normal thyroid or as little as 4000 rad in thyroids of patients who have had lymphangiograms.

Irradiation of the middle ear produces 5 percent and 50 percent incidences of serous otitis media at 5000 and 7000 rad, respectively. Dosages to the vestibular apparatus have produced a Ménière's syndrome at 5 percent and 50 percent levels of 6000 and 7000 rad, respectively.

Radiation effect on bone. Necrosis of bone in general and of the mandible in particular is frequent after high-dose radiation therapy, especially in treatment of lateral tumors treated with high doses and wedged pairs, of unequally weighted opposed lateral fields, or of en face electron beams. Such injury is termed "osteoradionecrosis." In uninjured bone, signs of radionecrosis appear above 7000 rad. The $TTD_{5/5}$ and $TTD_{50/5}$ for necrosis are about 6500 and 7500 rad. Orthovoltage photon beams, electron beams, and high-energy photon beams have energy preferentially deposited in soft bone tissue, increasing the probability of osteoradionecrosis for a calculated tumor dose.

The incidence of osteoradionecrosis is also influenced by dental condition. Patients with carious teeth in the radiation field or with dental extractions performed during or shortly after therapy have an increased incidence of osteoradionecrosis. This is best avoided by prophylactically extracting all bad teeth before radiation, treating the remaining teeth with fluoride, and allowing sufficient time for healing (usually 10 days to 14 days) before starting therapy.

Radiation effects on the gastrointestinal tract. Gastrointestinal effects of radiation therapy can be severe but are generally temporary. The esophagus reacts acutely, in a manner similar to the oral mucosa. Esophagitis appears two to four weeks into therapy and usually subsides completely as the mucosa regenerates. Chronic damage, including stricture that may be associated with ulceration, occurs 6 to 12 months after treatment as a result of submucosal fibrosis. The $TTD_{5/5}$ and $TTD_{50/5}$ are about 6300 and 7500 rad, respectively. In cases not responsive to dilatation partial resection may be required.

Rectal ulceration is negligible below 5000 rad but reaches a 5 percent level at 5500 rad. Above 8000 rad the rate of severe complications such as fistula, perforation, ulceration, and obstruction approaches 25 to 50 percent. In general, treatment planning should attempt to limit the rectal dose to 5500 rad. The volume of normal rectum treated to this dose can often be reduced by carefully selected treatment plans that decrease the rectal dose. These include rotational plans with wedges that omit the rectal area from the rotation, as are applicable for bladder and prostate tumors, lateral arc plans, as are useful for prostate plans, or merely careful blocking of rectal tissues in the lateral fields of "four-field" plans (anterior–posterior, posterior–anterior, and lateral fields).

Radiation effects on the bladder. The epithelium of the bladder and ureters follows kinetics similar to that of the skin with an acute syndrome including dysuria and frequency appearing shortly after therapy begins. Irradiated bladders are susceptible to infection, and this should be ruled out when these symptoms begin. Healing is usually rapid after therapy and, in the absence of infection management during radiation, should be symptomatic only without antibiotic prophylaxis.

Despite rapid resolution of the acute syndrome, chronic changes, including ulceration in regions of high dose and bladder contracture, especially if the entire bladder was irradiated, can appear. The same principles apply for treatment planning as for avoiding rectal complications. In addition, complications can be avoided by minimizing the amount of bladder treated. For instance, especially in the reduced field portion of prostate treatment, patients should be treated with a full bladder, in order to expand as much of it as possible out of the treatment portals.

Histopathologic changes include thinning transitional epithelium with dilated capillaries yielding a telangiectatic appearance. These changes are often associated with areas of high dose from radium for gynecologic tumors, usually near the ureters or bladder trigone. The $LD_{5/5}$ and $LD_{50/5}$ for localized and whole-bladder areas are 6500 to 7500 rad and 6000 to 7000 rad, respectively. Ureteral stricture appears at higher 5 percent and 50 percent dosages, 7000 and 8000 rad, respectively.

8.0 Systemic effects of radiation therapy

The systemic effects of radiation therapy can be divided into two parts. The first is the set of acute syndromes resulting from whole-body radiation, commonly called "radiation sickness." Second are the late effects of radiation including carcinogenesis and development of mutations.

Acute radiation syndromes. Animal experiments have provided the bulk of the data upon which our understanding of these syndromes rests. These are supplemented by anecdotal but extremely important human experiences such as those of Japanese atomic bomb survivors, those of therapists and patients exposed to radiation, and those of the victims of the limited number of radiation installation accidents. From these the general pathophysiology of "radiation sickness" has been well established, although for humans several important questions remain unanswered. Therapeutic radiation involves small doses to small volumes applied over a protracted period. Accidental radiation involves large doses to the entire body exposed in one instant. The difference between biologic effects of the two types of radiation is enormous.

Three distinct modes of death after high-dose, whole-body irradiation appear in animals. First is the central nervous system (CNS) syndrome, in which death occurs in a matter of hours after severe nausea and vomiting, disorientation, respiratory distress convulsions, and coma occur. Although the exact mechanism of CNS death is not fully understood, it is thought to involve an autolytic process in the nervous tissue itself. High doses of irradiation, 10,000 to 12,000 rad, appear to be needed in order to initiate this catastrophic process. Although damage to the gastrointestinal tract and marrow also occurs, the usual tissue responses, which normally take days to weeks, do not have time to mature.

At lower dosage levels, 500 to 1200 rad, death occurs because of the gastrointestinal syndrome, which is associated with extensive bloody diarrhea and gastrointestinal mucosal destruction. Death usually occurs between 3 and 10 days after exposure. At still lower dosages, 250 to 500 rad, the bone marrow is the organ whose failure ultimately causes death, usually several weeks later, when the mature cells in the circulation at the time of radiation finally die off. The precursor population, which has been sterilized by the radiation, is inadequate to replace mature cells, and the patient dies, usually from infection secondary to granulocyte depression and immune system deficiency, bleeding, or anemia from hemorrhage secondary to thrombocytopenia rather than from red blood cell depression.

The mean lethal dose, defined as the dose that kills 50 percent of subjects in a given number of days from whole-body exposure, is not precisely known in humans. In general, smaller mammals such as rats have higher $LD_{50/5}$ values, 840 to 1520 rad, than do larger animals such as sheep, whose range is 155 to 265 rad. It appears to take longer, about 60 days, for the full effects of radiation to manifest themselves in humans. From available data, the $LD_{50/60}$ for humans appears to be about 400 rad.

For persons receiving between 400 and 500 rad, close monitoring both without antibiotics and symptomatic drugs is advocated. If over 500 rad has been received, hemopoietic death is quite probable, although survivors at levels above this have been reported, and consideration should be given to hospitalizing such persons in a laminar flow-type unit in a pathogen-free environment after externally "sterilizing" them with antibiotics and antiseptic soaks. As a last resort, bone marrow transplantation can be considered.

In addition to radiation sickness with whole-body radiation, the syndrome is also observed in patients treated with segmented or regional therapeutic radiation. Thus patients receiving mantle radiation or treatment to the brain, head and neck, or peripheral extremities may develop anorexia, lassitude, general malaise, or fatigue. This nonspecific metabolic syndrome may be due to internal scatter of radiation or may be secondary to the release of some mediator substance from normal tissues exposed to radiation with secondary systemic effects.

"Radiation sickness" may develop with irradiation to any site and is not dependent upon exposure of the gastrointestinal tract.

Nonspecific life shortening is an effect induced in some animals after exposures to doses of radiation insufficient to cause mortality. Blood counts and weight return to normal, and gastrointestinal symptoms disappear. In one study, the exposed animals died sooner than controls. Physiologically, these animals behave like their older counterparts. In other experiments, however, animals irradiated at low dose rates were found to live longer than controls. A linear relationship between life shortening and radiation dose has been found in some species. For only one population of humans, American radiologists from 1945 to 1954, has life shortening been demonstrated. They were compared to other medical practitioners as controls. In contratrast, British radiologists from 1897 to 1957 appeared to live longer than the general population. The Japanese atomic bomb survivors also show no life shortening when cases of induced neoplasia are excluded. In conclusion, there is still a lack of substantial evidence to support the existence of nonspecific life shortening in humans.

Radiation carcinogenesis. The induction of tumors by x-ray is a well-estab-

lished entity that must be considered in all phases of nuclear and radiological technology. Monitoring for this may prove it to be one of the most important limiting toxicities of therapeutic radiology when used in multidisciplinary protocols, as recent experience with Hodgkin's disease treated by chemotherapy plus extended field radiotherapy has shown.

Small animals develop an increasing incidence of malignancy up to a maximum of about 300 rad after which the frequency falls back to "normal." Human experience consists of:

1. skin cancer in early radiologists
2. lung cancer in pitchblend miners
3. bone tumors in radium dial painters
4. liver tumors in patients examined with thoratrast
5. increased leukemia in Japanese atomic bomb survivors
6. thyroid cancers in children irradiated for enlarged thymus glands

In the induction of leukemia it is difficult adequately to assess risk as a function of dose rate as well as total dose. It has been calculated that at Hiroshima there was a leukemia risk of 1.52 cases per million persons exposed per year per rem ("radiation exposure in man") allowing a correction for different types of radiation having different biologic effects. The Nagasaki value was 1.82. These figures imply the untested assumption that incidence figures calculated for single larger doses could be extrapolated for protracted exposures at lower dose rates. They also assume both no threshold dose and a linear dose-response relationship. Without further data, such an extrapolation must be viewed with considerable skepticism.

Evidence suggests that the Japanese atomic bomb survivors and spondylytics have increased incidences of solid tumors as well as leukemias. The total risk may be as high as 6 cases per 10^5 patients exposed per rem, again making the previous assumptions. There is a latent period of 5 to 20 years for leukemias and up to 30 years for solid tumors.

Carcinogenesis associated with therapeutic radiation (as opposed to whole-body radiation) is a reality but has been observed infrequently, as compared to that induced by diagnostic or low-level radiation. It is probable that therapeutic doses, although capable of inducing cancer, also provide the dose that destroys carcinogenically converted cells. Thus, in radiation-treated carcinoma of the cervix, no increase in leukemia, in local (in-field) tumors, or in other visceral malignancies occurs, in spite of extensive high-dose radiation and long-term follow-up.

Radiation-induced chromosomal damage. Genetic effects of radiation have been well studied in animal systems and probably exist in humans. From present human data, however, it is difficult to estimate the genetic hazards of radiation exposure. For instance, no increase has yet been observed in the incidence of prenatal or perinatal malformation in the descendants of the Japanese exposed at Nagasaki and Hiroshima. Animal data, nevertheless, imply that the dose required to double the spontaneous mutation rate ("doubling dose") in humans probably lies between 10 and 100 rem. For acute exposure, a dosage of 30 rem has been suggested. If a man receives such a dose, conception should probably be deferred for two months. The period should probably be up to one year for women. Extrapolating from mouse data, one finds that the radiation to pregnant women will, in general, cause prenatal death if exposure occurs up to 10 days after conception and will probably cause multiple system abnormalities and/or neonatal death if exposure occurs from 11 to 41 days after conception. Analysis of the limited amount of human data (atomic bomb and pelvic x-ray patients) shows roughly that:

1. Dosages of up to 250 rad delivered before 2 to 3 weeks gestation will either cause resorption, abortion, or births without significant abnormalities.
2. From 4 to 6 weeks, severe multisystem abnormalities are expected.
3. From 11 to 16 weeks, stunted growth, microcephaly, and mental retardation are present.
4. From 16 to 20 weeks, milder versions of the above occur.
5. After 30 weeks, serious handicaps to early life are not evident, although later effects could be serious.

If a fetus receives over 10 rad in the first six weeks, a therapeutic abortion should be performed.

9.0 The interaction of radiation and cytotoxic drugs

Phillips has categorized four classes of drugs that interact with radiation, these are: (1.) radiation-protective agents that concentrate in sensitive tissues such as the integument, gastrointestinal tract, and bone marrow; (2.) radiation sensitizers that act on hypoxic tumor cells; (3.) radiation sensitizers that are incorporated into tumor DNA; and (4.) cancer chemotherapy drugs that sensitize tumor and normal cells to radiation, but which kill tumor cells as well. This discussion will focus on the fourth category because of its therapeutic implications.

Three categories of cytotoxic drugs and radiation interaction can be delineated. First, the DNA-binding agents, particularly Adriamycin and actinomycin D, interact synergistically with radiation, particularly in normal cells. The tissues of the skin, esophagus, heart, liver, and pelvic organs have all been reported to have acute inflammatory responses as a consequence of drug and radiation interaction. This interaction may be caused by the drug's inhibition of mechanisms for repair of radiation damage in normal cells. Upon exposure to radiation, the normal tissues experience an inordinate cell kill without regenerative capacity. Such effects are more prominent when the drug is administered concomitantly with radiation; if drug administration is delayed more than 21 days after completion of radiation, the normal organ tolerance to radiation is less affected. Nonetheless, drug exposure may produce acute skin flare in the portal of previous radiation.

Patient D, a 65-year-old woman with oat cell carcinoma, received combination chemotherapy, which included Adriamycin. She concomitantly received a dosage of 4500 rad to the mediastinum. Two weeks after completion of radiation, the patient complained of dysphagia, and a barium swallow demonstrated stenosis of the esophagus, which lay directly under the radiation therapy portal. Esophageal bouginage was required for the next eight months to maintain adequate lumen size for nutrition (Fig. 18.4).

Dose or schedule modification of the radiation and drug therapy are necessary to minimize the enhanced effect on normal tissues.

A second category of drug-radiation toxicity is the additive effect observed when radiation is applied to sites where the drug is toxic to normal tissues. Adriamycin cardiomyopathy may develop at lower cumulative doses than usual in patients receiving thoracic radiation; gastrointestinal toxicity secondary to 5-fluorouricil administration may be enhanced for patients receiving radiation therapy to the abdomen. Bleomycin employed in conjunction with radiation for treatment of esophageal carcinoma has been shown to result in an additive effect on the induction of pulmonary toxicity. Methotrexate encephalopathy may similarly be augmented in patients receiving cerebral

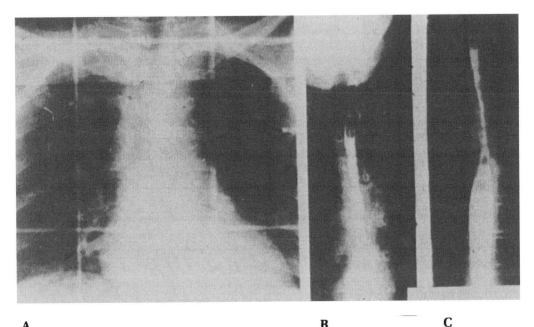

A
B
C

Fig. 18.4 Port films (A) (Patient D) who received concomitant radiation and Adriamycin and then developed severe stricture of the esophagus. (B and C).

radiation therapy. In general, the additive effect in this category occurs when the agents are delivered concomitantly, and recall is not observed.

An unusual drug-radiation interaction has been observed in patients receiving MOPP therapy following previous irradiation. Radiation pneumonitis is a common subclinical or clinical phenomenon in patients receiving mantle field radiation. Subsequent treatment with MOPP therapy, which involves corticosteroids, may result in exacerbation or clinical activation of previous radiation pneumonitis when steroids are withdrawn. The mechanism of this effect is unclear.

Carcinogenesis as a consequence of radiation and of chemotherapy has been discussed earlier. The development of second neoplasms in patients receiving both radiation therapy and chemotherapy is an important consideration in this era of combined modality therapy. The use of combined therapeutic modalities may promote substantially more cures for previously incurable cancers and will surely allow for the observation of delayed carcinogenic and other toxic effects. The data are most complete for combined modality therapy for Hodgkin's disease, for which radiation therapy and chemotherapy are commonly used. In an analysis of patients receiving chemotherapy only, radiation therapy only, and radiation therapy combined with intensive chemotherapy, the incidence of second malignancies was most prominent in patients receiving combined modalities. Second tumors did not increase significantly in patients treated with chemotherapy alone.

10.0 Complications of immunotherapy

Immunotherapy for cancer has involved trials with stimulants and potentiators of the normal host immune mechanism. The immune system normally acts as a surveillance system to prevent the im-

plantation and growth of neoplastic cells, which are constantly developing as a consequence of mutation or carcinogenic exposure. Theoretically, the various forms of immunotherapy are selective for tumor-cell kill and spare normal cells, thus minimizing or obviating visceral toxicity. Nonetheless, systemic and organ-related complications of the various forms of immunotherapy have been observed.

The major concern for potential adverse effects of immunotherapy is the theoretical concept that tumors could be potentiated and tumor growth augmented. The mechanism for such an effect is reasoned to be a consequence of immune stimulation of the formation of blocking antibodies, which could protect the tumor by coating tumor cells and preventing lymphocyte killer cells from tumor cell interaction. This theoretical possibility has never been demonstrated in clinical circumstances.

The major immune stimulant employed in clinical trials has been bacillus Calmette-Guerin. It has been applied intralesionally for cutaneous tumors, by scarification in proximity to regional lymph node sites, intradermally, orally, intravenously, and topically to serosal (pleural) and mucosal (bladder) surfaces. Depending upon the dose, the purity of the preparation, and the percentage of live organisms, bacillus Calmette-Guerin may be associated with a transient mycobacterial infection with fever and chills. This bacteremia may progress to implantation of the organism in visceral sites. Systemic mycobacterial infections are common, if not universal, with the intradermal and intralesional application of live bacillus Calmette-Guerin organisms, and granulomas and liver organisms have been identified in regional lymph nodes as well as in liver biopsy specimens. Occasionally, bacillus Calmette-Guerin may induce an allergic reaction with anaphylaxis and an associated coagulopathy. Finally, as a consequence of a local cutaneous application of the immunotherapy, secondary bacterial infection may develop locally and become systemic. A summary of complications of immunotherapy is presented in Table 18.5.

The methanol-extracted residue of bacillus Calmette-Guerin is a pure preparation of the cell wall of the microbacterial organism, which is generally applied intradermally. Local cutaneous reactions are the only adverse effect thus far reported with this residue. Cornybacterium parvum is administered, generally intravenously, as alcohol-killed organisms and is associated with fever and chills, and occasionally with hypotension.

Other experimental forms of immunotherapy include levamisole, an antihelminthic drug that is known to "turn on" T cells. Although purportedly innocuous, levamisole has been associated with aplastic anemia and other adverse effects.

11.0 Summary: the therapeutic index

The broad experience with complications of therapeutic modalities, including chemotherapy and radiation and the combined application of the two, must be viewed within the confines of the thera-peutic index. The multiplicity of adverse effects described in this chapter is observed in varying severity in most patients, depending upon a number of variables including host and tumor interaction and technical factors related to the drug or radiation. Improvements in technology and supportive measures may obviate or abrogate in part the adverse effects of therapy, but in all the clinician must balance possible adverse effects with the expectation of achieving a therapeutic goal. Attempts at cure in the face of unacceptable acute or chronic toxicity are unreasonable. Chemotherapy and radiation therapy could theoretically annihilate any tumor given sufficient dose, but the practical cost to the patient would be exorbitant.

Therefore, exploring new modalities of therapy that can decrease toxicity while increasing the antitumor effect are necessary. New chemotherapeutic agents are now sought, and alternative combinations of existing therapies are investigated. In addition, important advances must be made in the areas of supportive therapy and preventive therapy directed at protecting the patient's normal cells.

Table 18.5 Complications of Immunotherapy with Nonspecific Immune Stimulants or Potentiators (Bacillus Calmette-guerin, Methanal-Extracted Residue, Corynebacterium Parvum)

Minor	Fever and chills
	Local pain or secondary infection*
Major	Systemic mycobacterial infection
	Systemic bacterial infection
	Anaphylaxis
	Tumor growth stimulation

*Especially with scarification and intralesional application.

References

Aristizabal, S. A. et al. Adriamycin irradiation cutaneous complications. *Int. J. Radiat. Biol.* 2:325–331, 1977.

Aungst, C. W.; Sokal, J. E.; and Jager, B. C. Complications of BCG vaccination in neoplastic disease. *Ann. Intern. Med.* 82:666–668, 1975.

Bast, R. C.; Zbar, B.; Borsos, R.; and Rapp, H. J. BCG and cancer. *N. Engl. J. Med.* 290:1458–1467, 1974.

Belli, J. A., and Piro, A. J. The interaction between radiation and adriamycin damage in mammalian cells. *Cancer Res.* 37:1624–1630, 1977.

Bender, R. A., and Young, R. C. Effects of cancer treatment on individual and generational genetics. *Seminars in Oncology* 4:47–56, 1978.

Bloomer, W. D.; and Hellman, S. Normal tissue responses to radiation. *N. Engl J. Med.* 293:80–83, 1975.

Chabner, B. A. Second neoplasm: a complication of cancer chemotherapy (editorial). *N. Engl. J. Med.* 297:213–214, 1977.

Chabora, B. M.; Hopfan, S.; and Wittes, R. Esophageal complications in the treatment of oat cell carcinoma with combined irradiation and chemotherapy. *Radiology* 123:185–187, 1977.

Felix, E. L.; Jessup, J. M.; and Cohen, M. H. Severe complications of intralesional BCG therapy in an unsensitized patient. *Arch. Surg.* 113:893–896, 1978.

Goldsmith, M. A.; Slavik, M.; and Carter, S. K. Quantitative prediction of drug toxicity in humans from toxicology in small and large animals. *Cancer Res.* 35:1354–1364.

Hardy, T. J.; An, T.; Brown, P. W.; and Terz, J. J. Postirradiation sarcoma (malignant fibrous histiocytoma) of axilla. *Cancer* 53:118–124, 1978.

Mark, G. J.; Lehimgar-Zadeh, A.; and Ragsdale, B. D. Cyclophosphamide pneumonitis. *Thorax* 33:89–93, 1978.

Mindell, E. R.; Shah, N. K.; and Webster, J. H. Postradiation sarcoma of bone and soft tissues. *Orthop. Clin. North. Am.* 8(4):821–834, 1977.

Phillips, T. L. Chemical modification of radiation effects. *Cancer* 39:987–999, 1977.

Ritch, P. S. et al. Disseminated BCG disease associated with immunotherapy by scarification in acute leukemia. *Cancer* 53:167–170, 1978.

Rosenow, E. C., III. The spectrum of drug-induced pulmonary disease. *Ann. Intern. Med.* 77:977–991, 1972.

Roswitt, B.; Malsky, S. J.; and Reid, C. B. Radiation tolerance of the gastrointestinal tract. *Frontiers of radiation therapy and oncology,* J. M. Vaeth, ed., vol. 6, p. 160. Baltimore: University Park Press, 1972.

Rosenthal, S., and Kaufman, S. Vincristine neurotoxicity. *Ann. Intern. Med.* 80:733–737, 1974.

Rubin, P., ed. *Radiation biology and radiation pathology syllabus.* Baltimore: Waverly Press, Inc., 1975.

Schein, P. S., and Winokur, S. H. Immunosuppressive and cytotoxic chemotherapy: long-term complications. *Ann. Intern. Med.* 82:84–95, 1975.

Sostman, H. D.; Matthay, R. A.; and Putnam, C. E. Cytotoxic drug-induced lung disease. *Am. J. Med.* 62:608–615, 1977.

Weiss, H. D.; Walker, M. D.; and Wiernik, P. H. Neurotoxicity of commonly used antineoplastic agents. *N. Engl. J. Med.* 291:75–81 127–135, 1974.

Part VI   Rare and Uncommon Manifestations of Cancer

Chapter 19

Paraneoplastic Syndromes of Malignancy

J. Lokich

N. Anderson

1.0 Hormone syndromes in neoplasia

The production of humoral substances by tumors is common and may even be a universal concomitant to neoplasia. Tumors derived from endocrine glands may produce hormone immunochemically identical to the normal hormone and these hormones can be biologically active or nonfunctional. Carcinoma of the adrenal gland, for example, is associated with Cushing's syndrome in only 50 percent of patients while malignant parathyroid tumors are almost always functional (Table 19.1). Endocrine tumors are often benign and may be asymptomatic and nonfunctional, while the malignant tumors often retain the functional capacity of the gland and present with typical features of excess hormone production.

Endocrine tumors in one site may be associated with tumors in other component glands of the endocrine system (Table 19.2). Tumors comprising a multiple endocrine neoplasia syndrome are commonly benign. Thymic carcinoid tumors, however, which are observed particularly with type II multiple endocrine adenomatosis, and medullary carcinoma of the thyroid are usually malignant. The interrelationships among the various endocrine tumors are important considerations for early detection of cancer in the familial variants.

Pancreatic tumors are particularly important because they produce unique clinical syndromes and are often occult. The tumors of the component cells of the islets of the pancreas are exceedingly rare and often benign. When the tumor is malignant, the clinical course is often protracted, and survival can be considerable. Renal tumors also have been associated with the secretion of active physiologic substances. The literature contains isolated case reports of renal tumors that

Table 19.1 Tumors Derived from Endocrine Tissue

Endocrine Organ	Tumor	Product	Comment
Adrenal	Pheochromocytoma	Adrenalin	90% benign
	Cortical tumor	Cortisol	50% of malignant tumors functional
Thyroid	Papillary or follicular	T_3, T_4	Malignancy variable
	Medullary	Calcitonin	Familial and generally malignant
Pituitary	Multiple types	GH, ACTH, LH, FSH	Generally benign
Parathyroid		PTH	95% of malignant cases functional*
Endocrine-Exocrine Organ	Pancreatic islet cell		
Beta Cells	Insulinoma	Insulin	80% benign
Delta Cells	Zollinger-Ellison syndrome	Gastrin	50% benign
Alpha Cells	Glucagon	Glucagon	Predominantly malignant†
Alpha Cells	Werner-Morrison syndrome	Vasoactive intestinal peptide (VIP)	65% benign
D Cells	Somatostatinoma	Somatostatin	Benign‡ and familial

* 50 cases reported
† 27 cases reported
‡ 2 families reported

Table 19.2 Multiple Endocrine Neoplasia (or Adenomatosis) Syndromes and Associated Clinical Diseases

Type I: Werner's Syndrome
         Pituitary tumors
         Pancreatic islet tumors
         Parathyroid tumors

Type II: Sipple Syndrome
         Medullary cancer of the thyroid
         Pheochromocytoma
         Parathyroid tumors

Other Abnormalities
         Thymus tumor (carcinoid)
         Mucosal neuromas
         Carcinoid tumors (lung, gastrointestinal tract)

secrete erythropoeitin, prostaglandins, and renin. These tumors are most commonly benign.

Tumors that do not originate within endocrine tissue may also produce hormones. This "ectopic" production of hormones results in the clinical paraneoplastic syndrome. Nonendocrine tumors produce a hormone that is immunochemically similar to the normal hormone but which is much less commonly functional. For example, although lung cancer is associated with ACTH production in more than 80 percent of patients, Cushing's syndrome rarely occurs.

The mechanism by which nonendocrine tumors produce hormones may be related to the embryology of the tumor cell. Three theories attempt to explain the evolution of ectopic hormone-producing tumors. One theory proposes that sequestered remnants of potential endocrine tissue undergo neoplastic degeneration. For example, oat cell carcinoma, which is commonly associated with the production of hormones, is derived from the neural crest similar to the endocrine glands. Neurosecretory granules can be demonstrated within the oat tumor cell by electron microscopy. A second theory claims that the neoplastic cell hybridizes with a cell that has an endocrine potential and thus acquires the capability for hormone production. An epidermoid cancer in the lung, for example, may hybridize with a circulating or neighboring endocrine cell and incorporate the genetic material necessary to establish hormone synthesis. A third theory suggests that the neoplastic process reverses differentiation of the cell to the extent that operant genes that have the capability of inducing the protein synthesis necessary for hormone production are not repressed. This last theory accounts for the fact that tumors can produce more than one polypeptide and therefore may produce multiple concomitant endocrine syndromes.

The most common cancers to be associated with paraneoplastic syndromes are the small cell undifferentiated tumors, particularly those derived from the lung. These tumors, as indicated previously, are derived from Kulchitsky cells, which are descendants of neural crest cells and characteristically demonstrate neurosecretory granules. An important aspect of these tumors is their exquisite responsiveness to radiation and chemotherapy. In spite of the effectiveness of treatment, however, the long-term prognosis for patients with paraneoplastic syndromes is limited. For patients with oat cell tumors in whom a secretory product and a paraneoplastic syndrome is clinically demonstrated, the prognosis is worse when compared to patients similarly staged but without the ectopic hormone syndrome.

Five major ectopic hormone syndromes have been described: Cushing's syndrome, hyperparathyroidism, the syndrome of inappropriate ADH secretion (SIADH), thyrotoxicosis, and hypoglycemia. The nonendocrine tumors associated with these specific syndromes are of diverse origin, with the exception of thyrotoxicosis, which has only been reported in association with trophoblastic tumors (Table 19.3). The five syndromes are important because the clinical manifestations

Table 19.3 Tumors Associated with the Five Major Ectopic Hormone Syndromes

Syndrome	Associated Tumors*
Cushing's syndrome	Lung (oat cell), pancreas, prostate, thymus, thyroid
Hyperparathyroidism	Kidney, lung (epidermoid), breast, ovary, bladder
Inappropriate ADH (STADH)	Lung (oat cell)
Hyperthyroidism	Trophoblastic tumors (choriocarcinoma)
Hypoglycemia	Peritoneum, mesenchymal, mesothelioma, hepatoblastoma, stomach

*Listed in decreasing frequency

of the hormone excess may be the initial clues to the presence of cancer. Furthermore, the clinical syndrome and the secondary metabolic derangement may be life threatening. Specific treatment of the tumor, if effective, uniformly results in reversal of the clinical syndrome. Alternatively, treatment directed specifically at the metabolic derangement may be only temporarily effective in controlling the hormone excess. For example, fluid restriction in patients with inappropriate ADH secretion or the use of beta-blocking agents in patients with thyrotoxicosis is often effective. The automomy of the neoplastic tumor, however, allows for the production of tremendous quantities of the peptide mediator, which requires comparable doses of the antidote.

The antithesis of ectopic hormone production is hormone insufficiency, which is exceedingly rare. Hormone insufficiency is included in the paraneoplastic considerations because of its potentially life-threatening nature. Table 19.4 lists the three categories of hormone insufficiency, but only diabetes insipidus is well recognized and clinically important. The mechanism of hormone insufficiency is related to metastasis to the site of production of the hormone or insufficiency of the tropic hormone. Diabetes insipidus generally occurs as a consequence of breast cancer metastasis to the hypothalamus. Diabetes mellitus rarely occurs as a prelude to primary pancreatic carcinoma because it

is unusual for a tumor to replace totally all islet components of the pancreas. Clinical adrenal insufficiency has been previously reported with adrenal metastases although it is extremely uncommon. Nonetheless, hyperkalemia and hyponatremia in patients with extensive retroperitoneal tumor should suggest the possibility of adrenal replacement by tumor.

A number of clinical syndromes associated with nonendocrine tumors are presumed to be mediated through an ectopic hormone substance. No hormonal substance, however, has been isolated in any of the syndromes (Table 19.5). Two of the syndromes, myasthenia gravis and the nephrotic syndrome, may be related to an immune-complex mechanism with the host producing an antitumor antibody that subsequently combines with the tumor antigen and is deposited in the muscle end plates or the kidney. Hypertrophic pulmonary osteoarthropathy has been associated with the secretion of growth hormone in occasional patients, but this mechanism has not been substantiated, and the syndrome may be secondary to a host neurovascular reaction to the tumor. Abnormal liver function tests, predominantly of the liver enzymes, occur particularly with renal cell carcinoma, and may be observed in the absence of hepatic metastases. The major reason for assuming that these syndromes are associated with secretion of a hormone substance is that when the tumor is controlled,

Table 19.4 Hormone Insufficiency Syndromes Related to Cancer Metastasis

Syndrome	Pathologic mechanism	Comment
Diabetes insipidus	Metastasis to hypothalamus	Most common with breast tumor; treated with chlorpropamide
Adrenal insufficiency	Metastasis to adrenal gland	Most common with lung cancer; treated with corticosteroid replacement
Diabetes mellitus	Metastasis to pancreas	Uncommon except with primary tumor of the pancreas

Table 19.5 Cancer Syndromes Possibly Mediated by Tumor Secretory Products (or So-called Pseudoparaneoplastic Syndromes)

Clinical syndrome	Humoral substance
Myasthenia gravis	Curarelike substance or immune complexes
Neuromyopathy	Unknown
Cerebellar degeneration	Unknown
Hypertrophic pulmonary osteoarthropathy	Growth hormone
Nephrotic syndrome	Immune complex (cross-reacting tumor and antibody)
Hepatic enzymopathy	Unknown (possibly immune-complex mediated)
Cancer cachexia	Unknown
Pyrexia	Unknown

the syndrome generally disappears. Exceptions are the neurologic and myopathic manifestations of tumor. This group of syndromes is known as the pseudoparaneoplastic manifestations of cancer.

The paraneoplastic and pseudoparaneoplastic syndromes present important diagnostic and therapeutic problems. Management of the syndrome often, but not invariably, depends on effective therapy for the tumor, but pharmacologic therapy or control of the extreme physiologic effects of the excessive hormone may also be important in circumstances in which the tumor is insensitive to cytotoxic therapy.

2.0 Cushing's syndrome and ACTH-secreting tumors

The clinical manifestations of ACTH-producing tumors is a variant of Cushing's syndrome. Hypertension, hypernatremia, and hypokalemia are commonly observed in the absence of such typical physical features of the syndrome as centripetal obesity, striae, and moon facies. Approximately 150 patients with oat cell lung

cancer have been reported to have had Cushing's syndrome. However, 80 percent of patients with lung cancer of various histologic types have elevated ACTH levels in their circulating blood; this disparity indicates that the neoplastia-derived hormone is not biologically active in the large majority of patients. In addition to lung cancer, Cushing's syndrome has been reported in patients with prostatic cancer and other tumors derived from tissues that are remnants of the embryonic foregut. These tumors are often undifferentiated and histologically similar to the oat cell tumor.

Patient A, a 59-year-old white woman, was admitted for evaluation of profound lethargy and muscle weakness. She had been well until six weeks prior to admission, when she noted gradually increasing fatigue that interfered with her work as an assembly worker in a doll manufacturing factory. She also noted bilateral pedal edema for which she was placed on a diuretic. The fatigue was associated with profound muscle weakness of the lower extremities and gradually increased until she could no longer work. Both she and her husband noted the development of increased facial hair, a definite deepening of the color of her skin, and hyperpigmentation of her areolae. Physical examination revealed an ill-appearing, middle-aged woman with obvious fatigue.

The skin was very oily and generally hyperpigmented; the pigmentation was most pronounced over both areolae. There were a few early acneiform lesions of the face and a marked increase in coarse facial hairs. In other ways the body habitus was normal with no obvious redistribution of body fat. Profound muscle weakness of the quadriceps muscles was bilateral with early atrophy. Blood pressure was 140/80. Initial laboratory evaluation included a complete blood count that was normal except for only five percent lymphocytes; 1.2 mEq/L serum potassium; 146 sodium; 66 chloride; 64 bicarbonate; 7.63 arterial pH; 88 pO_2; 59 pCO_2; serum cortisol was greater than 60 mg/ dl (normal = 7 to 25). A diagnosis was not immediately apparent, and she was treated with large doses of intravenous and oral KCl up to 10 mEq/hr for eight days. This, in addition to the use of spironolactone (Aldactone), increased the serum potassium to 3.4 mEq/L. On the ninth hospital day a chest x-ray revealed complete collapse of the left-lower lobe; bronchoscopy revealed total obstruction of the left lower lobe bronchus by a large intrabronchial mass. Biopsy of the mass revealed small cell (oat cell) carcinoma of the lung.

A diagnosis of oat cell carcinoma with ectopic production of ACTH was made. By this time the patient was receiving 600 mg of spironolactone daily in four divided doses and 150 mEq of KCl in three divided doses; her serum potassium on this regimen was 2.8 mEq/L. Follow-up laboratory evaluation revealed: Hb 11.9 of gm; Hct of 36%; white blood cell count of 15,400/mm³ with six percent lymphocytes; platelets of 284,000/mm³; serum sodium of 143 mEq/L; potassium of 2.5;

chloride of 94; carbon dioxide of 39; blood urea nitrogen of 15; creatinine of 0.6 mg/ dl; blood glucose of 282 mg/dl; urine glucose of 3 +. An 8:00 A.M. serum cortisol was 35.0 mg/dl; 8:00 P.M. serum cortisol was 42.4 mg/dl; 24-hour urine for 17 ketosteroids was 40 mg (normal = 3.3 + 1.1); serum ACTH 3887 pg/ml (normal = 15 to 100). Liver, bone, and brain scans were all normal, but a metastatic series demonstrated severe osteoporosis. Cancer chemotherapy was initiated with a three-drug regimen of cyclophosphamide, lomustine (CCNU), and methotrexate. The lomustine and cyclophosphamide were given at 21-day intervals, and the methotrexate was given orally twice per week. She was discharged on 600 mg spironolactone daily and 150 mEq of KCl to maintain a serum potassium above 3.5.

Seventeen days later she was readmitted for evaluation of the effectiveness of the initial chemotherapy. Only minimal improvement appeared in her muscle weakness, and her lethargy persisted. Masculinization and hyperpigmentation were unchanged. Laboratory evaluation showed: Hb of 11.4 gm; Hct of 35%; white blood cell count of 6800/mm³ with 27% lymphocytes; serum sodium 137 mEq/L; potassium of 2.9; chloride of 92; carbon dioxide of 31; blood urea nitrogen of 16 mg/dl; creatinine of 0.7 mg/dl; blood glucose of 317 mg/dl; urine glucose of 3 +; serum cortisol was greater than 80 mg/dl (repeat time 2); serum ACTH was 280 pg/ml, serum thyroxine was 7.1 mcg/dl; serum TSH was 2.9. A chest x-ray revealed marked improvement from pretreatment x-ray, with resolution of left-lower lobe collapse but persistence of a four-centimeter perihilar mass on the left. Because of persistent hyperglycemia and hypokalemia, the patient was again discharged on spironolactone 600 mg daily, KCl 150 mEq daily, and Orinase (tolbutamide) after a second course of cyclophosphamide and lomustine (CCNU). Two weeks later she had regained some of her strength

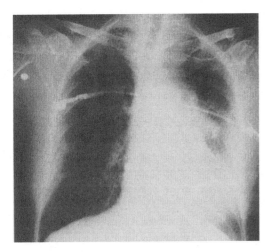 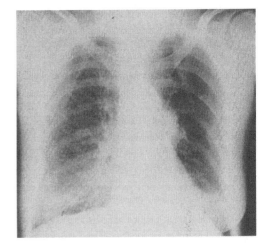

Fig. 19.1 Sequential radiographs (Patient A) with oat cell carcinoma and secondary Cushing's syndrome demonstrating hilar mass lesion (A) and subsequent regression (B).

and felt significantly improved although masculinization had not decreased. A repeat chest x-ray was almost normal with only a suggestion of a perihilar mass (Fig. 19.1). Her potassium was 5.1 mEq/L, and the spironolactone and KCl were decreased. In spite of resolution of the mass by radiographic follow-up, the metabolic abnormality persisted. Eight weeks after initiation of tumor therapy, her serum potassium suddenly rose to 7.8 mEq/L, and was controlled with only minimal supplement thereafter. The patient also developed a Pneumocystis carinii pneumonia, presumably secondary to the profound immunosuppression related to chronic endogenous hypersecretion of steroids.

ACTH-secreting tumors are generally primary in the lung and the clinical manifestations are the classic metabolic changes of hypokalemia and hyperglycemia.

The clinical manifestations of ACTH-secreting tumors are variable, but the most common presentation is hypokalemic alkalosis. Thus, patients present predominantly with secondary symptoms of hypokalemia including polyuria and muscle weakness. In addition, diabetes mellitus and hypertension are commonly observed. Masculinization and hyperpigmentation are distinctly unusual, however, and occur most commonly with chronic or slowly growing tumors. Similarly, osteoporosis requires a long period of steroid exposure to develop.

Cushing's syndrome is never secondary to cortisol secretion from the tumor but is always a manifestation of tropic hormone excess. The adrenal glands are therefore hyperplastic. Therapeutic adrenalectomy has not been employed, although ablative procedures for prostatic cancer have incidentally identified hyperplastic adrenal glands in patients with Cushing's syndrome. Therapy to correct the ectopic hormone syndrome focuses on eradication or control of the tumor itself. Oat cell carcinoma is a radiation- and drug-responsive tumor, and reversal of the ACTH syndrome can be accomplished with either chemotherapy or irradiation, although resistance develops promptly, and recurrence is followed by rapid deterioration. Another potential control for the syndrome is the application of metabolic inhibitors of cortisol synthesis, such as OPDDD (mitotane) or aminoglutethamide (Cytogren). This method, however, has not been reported, and its toxicity would presumably be prohibitive, as the antagonist dose required would be substantial in view of the autonomous nature of the tumor and its enormous production of tropic hormone. The resolution of biochemical abnormality may be observed over a protracted time in spite of rapid tumor response. For Patient A, large doses of spironolactone were necessary to maintain serum potasssium levels at eight weeks after initiation of treatment even when the tumor was barely evident radiographically. Delayed resolution of the syndrome may be related either to secondary autonomous adrenal gland function or to increased sensitivity of the hyperplastic gland, even to low levels of ACTH.

3.0 Syndrome of inappropriate ADH secretion (SIADH)

The clinical manifestations of inappropriate ADH secretion (SIADH) are hyponatremia and water intoxication with secondary cerebral deterioration. Patients with SIADH often present with nonspecific neurologic signs and symptoms, including confusion and disorientation. The SIADH may appear as the initial manifestation of a small, clinically occult tumor. Invariably, the primary tumor is a lung cancer, generally of the oat cell type. Confirmation of the syndrome may be determined by analysis of urine for excessive ADH levels, but more often SIADH is diagnosed by comparing urine and serum osmolality determinations, which are disparate in patients suffering from water intoxication due to SIADH.

Patient B, a 48-year-old white woman, was admitted to the hospital because of a serum sodium of 112 mEq/L. She had been well until one week prior to admission when she developed anorexia associated with mild nausea, polyuria, and polydypsia. She also noted severe leg cramps daily as well as easy fatigability, which was associated with insomnia. A dry, nonproductive cough present for 12 months became more pronounced, and her husband noted that her voice had become more "husky" in the preceding three weeks. She denied diarrhea, fever, chills, or weight loss. She had smoked one or two packs of cigarettes each day for 20 years until 10 years prior to admission, when she discontinued cigarettes altogether. Physical examination revealed a blood pressure of 144/70 mm Hg without postural changes. The mucous membranes were well hydrated and the skin had good turgor. Laboratory evaluation revealed the following: serum sodium of 112 mEq/L; potassium of 4.3; chloride of 80; carbon dioxide of 20; blood urea nitrogen of 5 mg/dl; creatinine of 0.4 mg/dl. Chest x-ray demonstrated an ill-defined mass in the lingula with fullness of the left hilum (Fig. 19.2). She was treated initially with normal saline intravenously administered; fluids were then restricted to 1000 cc per day. After an inconslusive bronchoscopy, she underwent an open-lung biopsy to establish a diagnosis. Using a Chamberlain incision, a biopsy of the pulmonary tumor was performed, and the diagnosis of small cell carcinoma with involvement of the left hilar nodes was established. Following the histologic confirmation of the diagnosis, laboratory evaluation and metastatic survey, including intravenous pyelogram, bone scan, liver scan, and brain scan, were performed; all were normal. Because of the inappropriately elevated urine osmolality (795 mOsm/L) and a normal renal and adrenal organ system, she was thought to have the SIADH secondary to small cell carci-

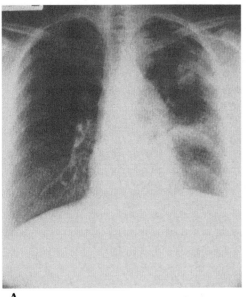

A

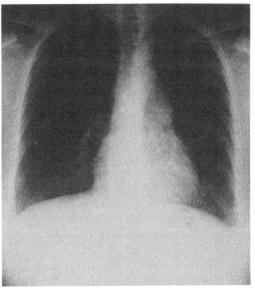

B

Fig. 19.2 Sequential radiographs (Patient B) with oat cell carcinoma and the inappropriate ADH syndrome demonstrating left parahilar mass and peripheral lung lesion in the upper and middle lung fields (A) with regression following chemotherapy (B).

noma of the lung. She was restricted to 500 cc of fluid per day, which resulted in a slight rise in the serum sodium to 122 mEq/L. Definitive antitumor treatment, however, resulted in rapid resolution of the tumor and secondary control of the SIADH. She received a regimen of cyclophosphamide, Adriamycin, and vincristine, and eight days following chemotherapy her blood urea nitrogen had risen to 9.0 mg/dl and the sodium to 135 mEq/ L. With each successive course of chemotherapy the serum and urine osmolalities continued to return to normal; she regained almost normal physical stamina with no hint of her previous symptoms. The chest tumor regressed completely on radiographs.

SIADH is the most common paraneoplastic syndrome.

Excessive ADH secretion by lung tumors is commonly observed if patients are screened routinely for detection of elevated ADH levels, but like ACTH and lung tumors, the clinical syndrome is uncommon. Most of the tumors secrete biologically inactive material immunologically cross-reactive to physiologic ADH. In patients with the syndrome, the monitoring of serum electrolytes is a useful measure for tumor growth and the effectiveness of therapy. Rapid reversal of the ADH syndrome may be effected by water restriction, but like the ACTH syndrome, the most definitive therapy is directed at control of the tumor. Radiation therapy directed at the localized tumor or systemic chemotherapy for disseminated tumor is commonly effective against oat cell cancer; therefore, initial control of the SIADH is often possible. The metastatic extension of the tumor is not often associated with exacerbation of the

SIADH. This phenomenon may be related to a lack of differentiation or a mutation of the tumor that develops with metastases. Although the correction of hyponatremia may occur rapidly, the osmotic imbalance may persist for some time. Symptomatic improvement invariably occurs with restitution of serum sodium.

Pharmacologic manipulation may be used to treat the SIADH. Lithium carbonate and demeclocycline have both been effective in reversing the syndrome even in the absence of tumor control. The mechanism of action for these drugs appears to be a peripheral block of ADH at the level of the renal tubule, and surprisingly low doses of either lithium or demeclocycline may be effective in reversing the syndrome.

4.0 Thyrotoxicosis and placental tumors

Thyrotoxicosis is an extreme hypermetabolic state clinically characterized by tremor, fever, and tachycardia. The nonendocrine tumors associated with the development of clinical hyperthyroidism are the trophoblastic tumors of either gestational or nongestational origin. It is possible that biologically inactive TSH is present in other tumors, but routine screening of patients with lung cancer and other tumors for elevated levels of TSH has not been conducted.

Thyrotoxicosis develops either secondary to a TSH product derived from the trophoblastic tissue or is an effect of human chorionic gonadotropin (HCG) itself, which may have biologic activities that include stimulation of the thyroid.

Patient C, a 26-year-old gravid 2, para 0, abortive 0 woman first came to medical attention during her 33rd week of pregnancy, when she suddenly developed anemia and lower extremity edema. Initial laboratory evaluation included the following: LDH 1092 Iu; bilirubin of 4.0 mg/dl; hematocrit of 23 percent, reticulocyte count of 9.0 percent. She was thought to have an acute hemolytic anemia, but a Coombs' antiglobulin test was negative, and serum heptoglobin was normal. She was transfused with packed red blood cells and observed closely.

At week 35, labor was induced because of persistent anemia and fetal distress. An emergency Caesarean section was performed and a healthy six-pound boy was delivered without complication. At surgery the patient's ovaries were noted to be massively enlarged, filling almost the entire lower abdomen. In addition, a very large hemorrhagic mass in the left lobe of the liver was observed. No biopsy was performed because of the possibility of hemorrhage. Postoperatively, a urinary gonadotropin level was reported at 225,-000 per 24 hours, and a serum determination of beta-subunit HCG was 940,000 IU/ml. The placenta was reinvestigated pathologically and found to be totally normal with no evidence of choriocarcinoma. Hepatic angiogram revealed the presence of multiple vascular lesions in the left and right lobes consistent with choriocarcinoma. A chest x-ray revealed the presence of a large, six-centimeter pleural-based mass consistent with metastatic disease. A partial left hepatectomy was performed to prevent hemorrhagic catastrophe. Pathologically the liver lesion was typical for choriocarcinoma.

Postoperatively, the patient experienced a sudden onset of bilateral headaches, disconjugate gaze, horizontal nystagmus, and cranial nerve palsies, all symptoms suggesting occult central nervous system tomographic metastases. A scan revealed massive dilatation of the ventricular system and a large cerebellar lesion in the left posterior fossa. Therapy with dexamethazone (Decadron), intrathecal methotrexate, and irradiation was initiated with resolution of neurologic symptoms. The patient also developed acute thyrotoxicosis with high-output cardiac failure. She had lid lag, mild exophthalmos, and tachycardia at a rate of 120 to 130 with a fine tremor at rest. Serum thyroxine was 27 mc/dl (normal = 4 to 11) and the TSH level was 12.0 (normal is undetectable). Throughout her illness, the TSH and thyroxine closely paralleled HCG levels and were almost as sensitive as HCG as markers of tumor response (Fig. 19.3). With a decreased HCG and thyroxine secondary to antitumor treatment, the clinical signs of hyperthyroidism became less evident but not totally absent. She required propranolol to counteract the peripheral effects of increased thyroid hormone. The patient developed severe leukopenia with secondary ab-

dominal sepsis, which necessitated a delay of almost eight weeks in chemotherapy, during which time the tumor recurred in the liver and the HCG rose precipitously. Upon reintroduction of chemotherapy, however, there was rapid clinical and biochemical improvement.

Thyrotoxicosis is a common association of trophoblastic tumors.

Thyrotoxicosis has many clincial manifestations ranging from the hypermetabolic state to lymphadenopathy and splenomegaly. When excessive TSH secretion

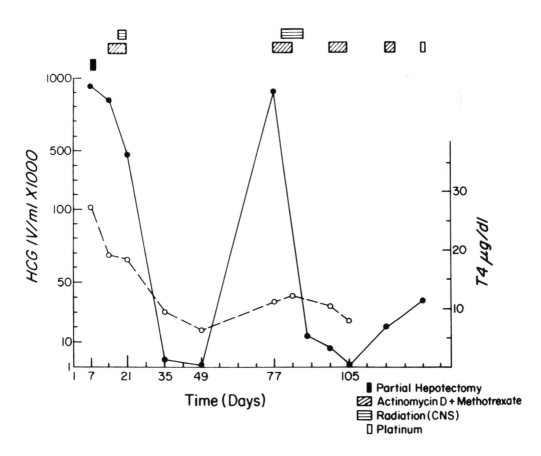

Fig. 19.3 HCG and T₄ levels in response to tumor-specific therapy for Patient C with choriocarcinoma and secondary hyperthyroidism.

develops in association with trophoblastic tumors, thyrotoxicosis is invariably manifested in its classic form. Occasionally, the hypermetabolic state may proceed to the extreme and result in high-output heart failure, but the clinical manifestations may be more subtle. Treatment of thyrotoxicosis depends first upon recognition of the metabolic derangement, as patients with progressive cancer often demonstrate many of the clinical features of thyrotoxicosis including weight loss, tremor, and tachycardia.

Trophoblastic tumors are especially responsive to chemotherapy even in the presence of metastases; therefore, tumor-specific therapy may control the thyrotoxicosis. In the absence of effective therapy, or if the tumor becomes resistant to treatment, either antithyroid drugs such as propylthiouracil or beta-adrenergic blockers may be useful

5.0 Hypoglycemia and mesenchymal tumors

In addition to the islet cell tumor derived from beta cells, which results in hypoglycemia secondary to autonomous insulin production, a group of nonpancreatic tumors is associated with hypoglycemia. These tumors primarily include mesenchyma-derived tumors involving the retroperitoneum and pleural-based tumors in the thorax. The indentification of an insulinlike substance secreted by these tumors has not been established, and the mechanism of hypoglycemia in these tumors is therefore unclear although the syndrome recedes with surgical removal of the tumor. The typical clinical features of hypoglycemia episodes are similar to those of exogenous insulin overdose and include a disordered mental state, diaphoresis, and immediate relief of symptoms in response to glucose administration. The intermittent and episodic pattern of the hypoglycemia is similarly characteris-

tic, suggesting that the secretory activity of the tumor is not completely autonomous.

Patient D, a 57-year-old insurance salesman, was admitted for evaluation of a rapidly enlarging abdominal mass and documented attacks of hypoglycemia. Six months prior to admission, his wife began noticing "strange behavior" characterized by prolonged periods of staring vacantly into space; these episodes occurred primarily before breakfast. At times he would take 20 minutes to put on his socks; all attempts by his wife to "break through" to him during such episodes were futile. His personality also changed, and he became forgetful and easily irritable. His personal administration of business matters, which had been previously very well organized and systematic, became progressively impaired until he could not easily locate certain business contacts. On at least one occasion during this time, his wife and son discussed the need for psychiatric hospitalization, feeling that he was "losing his mind." One month prior to admission he collapsed by his car while leaving work at night. He was taken by ambulance to a local hospital, where a blood glucose was measured at 42 mg/ dl. After an intravenous infusion of 50 percent dextrose, his mental status returned to normal, and he suffered no sequelae of the event. Glucose tolerance test (GTT) revealed the following: 59 mg/dl after fasting; 160 mg/dl after one-half hour; 219 mg/dl after one hour; 42 mg/dl after two hours. His physician told him that he suffered from "hypoglycemia" and placed him on a high-protein diet. His left leg swelling was attributed to gout.

Because of the persistence of recurring attacks of blurred vision, loss of mental acuity, dysarthria, and forgetfulness, which he thought were due to hypoglycemia, his wife arranged a schedule of frequent, small, high-glucose content feed-

ings. These included a 7:00 A.M. breakfast with juice, toast, and eggs; a 10:00 A.M. snack of coffee with sugar and roll: a 12:00-noon lunch; a 3:00 P.M. snack of fruit juice and cookies; a 6:00 P.M. dinner; an 8:30 P.M. snack of milk and fruit; an 11:30 P.M. snack of fruit juice and sugar; and a 3:00 A.M. snack of milk and toast with jelly. The sudden appearance of a "soccer ball"-sized abdominal mass and a 25-lb weight gain prompted reevaluation. Physical examination revealed a large, nontender, spherical 20 × 20-cm mass arising in the pelvis and filling the abdomen to the umbilicus. There were no bruits over the mass. The left leg had 4+ pitting edema to mid-thigh. Laboratory examination was normal except for a GTT, which demonstrated persistent hypoglycemia at five hours. In addition, barium enema demonstrated a mass deep in the pelvis with draping of the sigmoid around the mass; an abdominal echogram revealed a 21 × 12 × 25-cm mass arising from the pelvis with homogeneous echo pattern; and an arteriogram demonstrated hypovascularity of the lesion (Fig. 19.4). The patient underwent a laparotomy at which time a large ovoid mass, 25 × 16 × 16 cm and weighting 3600 gm was easily removed. The mass was well encapsulated and attached with a 3-cm pedicle in the retroperitoneum. It was identified pathologically as a spindle cell sarcoma of moderate pathologic grade. Intraoperatively, simultaneous blood glucose levels were obtained from the efferent arterial supply and the afferent venous drainage; the blood glucose levels were exactly the same. The tumor itself was devoid of significant insulin activity as measured by the insulin radio-immunoassay system; actual values were 0.0002 microunits/ml in the fatty portion and 0.0005 microunits/ml in the hemorrhagic portion. Within 15 minutes of removal of the tumor the blood glucose rose to 152 mg/dl.

Postoperatively, the patient did very well with no recurrence of hypoglycemia or hypoglycemic symptoms. He returned to a normal diet. The left leg edema resolved over 3 days, during which he underwent a vigorous, spontaneous diuresis that was thought to be a postobstructive fluid loss. He was discharged on postoperative day 12 with no complaints. On the day of discharge a repeat oral GTT with insulin and glucagon levels was performed. He was seen three months postoperatively and remained in excellent health. Although insulin was not identified in the tumor or in the patient's serum, nonspecific insulinlike activity was identified in both tissue and serum.

Hypoglycemic syndromes are commonly due to mesenchymal tumors of the abdominal cavity.

It has never been demonstrated that insulin is secreted by these tumors, possibly because the tumor may secrete an insulinlike substance that induces hypoglycemia but which is immunologically distinct from insulin itself. The tumor substance may facilitate the development of hypoglycemia by the inhibition of gluconeogenesis, and tumor extracts have been shown to induce hypoglycemia in animal model systems by such a mechanism. Although the tumors are frequently enormous, the theory that tumor consumption of glucose is the cause of the hypoglycemia has not been verified by quantitative metabolic studies or by measurement of arterial and venous glucose concentrations across the tumor bed.

The clinical management of hypoglycemia by pharmacologic manipulation with diazoxide, glucagon, or other hyperglycemic drugs has not been reported, but presumably these agents would have some measure of effectiveness, as they are not insulin antagonists but rather function independently of insulin to mobilize glucose peripherally. Common therapy

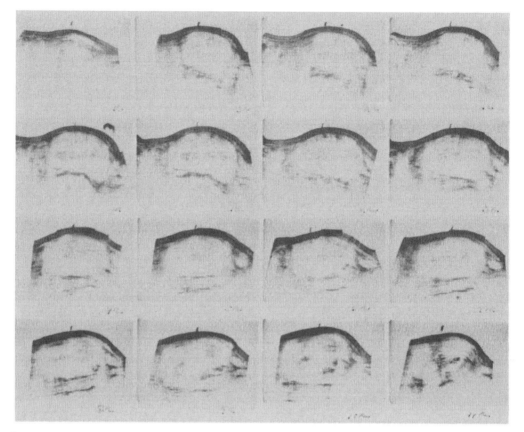

A

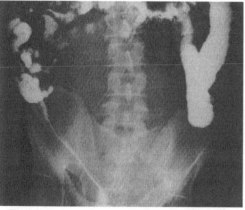

B

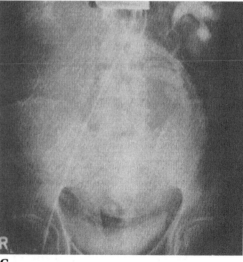

C

Fig. 19.4 Patient D with an intra-abdominal mass clearly demonstrated by ultrasound (A) and barium enema (B) with displaced bowel; arteriogram (right) reveals general hypovascularity of the mass lesion (C).

for hypoglycemia is the use of frequent feedings. The most effective management, however, is tumor removal, which is only occasionally possible. Of the 200 reported cases of mesenchymal tumor-associated hypoglycemia, more than 150 patients died either of the tumor or of its secondary effects.

6.0 Pseudoparaneoplastic syndromes

The clinical syndromes termed pseudoparaneoplastic are those in which a tumor substance has not been demonstrated, but in which control of the tumor is often associated with a reversal of clinical effects. Examples of pseudoparaneoplastic syndromes are indicated in Table 19.5. No tumor-specific substance or hormone mediator has been established, and the possibility of immune mechanisms, particularly autoimmune reactions, has been considered as the pathophysiologic mechanism of some of the syndromes.

The pseudoparaneoplastic syndromes are a heterogeneous group of secondary tumor effects with an ominous prognosis and rare reversibility.

Neurologic effects of cancer do not precisely fit the definition because the secondary neurologic syndromes are often not reversible, possibly because of a toxic effect on the neural tissue and the inability of the neural tissue to regenerate. The cerebellar degeneration syndrome, for example, typically demonstrates gliosis throughout the cerebellum, and even with effective tumor therapy for the associated lung tumor, the clinical picture rarely improves because the pathologic effects in the cerebellum are permanent.

Myasthenia in cancer patients is manifested as a proximal myopathy that progresses to an areflexic paralysis; it is almost exclusively associated with oat cell carcinoma. The syndrome is generally referred to as the Eaton-Lambert syndrome and may be the initial manifestation of an occult tumor, although the tumor generally is clinically detectable within a short time.

Patient E, a massively obese 42-year-old black woman and member of Jehovah's Witnesses, first presented with wheezing and cough. Bronchodilator therapy was ineffective; a chest x-ray showed a mass in the right hilum, and the patient was admitted for evaluation (Fig. 19.5). Physical examination was normal except for scattered wheezes and morbid obesity. The neurologic examination was normal and without muscle weakness. A bronchoscopy revealed only a narrowed right intermediate lobe bronchus; bronchial washings and sputum cytologies were repeatedly negative. A transbronchial lung biopsy and a node biopsy were also negative. She was discharged with no established diagnosis but with suspicion of primary carcinoma of the lung.

Three months after the right hilum mass was discovered, she was readmitted because of severe bilateral leg weakness prohibiting walking and standing. She was totally bedridden because of the weakness. Neurologic examination revealed a profound proximal muscle weakness in the lower and upper extremities, with no paresthesias or sensory abnormalities. Deep tendon reflexes were universally diminished without pathologic reflexes. An open-lung biopsy revealed the presence of small cell carcinoma (oat cell) with metastases to two hilar lymph nodes. An electromyogram (EMG) revealed the following (Fig. 19.6):

1. *Abnormally low amplitude action potential in the ulnar nerve (0.8 mV; normal-15 to 20 mV).*
2. *Repetitive stimulation at 1, 2, 5, and 10/sec produced no decremental or*

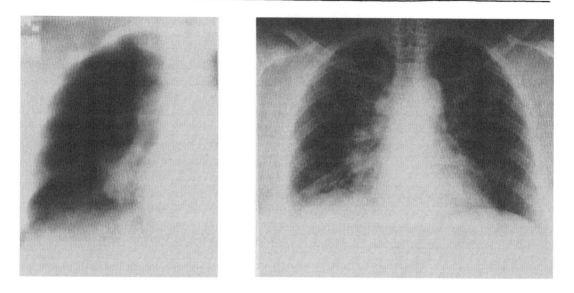

Fig. 19.5 Chest radiograph (Patient E)   and a left hilar mass (B).
demonstrating tomogram clarification (A)

incremental increase in muscle-action potential.

3. Repetitive stimulation at 20/sec produced a brief decrement followed by a 16 percent increase in muscle-action potential.

4. Repetitive stimulation at 50/sec produced an 84 percent increase in muscle-action potential amplitude.

5. Brief exercise was followed by an immediate but transient increase in muscle response from 2.0 mV to 10.0 mV (500%).

6. Tensilon (10.0 mg) produced no increase in muscle-action potential.

The EMG findings were considered classic for the Eaton-Lambert syndrome associated with small cell carcinoma of the lung. The patient was begun on guanidine hydrochloride 125 mg PO q.i.d., slowly increasing to 500 mg PO every four hours. Fifteen days after institution of guanidine therapy she was able to walk without assistance and showed a marked increase in general muscle strength. Repeat EMG revealed an increase in the baseline muscle amplitude to 2.8 mV, but this was still markedly reduced from normal values. Brief exercise increased the action potential to 6.0 mV for a 50 percent increase in the action potential. The tumor; however, failed to respond to therapy, and the patient died two months later with progressive paralysis.

The myasthenic syndromes associated with nonthymic malignancy are almost universally a consequence of oat cell carcinoma. This particular tumor is often associated with paraendocrine secretory syndromes and therefore the myasthenic syndrome is presumed to be due to a related mechanism. Autoimmune reactions, however, have also been implicated in the neuromuscular syndromes associated with bronchogenic cancer.

Hypertrophic pulmonary osteoarthropathy is a characteristic syndrome composed of periarticular pain in association with clubbed digits, and radiographic evidence of a tumor mass in the lungs with

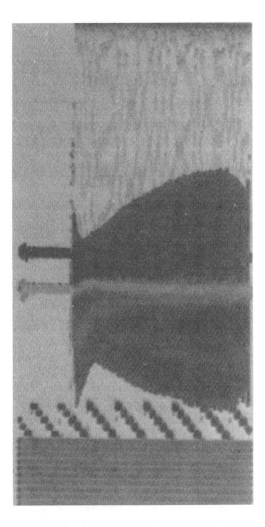

Fig. 19.6 Electromyogram revealing "fish-tail" appearance following repetitive stimulation with decrease in action potentials followed by rapid facilitation.

tumors and is extremely common with mesothelioma. It had been thought that the syndrome was related to growth hormone secretion. Studies have demonstrated, however, that these tumors do not secrete excessive growth hormone. The rapid resolution of the pain at tumor removal suggests that the tumor does secrete some ectopic substance that induces the osseous changes.

Hypertrophic pulmonary osteoarthropathy secondary to tumor is part of the differential diagnosis of arthritis or bone pain in cancer patients.

The nephrotic syndrome, which has been associated with lung cancer, colon cancer, and Hodgkin's disease, has been attributed to immunologic mechanisms. The immune mechanism is either the deposition of immune complexes composed of tumor antigen and host antibody or the production of a host antibody that is simply cross-reacting with the tumor and the end organ (kidney). The hepatic enzymopathy that has been associated particularly with renal cell carcinoma and which is manifested primarily as abnormal liver function tests in the absence of tumor metastatic to the liver may be mediated by immune-complex mechanisms. Removal of the primary tumor has resulted in improvement in the nephrotic syndrome and hepatic enzymopathy, respectively, and may be related to simple removal of the antigenic source.

Finally, cancer cachexia and cancer pyrexia are possible paraneoplastic syndromes of obscure mechanism. Pyrexia has commonly been associated with specific tumor types, particularly renal cell carcinoma, the lymphomas, and Hodgkin's disease, and a pyrogenic substance has been identified in the urine of some patients with Hodgkin's disease. Cancer cachexia remains a total enigma

periosteal elevation along the distal long bones. The pain syndrome may be observed in the absence of clubbing or standard radiograph changes, but the bone scan will reveal a typical pattern of symmetrical increased uptake along the cortical bone and the distal joints (wrists and ankles). The syndrome has been associated with both primary and secondary lung although tumor production of catabolic mediators or anti-anabolic mediators or substances that induce anorexia or taste distortion are possibilities.

7.0 Hormone insufficiency syndromes

Hormone insufficiency rarely occurs in cancer patients. As indicated previously, the two important clinical manifestations of hormone insufficiency are diabetes insipidus and adrenal insufficiency.

Patient F, a 51-year-old woman, had a radical mastectomy for breast cancer in 1972 with prophylactic radiation to the chest wall following surgery. Two years later she developed local cutaneous metastases, which were treated with irradiation. No problems occurred until August 1976, when she developed progressive polyuria and polydypsia associated with vomiting. She was placed on estrogen and prednisone therapy because of multiple bone metastases. At that time metabolic evaluation revealed a low urine specific gravity (1.003) and a urine osmolality of 116 mOs$_m$; the serum osmolality was 279 mOs$_m$. Serum electrolytes were normal. Following water deprivation, the patient had a weight loss of approximately four percent of body weight and specific gravity of the urine decreased from 1.003 to 1.000. Vasopressin was administered (five units subcutaneously), and the urine specific gravity rose to 1.017. The patient was subsequently placed on 200 mg chlorpropamide daily; her urinary output decreased from 7.0 liters to 1.2 liters daily. Evaluation, including tomographic scan for the presence of metastatic cerebral disease, was normal although bone metastases were present in the skull. There was no evidence of increased cerebral pressure or abnormalities of the sella turcica. The patient was maintained on chlorpropamide therapy for an additional year without evidence of deterioration of other endocrine function.

Diabetes insipidus in cancer patients is invariably due to a hypothalamic metastasis.

The management of diabetes insipidus in such patients may include radiation to the brain or hypothalamus in addition to the use of a peripheral effector. Extension of hypothalamis metastases to the posterior and anterior pituitary may thereby be prevented.

Adrenal insufficiency rarely occurs in the cancer patient, except as a consequence of steroid withdrawal in patients who have been on steroid replacement or pharmacologic corticosteroid therapy. Another potential cause of adrenal insufficiency is acute hemorrhage into the adrenal glands. Although adrenal insufficiency is rarely a consequence of metastasis to the gland, metastatic lesions within the glands are common in patients with lung and breast cancers.

Patient G, a 77-year-old man with a large cell undifferentiated carcinoma of the lung that had been treated with radiation, presented seven months later with a large mass lesion of the gingiva. The patient apparently had been unable to ingest food or fluids for approximately one week, during which time the tumor grew rapidly. Upon admission to the hospital, the patient was noted to be disoriented, confused, and extremely weak. In addition, he appeared to be clinically dehydrated. Blood pressure on admission was 140/40. Laboratory evaluation revealed blood urea nitrogen of 30 mg/dl, serum sodium of 135 mg/dl, and potassium of 6.8 mEq/L. The serum glucose was 40 mg%, and serum corisol was less than 5.0 pg/ml. The patient died suddenly, and at postmortem examination the adrenal glands were found to be completely replaced by tumor (Fig. 19.7).

Adrenal insufficiency should be suspected in any patient with hyperkalemia and malignancy.

8.0 Summary

The *tropic* hormone has been implicated for two of the paraneoplastic syndromes of malignancy: ACTH and TSH. The target hormone, that which directly induces the metabolic syndrome, is involved in the other syndromes. Although identifica-tion of neither PTH nor insulin within the tumor has been possible, the clinical syndromes are typical of hormone excess and recede with tumor removal. Lung cancer, specifically oat cell carcinoma, is the most common tumor to produce three of the metabolic syndromes (ACTH and ADH secretion and myasthenia). Increased PTH is the most frequent metabolic abnor-mality and is commonly associated with squamous cell tumors, especially of the lung. Thyrotoxicosis is observed with tro-phoblastic tumors and hypoglycemia is found with mesenchymal tumors.

The prognosis is ominous for patients with paraneoplastic syndromes in malig-nancy, because the tumors can rarely be excised definitively and are therefore incurable. The one exception is thyrotoxi-

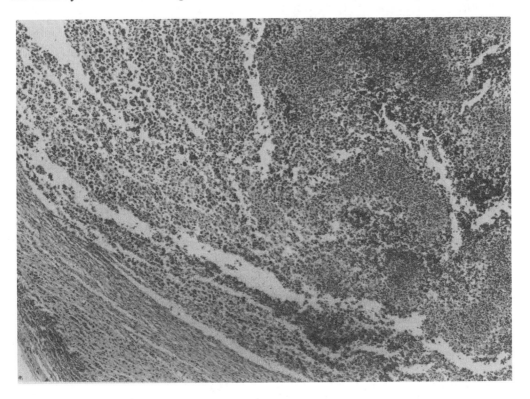

Fig. 19.7 Adrenal metastases (Patient G) indicating massive replacement of the entire adrenal gland with small rim of adrenal tissue at the inferior margin.

cosis associated with choriocarcinoma. Because choriocarcinoma is exquisitely responsive to chemotherapy, it is potentially curable. Each of the six metabolic syndromes represents a major, life-threatening complication of the underlying cancer. Furthermore, because therapeutic management of these cancer complications may be accomplished in the absence of tumor control, clinical recognition is important.

References

Anderson, N. R., and Lokich, J. J. Mesenchymal tumors associated with hypoglycemia: case report and review of the literature. *Cancer*, in press.

Anderson, N. R.; Lokich, J. J.; McDermott, W. V., Jr.; Trey, C.; and Falchuk, K. Gestational choriocarcinoma and thyrotoxicosis. *Cancer*, 44:304–306, 1979.

Bartuska, D. Humoral manifestations of neoplasms. *Seminars in Onccology* 2:405–409, 1974.

Block, M. B. et al. Multiple endocrine adenosis, type IIB. *JAMA* 234:710–714, 1975.

Baylin, S. B. The multiple endocrine neoplasia syndromes: implications for the study of inherited tumors. *Seminars in Oncology* 5:35–45, 1978.

Bolande, R. P. The neurocristopathies. *Hum. Pathol.* 5:409–429, 1974.

Brain, L., and Norris, F., Jr., (eds). The remote effects of cancer on the nervous system. p. 230 in *Contemporary Neurology Symposia I*: 1970.

Broder, L., and Carter, S. Pancreatic islet cell carcinoma: clinical features of 52 patients. *Ann. Intern. Med.* 79:239–257, 1973.

Corrin, B.; Gilby, E. D.; Jones, N. F.; and Patrick, M. B. Oat cell carcinoma of the pancreas with ectopic ACTH secretion. *Cancer* 31:1523–1527, 1973.

Ellison, E., and Wilson, S. The Zollinger-Ellison syndrome updated. *Surg. Clin. North. Am.* 47:1115–1124, 1976.

Forrest, J. N., Jr. et al. Superiority of demeclocycline over lithium in the treatment of chronic syndrome of inappropriate secretion of anti-diuretic hormone. *N. Engl. J. Med.* 298:173–177, 1978.

Ganda, O. et al. "Somatostatinoma": a somatostatin-containing tumor of the endocrine pancreas. *N. Engl. J. Med.* 296:963–967, 1977.

Graham, D.; Johnson, C.; Bentlif, P.; and Kelsey, J. Islet cell carcinoma, pancreatic cholera and vasoactive intestinal peptide. *Ann. Intern. Med.* 83:782–785, 1975.

Haefliger, J. M. Dubied, M. C.; Vallotton. Excrétion journaliére de l'hormone anti-diuretique lors de carcinome bronchique. *Schweiz. Med. Wsch.* 107:726–732, 1977.

Hall, T. C., et. Paraneoplastic syndromes. *Ann. N.Y. Acad. Sci.* 230:577, 1974.

Hall T., ed. Paraneoplastic syndromes. *Ann. N.Y. Acad. Sci.* 230:147–208, 533–546, 1974.

Lari, M. M. Long-term survival in islet-cell carcinoma of the pancreas. *Resident and Staff Physician* 107–111, June 1968.

Omenn, G. S. Ectopic polypeptide hormone production by tumors (editorial). *Ann. Intern. Med.* 72:135–138, 1970.

Schein, P. Chemotherapeutic management of the hormone-secreting endocrine malignancies. *Cancer* 30:1616–1626, 1972.

Chapter 20

Tumor of Unknown Origin (TUO)

J. Lokich

1.0 Definition and background

Primary cancer of unknown origin constitutes a substantial number of the cases seen at referral centers. Most therapeutic decisions are based on the precise definition of the tissue of origin of the primary tumor, and the problem is therefore important in clinical management. The unknown primary tumor, designated by the acronym TUO, for "tumor of unknown origin," is defined as a malignant tumor of any organ system (integument, liver, bone, lung,) characterized histopathologically (i.e., the tissue diagnosis is established) and representing a metastatic lesion in that primary tumors of that organ system can be excluded. An important corollary to this definition of TUO is that routine screening by physical examination and standard radiographs must fail to demonstrate the primary source of the lesion. This corollary restricts the definition and excludes patients whose lesions are obviously diagnosed with chest x-ray, breast examination, or contrast studies of the bowel. The primary lesion may (1) be too small to be capable of detection by routine clinical means; (2) be localized to an occult site such as the retroperitoneum; or (3) have undergone spontaneous involution thus becoming impossible to identify. It is well established that 10 to 30 percent of patients with TUO may not have a primary tumor established even at postmortem examination. The primary tumor may remain unknown because the disseminated tumor incorporates and obscures the primary, precluding localization. Isolated anecdotal cases of microscopic foci of primary testicular, ovarian, gastric, or breast cancers in the presence of widespread metastases have been reported, but these are rare. Spontaneous involution of choriocarcinoma or malignant melanoma has been observed but account for only a small portion of patients for whom a primary tumor is not found.

The evaluation of the patient with a TUO has developed substantially with the availability of new techniques for pathologic analysis, including histochemistry, immunologic definition of cell wall properties, and electron microscopy of intracellular organelles. Furthermore, new radiologic techniques such as computed tomography and radionuclide scanning aid in localizing primary tumors. Because new therapeutic methods involving radiation, chemotherapy, and combined modality therapy have led to advances in tumor-specific therapy, identification of the specific origin of a tumor has achieved paramount importance. The basic principle developed here is that, in the absence of a defined primary tumor, therapeutic management should be determined by the most favorable, treatable option. Nonetheless, the expanding list of potentially treatable tumors dictates a comprehensive search for the primary origin of a metastatic tumor, guided by cost effective prudence.

The diagnosis of TUO is contingent on histopathologic confirmation of malignancy and the exclusion of a primary tumor of that site.

The importance of obtaining a histopathologic diagnosis before undertaking an exhaustive search for a presumed primary tumor at other sites cannot be overemphasized. The identification of benign disease may obviate an extensive and potentially uncomfortable evaluation, sometimes including arteriography and barium enema. The sequential steps in the diagnostic search should be conditioned by the sensitivity to treatment of the sought-after primary tumor. Tumors with a low response rate and lack of specific therapy need not be identified since the tumor is, by definition, metastatic and incurable, but tumors for which specific treatment is available and may, in fact, be curative must be identified (Table 20.1).

This chapter will place in perspective

Table 20.1 Classification of Tumors by Available Therapy

Tumor Type	Therapy
A. Tumors for which specific systemic therapy is available	
Breast	Hormones
Ovary	Alkylating drugs
Lymphoma	Combination chemotherapy
Prostate	Hormones
Oat cell carcinoma	Combination chemotherapy
Neuroendocrine	Streptozotocin, thyroid extract
B. Tumors for which some form of systemic therapy may be effective	
Melanoma	Dacarbazine (DTIC)
Gastrointestinal cancer	5-Fluorouricil
Head and neck cancer	Methotrexate
Soft tissue sarcoma	Adriamycin
C. Tumors for which no effective therapy is established	
Renal cell carcinoma	
Bronchogenic carcinoma	

the diagnostic work-up of the patient with a TUO presenting in the six visceral sites: lung, bone and bone marrow, skin, lymph node, liver, and miscellaneous or uncommon sites. At each site, the most common metastic primary tumors as well as the appropriate diagnostic evaluation will be reviewed. The diagnosis of a TUO involves two important clinical questions with implications for therapy. First, is the lesion solitary or one of multiple lesions? Solitary lesions may be operable for therapeutic as well as for diagnostic purposes. Second, does the lesion represent a metastases from a previous malignancy, or is it a new primary tumor? Definitive surgical therapy is indicated in the latter circumstance, and it may involve a distinctive, surgical approach. The final common issue in the approach to the diagnosis of TUO is the sensitivity to treatment of the tumor to be identified.

Therapy for a TUO is determined primarily by considerations of the tumor most sensitive to treatment and secondarily by the most likely site of origin.

2.0 Histopathologic evaluation

The histopathologic classifications of tumor types are indicated in Table 20.2. The three basic tumor categories are mesenchymal tumors, including soft tissue and osseous sarcomas; lymphomatous disease, including Hodgkin's disease and the multiple variants of non-Hodgkin's lymphoma; and epithelial tumors, including the adenocarcinomas and epidermoid carcinomas. Combinations of epithelial and mesenchymal tumors are common and reflect the totipotential differentiation of many tumors. Such mixed tumors may be designated carcinosarcomas or adenosquamous tumors and are associated most often with lung, uterine, ovarian, and

Table 20.2 Histopathological Classification of Tumors

Epithelial Tumor
  Epidermoid (squamous)
  Transitional cell
  Adenocarcinoma (glandular)

Mesenchymal Tumor
  Connective tissue, including
    fibrosarcoma and liposarcoma
  Neural tissue
  Vascular tissue
  Muscle tissue
  Mesothelial tissue
  Osseous and cartilage tumors

Lymphoma Tumors
  Non-Hodgkin's lymphoma
    Lymphosarcoma
    Histiocytic lymphoma
    Mixed types
  Hodgkin's disease

Mixed Tumors
  Carcinosarcomas
  Adenosquamous tumors
  Collision tumors (special variant)

---

thyroid origin. A special type of mixed tumor is the collision tumor, representing two separate malignant diseases with metastases of one to the other. Collision tumors occur most commonly with lesions metastatic to primary renal tumors.

The importance of establishing the histopathologic type of cancer is that the pathology may indicate the tumor source and so focus the search for the primary tumor.

The first clinical step in the management of TUO is to obtain a histopathologic diagnosis.

For example, epidermoid carcinomas most commonly emanate from the squamous epithelium of the head and neck, lung, upper esophagus, or from the external genitalia and perianal area. In addition, squamous cell carcinomas may originate from the integument (skin) and from the transitional epithelium of the bladder, ureter, and renal pelvis in which case the epithelium has undergone differentiation. Epidermoid tumors of the gastrointestinal tract, breast, and other sites have also been described.

The adenocarcinoma tumors are glandular lesions that can arise from many organ systems, including breast, lung, gastrointestinal tract and accessory organs, ovaries, and unusal sites such as the maxillary sinuses and sweat or sebaceous glands. The sites of origin of glandular carcinomas may be distinguishable from one another pathologically, in most, but not all instances. Special histochemical stains for the presence of mucin secretion help to distinguish a glandular carcinoma of the stomach, for example, from a carcinoma of the breast, but the distinction is not universal, and breast tumors may be mucin secreting as well.

Mesenchymal tumors include the soft tissue sarcomas and osseous sarcomas and incorporate the following subtypes: fibrosarcoma, fibrous histiocytoma, liposarcoma, rhabdomyosarcoma, leiomyosarcoma, synovial sarcoma, chondrosarcoma, tumors of the vascular and nervous structures (hemangioendothelioma, angiosarcoma, hemangiopericytoma) neurolemmoma, and granular cell myoblastoma (schwannoma). Specific identification of the type of mesenchymal tumor is often not possible, and simple designation of spindle cell sarcoma or undifferentiated sarcoma is then used. The crucial distinction from the other histopathologic types of cancer, however, focuses attention on the connective tissue, skeletal structures, and mesenchymal tissue in the search for the primary tumor.

The designation of "undifferentiated" tumor may imply the inability to distinguish the mesenchymal, lymphomatous, or carcinomatous lesion. More commonly, this pathologic designation refers to lack of maturation of carcinomas and is equivalent to the anaplasia terminology. The use of the term "undifferentiated" should be supplemented with one of the three categories of tissue origins for tumors: sarcoma, lymphoma, carcinoma, and in the latter case should specify small cell or large cell. All tissues or visceral sites in the body are capable of developing undifferentiated tumors, and therefore the primary site is not determined by this histopathologic diagnosis. The problem of the TUO is magnified when the histopathologic diagnosis is undifferentiated tumor. Thus, a more precise definition of tumor pathology must be found. The guiding principle is to obtain additional tissue for the studies listed in Table 20.3

Electron microscopy, which requires special tissue preservation in gluteraldehyde, is essential to differentiate three tumor types: (1) oat cell carcinoma with round neurosecretory granules; (2) malignant melanoma with ovaloid melanogen granules; and, (3) characteristic neurosecretory granules associated with endocrine-type tumors (Fig. 20.1).

Electron microscopy is an important tool in the analysis of undifferentiated tumors to identify melanoma, oat cell carcinoma, and neuroendocrine tumors.

The identification of desmosomes or intracellular bridges is also more easily identified by electron-microscopic examination (Fig. 20.2).

Lymphomas may be identified and characterized by the types of lymphocytes within the tumor; specifically, B cells are identified by the presence of immunoglobulin receptors and T cells by the capability of the lymphocytes to form rosettes in specific in vitro systems. This latter technique requires fresh tissue.

Table 20.3 Pathological Studies of Tumor Tissue in "Undifferentiated" Tissue

Study	Objective
Electron microscopy	Identify melanosomes, neurosecretory granules, "oat cell" granules
Lymphoma cell wall markers	Identify types of lymphoma, including T, B, or null cell lymphoma
T cell rosettes Surface immunoglobulin	
Cell membrane receptors	Estrogen receptors in breast cancer, uterine cancer, and possibly melanoma. Androgen receptors in prostatic cancer
Histochemical stains	
PAS	Ewing's sarcoma
Mucincarmine	
Grimelius	Neuroendocrine tumors
Fontana	Carcinoid tumors
Esterase	Myeloblastoma

Lymphoma is the most treatable "undifferentiated" tumor and may be definitively identified pathologically by T or B cell characteristics.

Cell membrane receptor proteins have been identified for normal and malignant tissue that presumably function teleologically as transport systems. Hormone receptor proteins are the most well studied and have a specific diagnostic role as well as providing a therapeutic guide. Estrogen receptor protein (ERP) is specific for malignant tissue derived from the breast although ERP has been identified in small quantities in other tumors. Progesterone receptors, glucocorticoid receptors, and other nonhormone receptor proteins may play an important role in the future both for diagnosis and therapeutic consideration.

Histochemical staining, for example, for the presence of mucin secretion by mucicarmine stain or mucopolysaccharides by PAS staining with diastase is available using standard techniques for identifying specific tumors (Table 20.3). The Grimelius stain is particularly useful in the identification of neuroendocrine tumors.

Patient A, a 72-year-old man, presented with thoracic spinal cord compression and underwent decompression laminectomy. An undifferentiated tumor, "probably epithelial," was removed, and the patient received local radiation for a presumed lung primary. Two years later on routine follow-up the patient presented with a supraclavicular mass, and biopsy demonstrated the same tumor. Electron microscopy examination failed to demonstrate any features of epithelial tumors, and the patient was treated for a diagnosis of possible lymphoma by chemotherapy. Complete regression of retroperitoneal and all other adenopathy was demonstrated.

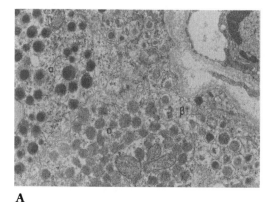

A

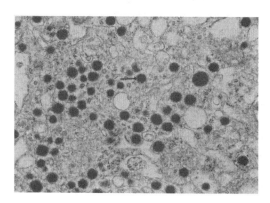

B

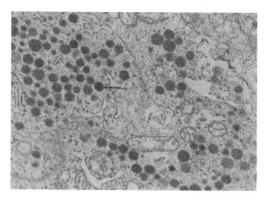

C

Fig. 20.1 Electromicrograph of a normal pancreatic islet demonstrating alpha (a), beta (b) and delta (d) granules. (magnification x2400) (A) Electromicrograph of two distinctive islet cell tumors glucogonoma with alpha granules (B) and somatostatenoma with delta granules (C).

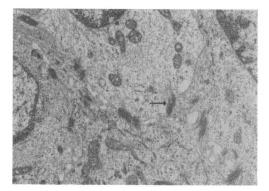

Fig. 20.2 Electromicrograph of undifferentiated carcinoma demonstrating intercellular bridges (arrow) or desmasomes. (magnification x1900)

Patient B, a 75-year-old woman, developed an anterior chest wall mass at the uppermost edge of the left breast. Biopsy and pathologic analysis revealed "poorly differentiated tumor consistent with primary breast tumor." The patient noted that some five years previously she had had a melanoma removed from the inner canthus of her right eye. Chest radiograph now revealed multiple pulmonary nodules, and brain scan demonstrated a frontal lobe lesion. Electron microscopic reexamination of the "primary" tumor in the breast revealed the characteristic melanosomes, and estrogen receptor protein assay failed to demonstrate the presence of the receptor.

These two cases illustrate the application of special pathologic studies in evaluating the undifferentiated or poorly differentiated tumor. The pathologic evaluation of the tumor tissue is crucial in establishing guidelines for the search for the primary tumor, and repeat biopsy is an important procedure for its definition. When the frozen section is classified as undifferentiated, the tumor tissue should be both frozen and preserved in all the appropriate solutions, including gluteraldehyde, to insure the availability of maximum information.

3.0 Serologic and biochemical tumor markers

With few exceptions, no tumor-specific tests are available for evaluating the patient with TUO. Three serologic or biochemical categories have been studied, including: enzymes, hormones, and tumor-associated antigens. Enzyme assays are not specific and merely reflect a secondary effect of the tumor on the organ involved. Acid phosphatase, which is directly tumor secreted and traditionally associated with prostatic carcinoma, is also elevated in patients with Gaucher's disease, but, more importantly, acid phosphatase is elevated in fewer than 40 percent of patients with metastatic prostatic cancer. Thus, screening by acid phosphatase is not always helpful. Regan isoenzyme of alkaline phosphatase has similarly been associated with ovarian cancer, but the correlation is not specific.

Hormone secretion may be specific for endocrine tumor, but distinction among hyperplasia, adenoma, and carcinoma is not possible by measuring blood levels. Furthermore, an endocrine syndrome may be incidental to the presence of a cancer.

Patient C, a 75-year-old woman, developed ovarian cancer and was treated successfully with chemotherapy. Extreme nausea and an unusual sensitivity of the tongue to hot or cold liquids prompted a systemic evaluation. The patient was discovered to have incidental primary hyperparathyroidism (PTH 11 pg/ml, Ca 12.7 mg%, PO$_4$ 2.0 mm/ml, and Cl 105 mg%), which was controlled with diuretic therapy only.

Another category of hormone secretors are the paraneoplastic nonendocrine tu-

mors (Table 20.4). The most common tumor to be associated with secretion of ectopic hormones is lung cancer, and particularly oat cell carcinoma. Such tumors have been associated with antidiuretic hormone secretion (ADH), parathormone (PTH) secretion (particularly with epidermoid carcinomas), ACTH, TSH (particularly with gestational tumors), HCG, calcitonin, and many others. The important point is the lack of correlation of circulating hormone levels with quantitative tumor burden; in less than 10 percent of patients is the elevation significant. Furthermore, the presence of the hormone in the circulation does not correlate with the clinical syndrome. Thus, immunologically detectable hormone may not be biologically functional hormone.

Tumor-specific proteins have been sought in order to attempt to detect early cancer in large populations. One of the earliest of these proteins was carcinoembryonic antigen (CEA) and alphafetoprotein (AFP). It has become clear that these

Table 20.4 Ectopic Hormonal Tumor Markers Associated with Nonendocrine Tumors

Tumor Marker	Site of Tumor
ACTH	Lung*
PTH	Lung†
Insulin	Lung
Glucagon	Pancreas
Gastrin	Stomach
Calcitonin	Lung, breast
Placental Proteins	Lung
HCG	Choriocarcinoma
Infrequent Tumor Markers	
Prostaglandin, erythropoietin, renin	Kidney
MSH, TSH, ADH	Lung, ovary

*Predominantly oat cell type
†Predominantly epidermoid type

tumor-specific proteins are actually linked with a number of tumors and are perhaps more appropriately named "tumor-associated proteins." Thus, CEA is present in patients with breast cancer, lung cancer, bladder and prostate cancer, colon cancer and other gastrointestinal tumors. Similarly, AFP is present in patients with nasopharyngeal carcinoma and germinal tumors of the testes in addition to the more commonly known association with hepatomas.

4.0 Pulmonary TUO

The most common cause of radiographically detected discrete lesions of the lung is bronchogenic cancer, even when a pulmonary lesion develops in a patient with a previously diagnosed malignancy of another site. Thus, in a review of patients with metachronously discovered pulmonary lesions and who had either a prior colon cancer or a prior breast cancer, the confirmed diagnosis of the lung lesion was primary lung cancer in 50 percent and 65 percent, respectively.

Solitary pulmonary lesions in patients with previous breast cancer should be evaluated for other sites of metastases.

The point is that a new lung lesion should prompt a search for other sites of metastases in patients with a prior malignancy. In this instance, the clinician is not searching for the primary tumor but is excluding other sites of disease. If the lesion is solitary, the likelihood of a new primary tumor increases.

Clinical and radiographic criteria to distinguish primary and metastatic malignancy in the patient with pulmonary lesions suggest one or the other but are not necessarily conclusive (Table 20.5). Metastatic lesions rarely produce endobronchial lesions. Nonetheless, positive sputum cytology may be observed in the patient with metastatic disease to the lung. Metastatic lesions to the lung rarely produce parenchymal lesions in association with mediastinal or hilar adenopathy. This reflects the fact that metastatic lesions generally are either hematogenous or lymphatic in their pathways of dissemination but are not both. Furthermore, metastatic lesions uncommonly implant through the hematogenous route and subsequently metastasize to the lymph nodes. One common aspect of lesions metastatic to the lungs is their spherical configuration, which, in conjunction with their multiplicity, almost always implies a metastatic origin; the primary lesions of the lung usually have irregular borders, and are generally solitary.

Advances in diagnosing pulmonary lesions have occurred with the advent of radiologically assisted techniques of obtaining tissue. Percutaneous transthoracic needle biopsy for obtaining cytologic specimens and the fluoroscopically guided transbronchial brush biopsy are but two of the new techniques. In addition, mediastinoscopy, sputum cytology, and scalene lymph node biopsy may be used. The choice of the approach depends upon the anatomical location of the lesion, the suspected clinical type of malignancy, and the potential morbidity of the procedure. For example, in patients with pulmonary insufficiency, the transcutaneous needle aspiration should be avoided because of the high incidence of secondary pneumothorax. Metastatic lesions involving the parenchyma are not accessible with the transbronchial approach generally, unless the lesion is cavitating and communicating with the bronchus.

A primary consideration in the treatment of lung lesions is the possibility for cure by thoracotomy and primary resection. Thoracotomy is a therapeutic as well as a diagnostic procedure for both primary lung cancer and metastatic tumor in the lung. Solitary and unilateral metastatic

Table 20.5 Clinical and Radiologic Criteria for Distinguishing Primary Bronchogenic Versus Metastatic Lesions to the Lung

Criterion	Primary Tumor Characteristic	Metastatic Tumor
Sputum cytology	40%	5%
Mediastinal or hilar adenopathy	Common	Rare*
Configuration	Variable	Generally spherical
Number of lesions	Generally solitary and confined to a single lung	Often multiple and involving both lungs

*In the absence of a parenchymal lesion, mediastinal adenopathy may represent metastases from urogenital cancer, lymphoma, or gastrointestinal cancer.

lesions may require thoracotomy to control disease. The specific requirements for therapeutic thoracotomy for pulmonary metastatic disease are (1) presence of a long disease-free interval, (2) slow growth rate, and (3) solitary metastases in the lungs without other sites of metastases. Therapeutic thoracotomy without previous diagnostic procedures is therefore recommended for a new lesion in a patient with or without a prior history of cancer.

Patient D, a 50-year-old woman, had a radical mastectomy for breast cancer at the age of 45. For five years she had been well, but on routine annual examination a discrete pulmonary nodule was observed on chest x-ray. The patient underwent bone scan, liver scan, and upper- and lower-GI series; all were normal. At thoracotomy a two-centimeter epidermoid carcinoma was removed.

The patient had a discrete solitary peripheral lesion that was surgically "curable" whether it represented a benign lesion, a primary lung cancer, or metastases from the previous breast cancer. The diagnostic evaluation required thoracotomy, and although the evaluation of other sites of metastases is appropriate, the search for other primary sites is not. In contrast patients with lung cancer inoperable for cure or with prior history of breast cancer and poor prognostic features should not undergo thoracotomy. (See patient E)

Patient E, a 72-year-old woman, had a Stage II breast cancer and 18 months later developed cough, dyspnea, and a right paratracheal mass. The patient received preoperative radiation on the presumption that the tumor was a primary inoperable lung cancer and underwent thoracotomy. The tumor was histologically identical to the previous breast cancer.

Almost all tumors are capable of metastases to the lungs, but no clinical or radiographic clues indicate the tumor type or site of origin. Some conservative generalities, however, are pertinent: (1) lesions metastasizing to the lungs form spherical opaque lesions without central cavitation; (2) lymphangitic metastases to the lungs are more common with breast cancer and gastric cancer and atypical of other forms of malignancy; (3) the most rapidly growing lung metastases are the testicular tumors and mesenchymal tumors; (4) pleural-based tumors usually represent metastases from breast cancer or ovarian cancer and lead to effusion with or without detectable malignant cells; and (5) large tumor masses (> 5 cm) are often slow growing metastases from sarcomas.

The most critical step in evaluating the patient with a pulmonary shadow and no previous malignancy is obtaining a histologic diagnosis (Table 20.6). The presumption that a lesion represents a malignancy and therefore requires a search for primary site before the histological

---

Pulmonary lesions in the patient without previous cancer should undergo thoracotomy only after ascertaining that other sites of metastases do not exist.

---

diagnosis is generally unwarranted. Even after establishing the diagnosis the metastatic work-up should be precise and focused. For example, adenocarcinoma in the lung represents 20 to 30 percent of all histologic types of lung cancer and

should not be presumed to be metastatic from another site without additional information. Therefore, routine radiographic evaluation of the colon and upper gastrointestinal tract should not be performed, but appropriate staging by radiographic studies to determine the extent of disease, based on the common metastatic pathways, is indicated.

5.0 Osseous TUO

The two components of the osseous system are the calcified cortex of the bone and the intramedullary cavity. These components have separate biologic and clinical characteristics and are discussed separately. The distinction between primary tumors of the bone and secondary metastatic lesions to the bone is less often a clinical problem for a TUO than for lesions of the lungs. Radiographic and clinical features readily distinguish primary bone lesions from metastatic lesions with

---

Table 20.6 Summary of Clinical Approach to Pulmonary TUO Lesions

1. Obtain histological diagnosis.
    a. Prior malignancy—if disease-free interval is greater than one year, and the lesion is solitary, thoracotomy should be performed.
    b. No prior malignancy—sequential diagnostic studies to include bronchoscopy and sputum cytology, particularly if the lesion is only marginally curable by surgery.
    c. In both instances, rule out distant or other sites of metastases.
2. Search for the primary tumor is defined by histologic type.
    a. Epidermoid or undifferentiated—no further studies.
    b. Adenocarcinoma—no further evaluation, unless ancillary data suggest primary tumor in gastrointestinal tract (e.g., guaiac-positive stool).
    c. Lymphoma—initiate staging procedures.
    d. Mesenchymal tumor—bone evaluation.
    e. Clear cell tumor—evaluate for primary tumor of renal, adrenal, and respiratory systems.
3. Therapy.
    a. Curative resection if lesion is primary lung tumor or a solitary metastasis with a disease-free interval greater than one year.
    b. Systemic therapy, usually chemotherapy based on primary site of origin.

the exception of metastatic mucin-secreting adenocarcinomas, which may mimic primary bone tumors.

Patient F, 69-year-old man, presented with a large pulmonary mass. Evaluation for potential sites of metastases revealed a lesion of the left femur; a biopsy was performed. Radiographically and pathologically, the lesion appeared to be a chondrosarcoma, and the lung mass was presumed to be a metastatic lesion. At thoracotomy and subsequent excision of the femur lesion, the tumor was interpreted pathologically as a mucin-secreting tumor of the lung.

Metastatic lesions may mimic primary bone malignancy if the tumor is mucin secreting.

Cortical bone lesions. Metastatic lesions within the cortex are generally osteoblastic or osteolytic. Five tumor types produce osteoblastic lesions; these include tumors of the breast, prostate, lung, thyroid, and lymphomas. Such lesions are not entirely osteoblastic but are a mixture of osteolysis with an osteoblastic response to the tumor. In prostatic cancer, osteoblastic response predominates, while in breast cancer the osteolytic component more often predominates. Osseous lesions occur most commonly in the axial skeleton, and metastasis beyond the proximal bone structures is unusual. The differential diagnosis of blastic lesions includes osteopoikelosis, osteomyelitis, and all benign diseases resulting in secondary bone reaction. Osteolytic lesions may be so subtle as to be interpreted as osteoporosis. For example, multiple myeloma is frequently recognized in the premorbid state as osteoporosis without the characteristically circumscribed "punched out" lesion.

The diagnosis of bone lesions and TUO must focus on the remediable tumors.

The first step is to determine with bone scan whether the lesion is solitary or multiple.

Bone lesions should be evaluated by establishing the number of lesions, obtaining a biopsy of the most accessible lesion, and focusing on treatable tumors.

Two important benefits accrue from identifying other sites of disease. First, another lesion site may be more accessible to biopsy; second, additional lesions may be discovered in weight-bearing areas that require prophylactic therapy. The potential primary sources of bone lesions that may be occult include breast and renal cell cancer. Mammograms and abdominal ultrasound are, respectively, the preferred means for identifying the primary tumor. Renal tumors cannot be considered treatable, however, since therapy for metastatic disease is ineffective.

Patient G, an 80-year-old woman, presented with a mixed osteoblastic-osteolytic lesion of the clavicle and secondary pathological fracture. Biopsy revealed clear cell carcinoma, and an intravenous pyelogram was performed. Renal failure with blood urea nitrogen of 100 mg% developed 10 days following the radiographic procedure.

The use of intravenous pyelography has major risk of complications, is uncomfortable, and the benefit of identifying a primary renal tumor is minimal.

Bone marrow metastases. Tumor within the marrow cavity is almost uniformly observed in association with cortical bone lesions. Tumors rarely metastasize to the marrow only. The presence of tumor within the marrow cavity is clinically important in that the marrow stem cells may be reduced, compromising therapy by reducing tolerance to chemotherapy or radiation. The most common tumors to metastasize and be detected in the bone marrow are such solid tumors as breast, lung, prostate, and melanoma, and primary tumors of the bone marrow such as leukemia, lymphoma, and myeloma.

Typically, the patient develops a leukoerythroblastic peripheral blood picture (nucleated red blood cells, immature white blood cells), but thrombocytopenia and/or leukopenia may also be observed. Bone marrow biopsy in at least two separate sites is required to determine the presence of the tumor. This dual site technique decreases the likelihood of sampling error. In addition to the biopsy, an aspirate (fluid phase) is obtained in order to evaluate the cytologic features of the cells. Occult tumors to the marrow are presumed to originate from breast cancer, the most successfully treated tumor, and therefore may be treated as such.

Patient H, a 59-year-old woman, had anemia for one year and was treated with iron. A bone marrow aspirate revealed clumps of tumor cells, although the metastatic radiographs of bone were normal. Mammograms established a two-centimeter lesion in the outer quadrant of the left breast that, on biopsy, was a carcinoma. The patient was treated with che-motherapy for breast cancer and had a reversal of the anemia for five years.

Breast cancer, which is occult, is a common tumor affecting bones or bone marrow, and it is the most sensitive to treatment.

Detection and diagnosis of bone metastases. Complaint of bone pain generally raises the possibility of bone metastases. The radionuclide scan may detect osseous lesions earlier than the standard radiographs, although false-negative scans may be observed in patients with such nonreactive neoplastic disease as multiple myeloma or with symmetrical metastases. The specific radiographic appearance of a bone lesion does not alone diagnose tumor, but some special features may occasionally be useful (Table 20.7).

Patient I, a 52-year-old woman, had breast cancer and underwent radical mastectomy and postoperative radiation therapy in 1956. Fourteen years later the patient developed pain over the scapula, and an osteolytic lesion of the scapula was noted. Although initially thought to represent metastases from the previous breast tumor, the radiologic examination re-

---

Table 20.7 Summary of Clinical Approach to Osseous TUO Lesions

1. Determine the extent of osseous involvement (bone scan and standard radiographic bone series) to determine if lesion is solitary or multiple.
2. Obtain histologic diagnosis.
3. Search for primary lesion for the most common tumors metastasizing to bone (lung, breast, and prostate) and focus on the most treatable tumor (prostate in men and breast in women).
4. Therapy should be directed at local palliation, and systemic therapy is deferred until a primary source is defined. For primary tumors of the bone (reticulum cell sarcoma, Ewing's, osteogenic sarcoma) therapy to the bone lesion should be definitive.

vealed an expansile lesion suggesting a radiation-induced osteogenic sarcoma. A fore-quarter amputation was performed upon histologic confirmation of the sarcomatous nature of the tumor.

6.0 Hepatic TUO

The liver is one of the most common sites for metastatic implants, because of the tremendous blood supply to the hepatic architecture through the arterial and venous system. Identifying the primary source for hepatic lesions is frequently problematic. Hepatoma, which is generally diagnosed by pathologic study and classification of one of two variants, must be excluded. Serum alphafetoprotein is elevated in at least 50 percent of hepatoma

patients and is occasionally helpful. The major group of metastatic tumors to be considered are the adenocarcinomas, but the distinction between adenocarcinoma of the breast or stomach and colon or ovary is often difficult. Therefore, the search for a primary tumor often focuses on these four tumors as well as on tumors of the lung or pancreas.

One clinical consideration is the frequency with which the tumors metastasize to the liver. The incidence of liver metastases in patients with a variety of primary tumors is indicated in Table 20.8. Colon, breast and lung cancers are the most common tumors and are therefore more statistically likely to be the primary source of the hepatic metastases. Of all tumors, however, only breast, ovarian, and possi-

Table 20.8 Relative Incidence of Hepatic Metastases by Primary Site

Site	Percentage of clinical hepatic metastases	Relative frequency of hepatic metastases	
		Major Group	Subgroup
Gastrointestinal		1	
Esophagus	60%		4
Stomach	80		2
Small Intestine	60		3
Colon-rectal	45		1
Accessory Organ		3	
Gallbladder	100		2
Bile Duct	100		3
Pancreas	80		1
Nongastrointestinal		2	
Lung	30		1
Breast	30		2
Melanoma	40		3
Special Category			
Carcinoid	80*		
Ovary	80†		

*Often solitary site of metastases
†Generally surface implants without parenchymal invasion

bly gastric cancer are potentially amenable to systemic therapy.

The distribution pattern of the hepatic lesion is useful diagnostically and therapeutically. For example, gastric and pancreas carcinoma often invade the liver contiguously. Ovarian cancer, however, does not usually invade the liver but is associated with implants on the liver surface. When metastases from a variety of primary tumors are confined to the liver, hepatic infusion with cytotoxic drugs, hepatic artery ligation, or even partial hepatectomy may be considered therapeutically.

Diagnostic evaluation of hepatic metastases. Diagnostic evaluation of the liver employs radioisotope scanning and ultrasonography. Radionuclide scanning is of three types. The Rose-Bengal scan measures hepatic secretory function; the sulfur-colloid or technetium scan identifies and evaluates parenchymal architecture and anatomy; and the gallium citrate scans permit specific quantitation of tumor. The latter scan may be most helpful in malignant melanoma that appears selectively to accumulate gallium particles. An important aspect of scanning is that scans are rarely positive without liver function test abnormalities or hepatomegaly and therefore are not advisable for routine screening.

Ultrasound distinguishes cystic from solid lesions within the liver and may supplement radionuclide scans in searching for small lesions within the liver and in evaluating simultaneously the retroperitoneum and the pancreas as possible primary sites. Angiography is the most specific and comprehensive diagnostic tool in evaluation of the liver but is accompanied by significant patient morbidity.

Tumor metastatic to the liver is generally an adenocarcinoma. The presence of the tumor in the liver establishes that the lesion is incurable, and the subsequent investigation should focus on locating such potentially treatable tumors as breast cancer. An extensive work-up is not always necessary since it may not provide additional information for therapy (Table 20.9).

Patient J, a 49-year-old woman, presented with right-shoulder pain and difficulty bending for low tennis returns. On examination, she had an enlarged liver with nodules. The stool was benzidine-negative. Barium enema demonstrated an asymptomatic lesion in the right colon. Surgery was not undertaken, and the patient was treated with hepatic infusion therapy.

Table 20.9 Summary of Clinical Approach to Hepatic TUO Lesions:

1. Obtain a histologic diagnosis either with closed liver biopsy or with laparoscopy-guided biopsy.
2. Estimate extent of disease within the liver to determine possibility of infusion or resection.
3. Search for the primary tumor using routine methods only: ultrasound scanning (pancreas), chest x-ray (lung), breast exam, or mammogram.
4. Therapy may involve laparotomy only if
   a. it can involve hepatic infusion, and surgical placement of the catheter is necessary.
   b. palliation of bleeding or obstructing lesion in gastrointestinal tract is necessary.

Patient K, a 45-year-old man, developed early satiety and was found to have an enlarged liver by examination. Ultrasound demonstrated a lesion of the pancreas, and the patient had a cytologic biopsy with ultrasonic guidance. The liver was found to be the major symptomatic site of the disease and infusion therapy was initiated.

These two cases illustrate that detection of the primary tumor may not influence therapy and that diagnostic procedures to confirm the histologic diagnosis may be hazardous. Both patients had incurable lesions mandating localized treatment of the liver, and the primary tumor was identified without recourse to an operation. The treatment most likely to assuage the local symptoms was instituted without regard for the primary site.

7.0 Cutaneous TUO

The most common tumors to metastasize to the skin are breast cancer and lung cancer, which reflects in part the relative frequency of these tumors in the general population. Skin metastases, however, may derive from any primary site. The origin of cutaneous metastases is seldom a clinical mystery; the primary tumor is either obvious, or the history of prior malignancy indicates the source. Furthermore, the distinction between primary tumor and metastases is not an issue, since the primary skin cancers (epidermoid and basal cell) are clinically and pathologically specific. Primary tumors arising from the skin adnexae (sebaceous and sweat gland tumors) are also pathologically distinctive. The exception is malignant melanoma that, if amelanotic and poorly differentiated, may be difficult to distinguish from metastasis from an extracutaneous visceral site.

The common cutaneous sites of metastases include the scalp, abdominal wall, umbilicus, and buttocks. Tumors in the skin may be within the dermal layers, the subcutaneous tissues, or both. The site of the lesion as well as the depth or level of the lesion may be helpful in finding the primary site. Scalp lesions are frequent cutaneous sites of metastases from breast cancer, lung cancer, and leukemia. Abdominal wall lesions are a typical site of metastases, and implantation of tumor in the umbilicus or periumbilical area is especially common. This latter tumor has been named as a physical sign in clinical diagnosis for "Sister Marie Joseph" and is commonly associated with intra-abdominal malignancy and with pancreatic carcinoma in particular. Ovarian tumors may become palpable within the subcutaneous tissue, related to paracentesis for ascites, and secondary implantation in the needle track. Metastatic tumors of the buttock have been reported from primary sites in the gastrointestinal tract and soft tissue sources proximal and distal to the buttocks. A major category of skin metastases is that associated with the hematologic tumor and especially acute monocytic leukemia and reticulum cell sarcoma. Leukemic infiltration is ordinarily superficial, and the multiplicity of lesions may suggest a nonspecific dermatitis.

Lesions of the skin and subcutaneous tissue are easily excised for biopsy, and histologic diagnosis is obtained early. The distinction between dermal metastases, which involve the superficial skin layers with clinical erythema of the overlying skin and induration, and subcutaneous lesions, which are palpable but do not produce secondary changes in the dermis, is important. Malignant melanoma, a primary skin tumor, is commonly confined to the subcutaneous tissue. Mesenchymal tumors also arise within subcutaneous tissue but without skin involvement. Breast cancer, on the other hand, frequently involves the dermal layers and without cutaneous extension. Extensive dermal or lymphatic permeation in breast cancer produces a characteristic picture referred to as an en cuirasse appearance. (Table 20.10)

8.0 Lymph node TUO

Identification of the primary tumor in patients with lymph node lesions is generally not problematic because the area of lymph drainage is generally contiguous with the site of the primary cancer. Nonetheless, occult primary disease may be present and/or a distant primary tumor not associated with the direct lymphatic drainage may be the ultimate source. Cervical lymph nodes are generally associated with manifest or occult carcinoma of the oral cavity or lungs; axillary lymph nodes with breast cancer lesions; and inguinal lymph nodes with lesions of the genitalia or perineum. Other lesions of the extremities to result in axillary or inguinal lymphadenopathy are melanoma and sarcoma. Each of the surface lymphatic drainage areas (cervical, axillary, and inguinal) represents a distinct type of diagnostic evaluation.

Cervical lymph nodes. The anatomic site of the lymph node abnormality and the number of lymph nodes involved is often important. For example, supraclavicular nodes in the scalene fat pad are linked to primary pulmonary neoplasms, particularly if the nodes are not contiguous with other nodal areas. High cervical nodes in the anterior chain are usually associated with tonsillar or intraoral cancer. Multiple node involvement, particu-

larly if bilateral, suggests a lymphoma-type disease.

Histopathologic classification is necessary to identify the pathologic class of tumor. Undifferentiated tumor (large and small cell) may be distinctive and specific for lung origin. Epidermoid carcinoma is a pathologic type that, although common as a pulmonary neoplasm, is also the most common tumor in the intra-oral cavity. In the presence of a normal chest x-ray, a search for an intraoral lesion is crucial.

Patient L, a 53-year-old man, had a high cervical node discovered on routine examination. Although the oral examination was normal, the chest x-ray revealed a hilar mass. Biopsy of the cervical node revealed epidermoid carcinoma similar to the tumor removed later at pulmonary resection. The patient subsequently developed multiple cervical nodes and pulmonary recurrence.

In this case the primary diagnosis was lung cancer, but because the lung lesion was not contiguous with low cervical nodes, the surgeon felt the two lesions were separate tumors. The epidemiologic factors associated with oral cancer and lung cancer may be compelling reasons to treat the two lesions as individual primary tumors. When the oral cancer, particularly, is diagnosed first, the subsequent development of pulmonary lesions can represent a new primary or metastases.

Patient M, a 57-year-old man with laryngeal cancer in 1973, had a partial laryngectomy and neck dissection. Four years

Table 20.10 Summary of Clinical Approach to Cutaneous TUO Lesions

1. Obtain a histologic diagnosis including special stains and preservatives (gluteraldehyde) if the lesion is subcutaneous or atypical.
2. Avoid wide excision until histologic diagnosis is established.

later he presented with multiple pulmonary lesions, predominantly on the pleural surface with effusion. Pleural biopsy revealed epidermoid carcinoma consistent with the primary laryngeal tumor.

In the absence of a defined lesion in the oral cavity, blind biopsy at the base of the tongue, in the tonsillar fossa, and in the naso- and retropharynx, is a critical diagnostic procedure. Primary tumors of the nasopharynx are submucosal and therefore often not obvious on the standard nasopharynx examination. When the primary tumor is not identified, treatment is regional (radiation or surgery) and offers a cure in 20 percent of patients with solitary nodal metastases of epidermoid type.

Patient N, a 24-year-old woman, developed right cervical swelling at the mid-level of the sternomastoid muscle. Biopsy revealed epidermoid carcinoma. Blind biopsy of the nasopharynx followed a normal intraoral examination. The pathologic specimen revealed features typical of nasopharyngeal carcinoma, and the patient was treated with radiation to the neck and nasopharynx.

Unusual tumors associated with lymphadenopathy in the cervical area include adenocarcinoma of the sinuses and neurosthesioma or tumors of the olfactory ridge.

Axillary lymph nodes. The presence of isolated lymph node metastases in the axillary group is most often linked with breast cancer. In fact, even in the absence of a palpable, mammographically identifiable lesion in the breast, mastectomy may be necessary, and discovery of an occult primary tumor possible only by extensive sectioning of the breast tissue. Surface markers, such as ERP on the lymph node tissue, may be diagnostic because neoplastic lesions of the breast have been

shown to contain ERP in approximately 50 percent of patients.

Identification of the primary breast cancer is important since this tumor is not only treatable but also potentially curable. Mammography should include xerography and possible thermography, and ultrasound of the breast may distinguish cystic lesions and guide aspiration of cysts. Even in the absence of an identifiable primary breast tumor, surgery is probably warranted.

Inguinal lymph nodes. The primary malignant lesion resulting in inguinal lymphadenopathy is almost always obvious. The search should focus on the genitalia and perineal area and considerations should include anal carcinoma, penile and vaginal carcinoma, cervical cancer, and less commonly, bladder and prostate cancers. These lesions may be distinguished in part by histologic review. Metastases from distant sites to the inguinal area are rare, and the search for primary disease, most commonly breast or lung, should be pursued only in the absence of local primary lesions (Table 20.11).

Patient O, a 54-year-old woman, had a breast cancer and multiple bone lesions when she developed inguinal adenopathy. A surgical excision revealed adenocarcinoma pathologically similar to the primary tumor in the breast that was ERP-positive. The patient subsequently underwent a successful adrenalectomy.

9.0 Uncommon sites of metastases

In addition to the five general categories of common metastatic sites, metastases may develop in atypical sites and present as an unknown primary tumor. The categories of metastatic lesions and the most common primary sites in this category are listed in Table 20.12. Unknown primary

Table 20.11 Summary of Clinical Approach to Lymph Node TUO Lesions

1. The primary lesion is almost always anatomically contiguous with the pathologic lymph node.
2. In the absence of an obvious regional clinical lesion, the search should still focus on occult regional primary with blind biopsy.
3. Local treatment may be undertaken, even in the absence of a primary tumor, with expectation for cure, particularly for cervical and axillary lymph node lesions.

lesions identified at atypical sites may represent (1) synchronous metastases with an occult primary, (2) metachronous metastases, or (3) multiple primary tumors. The atypical sites are all visceral, and therefore the possibility of a primary carcinoma is an important aspect of these miscellaneous TUO lesions.

Central nervous system lesions. These lesions may be divided into cerebral le-

sions and spinal cord lesions. Metastases from extra-central nervous system tumors are usually multiple. Lung, breast cancer, melanoma, and renal cell carcinoma all produce cerebral and spinal cord metastases.

Ophthalmic lesions. Tumors commonly metastasizing to the eye include breast and lung cancer. The lesions are most often retro-orbital or implanted on the re-

Table 20.12 Site of Metastases for TUO and Most Common Source of Primary Tumor

Site of Metastases	Most Common Source of Primary Tumor
Lung	Breast, lung, sarcoma, genitourinary tract
Bone	Breast, lung, prostate
Liver	Gastrointestinal tract, lung, breast
Lymph node	Melanoma, lymphoma, regional tumors
Skin and subcutaneous tissue	Breast, lung
Uncommon sites	
Brain	Lung, breast, melanoma, kidney
Ophthalmic	Melanoma, breast, lung
Gastrointestinal tract	Melanoma, lymphoma
Genitourinary tract	Lymphoma, lung, breast, regional tumors
Kidney	
Ovary	
Testicle	
Penis	
Endocrine origins	Renal cell, breast, lung
Thyroid	
Adrenal	
Pituitary	

tina and are clinically manifested as a secondary decrease in visual acuity and proptosis. Tissue diagnosis is seldom possible or warranted in this setting, and empirical therapy with radiation is indicated.

Gastrointestinal lesions. Malignant melanoma is the most common tumor to metastasize to the gastrointestinal tract and produces a typical radiographic appearance (bull's-eye sign) (Fig. 20.3) and gastrointestinal bleeding. Other tumors to metastasize to the bowel include lymphomas, leukemia, breast cancer, and lung cancer, but these tumors infrequently develop clinical manifestations.

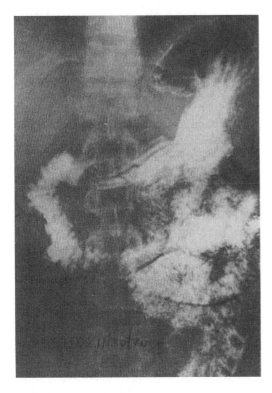

Fig. 20.3 *Upper GI series in a patient with metastasis to the small bowel demonstrating typical bull's-eye lesion in the second portion of the duodenum.*

Renal lesions. The kidney is an unusual site for metastases but is the most frequent site of "collision tumor" or metastases to a primary tumor. The rarity of kidney metastases is unexplained, and the vast majority of renal lesions represent primary tumors.

Ovarian lesions. The most common tumor to metastasize to the ovary is breast cancer. Breast cancer is associated with an increased incidence of primary ovarian cancer, and the two tumors may be histologically similar in appearance. Therefore, a lesion in the ovary can be a new primary tumor, and histopathological comparison of the primary breast lesion and the ovarian lesion is essential. Other common ovary tumors easily distinguished by pathology are lymphoma and leukemia.

Penile and testicular lesions. The most common tumor to metastasize to the penis and urethra is prostatic cancer. Rectal cancer has also been reported to implant along the penile urethra and cause clinical urinary obstruction or prostatism. Metastases to the testicles are extremely rare and are usually associated with the lymphomas and leukemias.

Endocrine gland lesions. A variety of tumors appear to have a propensity to metastasize to the endocrine glands. Lesions metastasizing to the thyroid are predominantly renal cell carcinoma; lesions metastasizing to the pituitary are most often breast cancer and lung cancer; lesions metastasizing to the adrenal gland are usually breast cancer. Such lesions rarely interrupt endocrine function but are mere oddities in the distribution of metastases.

Breast lesions. The most common tumors to metastasize to the breast are malignant melanoma, lymphoma, and breast cancer. In each instance, surgery should be restricted, and radical mastectomy is not required.

10.0 Solitary metastases

Solitary metastases are defined as metachronous lesions that develop in patients with known prior malignancy. The identification of such a lesion necessitates determination of the extent of disease (staging) to rule out the presence of tumor in other sites and to insure the solitary nature of the lesion. The lesion may then be surgically excised, based on the rationale that the singular site of disease is potentially curable and/or that the "solitary metastases" may indicate a new primary lesion with potential cure.

Such a rationale is often excessively optimistic because the overwhelming majority of such patients have disseminated disease. More reasonable therapy for solitary metastases is to monitor the lesion through a period of observation during which time the growth rate of the lesions may be established and a reasonable estimate of the biological activity of the tumor determined. The principles developed by Joseph for determining tumor doubling times in patients with pulmonary metastases are particularly appropriate (1971). Lesions with short doubling times are aggressive tumors, and during a period of observation other lesions often appear and preclude surgery.

Another rationale for surgical excision has been based on the "debulking" of tumors to make them more amenable or responsive to chemotherapy or radiation. Furthermore, removal of the tumor prevents subsequent metastatic seeding to other sites. The role of "debulking" in increasing tumor sensitivity to therapy has not, however, been established. A major controversy concerning whether metastatic lesions can metastasize to other sites is ongoing.

11.0 Synchronous primary tumors: Either/or metastases

Multiple primary tumors are well known in clinical oncology. The high incidence of second tumors in patients with prior malignancy and the accelerated incidence of third primary tumors in patients with two prior malignancies has been reaffirmed and confirmed by statistical epidemiologic studies. All this evidence raises the possibility of second primary tumors in the evaluation of new lesions in patients with prior malignancies.

Lesions at two sites may represent two synchronous primary tumors; alternatively, the lesions may represent a metastases from a single tumor. The vast majority of such lesions are not dual synchronous primary tumors; therefore, when patients have lesions at two sites, the primary tumor may be assumed to originate in one or the other site.

Patient P, a 72-year-old man, presented with undifferentiated tumor of the lung that was treated with local resection. Six months later the patient presented with a large lesion of the gingiva. Biopsy revealed the tumor to be consistent with the original lung primary, but it was considered that the gingival lesion was primary and had metastasized to the lung.

Patient Q, a 75-year-old man, presented with a five-year history of a carcinoma of the salivary gland. The tumor had been treated intermittently with radiation therapy and local surgical excision. The patient developed multiple pulmonary nodules, a lesion on the floor of the mouth separate from the previous intra-oral tumor, and multiple brain metastases. The presumption was that the tumor of the salivary gland had been totally controlled and that the metastatic lesions represented metastases from a new primary in the pulmonary parenchyma.

The distinction between metastases and primary tumors is not always clear-cut, but it is an overriding issue because, by definition, metastatic disease is incurable, whereas two primary sites are potentially individually curable.

12.0 Basic Rules of evaluation and therapy for TUO

The patient presenting with a lesion in one of the sites discussed in this chapter is potentially subject to extensive diagnostic search for the primary lesion. While the diagnostic evaluation may overlap into a staging work-up, this is unwarranted and often unnecessary. The do's and don't's in the clinical evaluation of the patient with a TUO are summarized in Table 20.13. The principles are based on the concept that the diagnostic work-up should focus on the best possibilities for therapy and on the clinical and biologic behavior for the primary tumor.

The problem of the unknown primary tumor or TUO is a common clinical circumstance, and the diagnostic work-up is often confused or "shot-gun." For a patient with a synchronous primary lesion that is clinically occult, the diagnostic work-up must be based on both the histopathologic type of tumor and the potential for tumor-specific therapy. For metachronous lesions, the presumption of a new primary tumor must be considered in order to provide optimal potential for cure since recurrence of the original tumor implies incurability. The goal in evaluating a TUO is determining the appropriate therapy.

13.0 References

Comess, M. S.; Beahrs, O. H.; and Dockerty, M. D. Cervical metastases from occult carcinoma. *Surg. Gynecol. Obstet.* 104:607, 1957.

Copeland, E. M., and McBride, C. M. Axil-

Table 20.13 Diagnostic Work-up and Schematic Flow Evaluation of Patient with TUO

Do	*Don't*
Establish a histologic diagnosis of malignancy.	Assume diagnosis of malignancy, search for primary tumor, or evaluate for metastases especially if the TUO is solitary.
Evaluate with special pathologic studies.	Pan-scan the body by "run the bowel," computed tomography, IVP, thyroid scan, uterine dilatation, and curettage

Assume primary tumor is maximally treatable.
   New primary cancer in patient with prior malignancy
   Lymphoma in patient with undifferentiated malignancy
   If adenocarcinoma, breast or ovary in women and prostate in men.	

lary metastases from unknown primary sites. *Ann. Surg.* 178:25, 1972.

Fitzpatrick, P. J., and Kotalik, J. F. Cervical metastases from an unknown primary tumor. *Radiology* 110:659, 1974.

France, C. J., and Lucas, R. The management and prognosis of metastatic neoplasms of the neck with an unknown primary. *Am. J. Surg.* 106:835, 1963.

Golomb, H. M., and Thomsen, S. Estrogen receptor: therapeutic guide in undifferentiated metastatic carcinoma in women. *Arch. Intern. Med.* 135:942, 1975.

Holmes, F. F., and Fouts, T. L. Metastatic cancer of unknown primary site. *Prog. Clin. Cancer.* 5:24, 1973.

Jess, R. H., and Neff, L. E. Metastatic carcinoma in cervical nodes with an unknown primary lesion. *Am. J. Surg.* 112:547, 1966.

Joseph, W. L.; Morton, D. L.; and Adkins, P. C. Prognostic significance of tumor doubling time in evaluating operability in pulmonary metastic disease. *J. Thorac. Cardiovasc. Surg.* 61:1, 1971.

MacComb, W. S. Diagnosis and treatment of metastatic cervical cancerous nodes from an unknown primary site. *Am. J. Surg.* 124:441, 1972.

Martin, H., and Morfit, H. M. Cervical lymph node metastases as the first symptom of cancer. *Surg. Gynecol. Obstet.* 78:133, 1944.

Moertel, C. G., et al. Treatment of the patient with adenocarcinoma of unknown origin. *Cancer* 30:1469, 1972.

Richardson, R. G., and Parker, R. G. Metastases from undetected primary cancers. *West. J. Med.* 123:337, 1975.

Smith, P. E., et al. Metastatic cancer without a detectable primary site. *Am. J. Surg.* 113:633, 1967.

Westbrook, K. C., and Gallagher, H. S. Breast carcinoma presenting as an axillary mass. *Am. J. Surg.* 122:607, 1971.

Whiteside, T., and Rowlands, D. T. T-cell and B-cell identification in the diagnosis of lymphoproliferative disease. *Am. J. Path.* 88:754, 1977.

Index